Cellular Pathology of Glandular Lesions and Uncommon Neoplasms of the Cervix

W. Glenn McCluggage • John Tidy
John H.F. Smith

Cellular Pathology of Glandular Lesions and Uncommon Neoplasms of the Cervix

Springer

W. Glenn McCluggage
Department of Pathology
Royal Victoria Hospital
Belfast
UK

John H.F. Smith
Department of Histopathology
and Cytology
Royal Hallamshire Hospital
Sheffield
UK

John Tidy
G18
Royal Hallamshire Hospital
Sheffield
UK

ISBN 978-1-4471-6944-4 ISBN 978-1-4471-2210-4 (eBook)
DOI 10.1007/978-1-4471-2210-4
Springer London Heidelberg New York Dordrecht

Softcover reprint of the hardcover 1st edition 2014

Printed on acid-free paper

Springer is part of Springer Science+Business Media (www.springer.com)

Contents

Introduction

Cervical histopathology specimens, mainly punch biopsies and loop excisions but also hysterectomy specimens, form a significant proportion of the workload of many surgical pathology laboratories. Most biopsies are performed because of an abnormality detected in a cervical cytology specimen taken during the course of an organised population cervical screening programme. The majority of biopsies are performed because of a suspected squamous abnormality. Although there can be problems in interpretation, the differential diagnosis of squamous lesions is relatively limited, and most cases are straightforward. Cervical glandular lesions are much less common than squamous lesions, but they result in a disproportionate number of diagnostic problems in both cytological and histological specimens. This book concentrates on cytological and histological aspects of cervical glandular lesions with a complementary chapter on the colposcopy and management of glandular neoplasia. Benign, premalignant and malignant cervical glandular lesions are covered. The former are characterised by a wide range of lesions which may be difficult to distinguish from premalignant and malignant glandular lesions. The full spectrum of premalignant and malignant cervical glandular lesions is expanding with the description of new entities. Although most premalignant and malignant cervical glandular lesions are human papillomavirus (HPV) associated, it is now well established that there are a number of different morphological types of non-HPV-related cervical adenocarcinomas, and these will increase in importance with the reduction in HPV-related cervical preneoplastic and neoplastic lesions secondary to the introduction of HPV vaccination programmes. We have also included chapters on the cytological and histological aspects of uncommon cervical neoplasms which, although rare, result in disproportionate difficulty for the pathologist. Although most lesions can be readily diagnosed using conventional haematoxylin and eosin preparations, immunohistochemistry may provide significant assistance in certain scenarios, and the value of markers is emphasised at relevant points. The majority of the cytology illustrations are photomicrographs of liquid-based cytology preparations reflecting contemporary British, and increasingly international, practice.

It is our hope that this book will be an easy-to-use practical guide which will be of value to consultant and trainee pathologists both specialist and generalist as well as other health care professionals involved in the management of cervical lesions. The many images included to complement the text are all in colour.

Belfast/Sheffield, UK
2014

W. Glenn McCluggage
John H.F. Smith

1 The Normal Cervix

John H.F. Smith

Abstract
In this chapter the anatomy and appearance of the normal cervix in histology and cytology specimens will be described with particular emphasis on glandular tissue.

Keywords
Cervix • Endocervix • Squamocolumnar junction • Squamous metaplasia • Transformation zone • Metaplasia

Structure and Development

The cervix is a fibromuscular organ, 3–4 cm in length and approximately 2.5 cm in diameter, lined and covered on the outer aspect by epithelium. It forms the inferior part of the uterus and projects into the vagina. Anatomically it is divided into the portio vaginalis which is that part which projects into the vagina and the supravaginal portion. It is continuous above with the body of the uterus at the uterine isthmus where there is a fibromuscular junction, the internal os, separating the fibromuscular tissue of the cervix from the muscular tissue of the body of the uterus.

The passage between the uterine cavity and the vagina is via the endocervical canal, which is continuous with the endometrial cavity above at the level of the internal os and the vagina below at the external os. The portion of the cervix lying exterior to the external os and in continuity with the vagina is called the ectocervix. The endocervical canal is approximately 3 cm long, fusiform in shape, and flattened from front to back. It measures between 6 and 8 mm in width at the widest point but cyclical changes result in alterations in the dimensions of the canal, in tissue vascularity and in the quantity and biophysical characteristics of mucus secreted by endocervical cells [1, 2]. Mucus secretion with increased vascularity, congestion and stromal oedema predominate during the proliferative phase of the menstrual cycle and reach a peak at ovulation in order to provide an ideal environment for the passage of spermatozoa.

The cervix varies in size and shape depending on a woman's age, parity and hormonal status. In nulliparous women it is barrel-shaped with a small circular external os but it changes shape and size during pregnancy and during delivery and labour, such that the multiparous cervix is larger than that found in nulliparous women and the external os appears as a wide, gaping transverse slit.

W.G. McCluggage et al., *Cellular Pathology of Glandular Lesions and Uncommon Neoplasms of the Cervix*,
DOI 10.1007/978-1-4471-2210-4_1, © Springer-Verlag London 2014

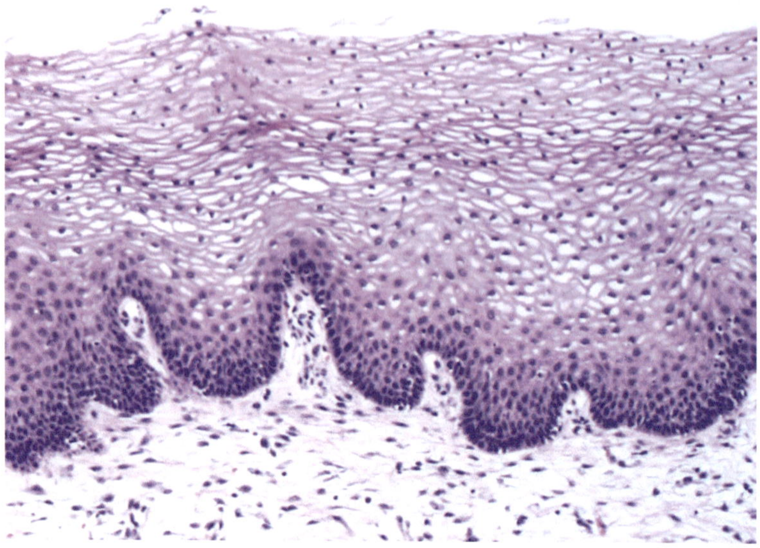

Fig. 1.1 Normal squamous mucosa of the ectocervix

Cervical Epithelium

The cervix is covered by both stratified non-keratinising squamous epithelium and columnar mucin secreting epithelium and these two types of epithelium meet at the squamocolumnar junction.

Squamous Epithelium

The ectocervix is covered by stratified non-keratinising glycogen-containing squamous epithelium. Histologically this epithelium is composed of a basal layer, a parabasal layer, an intermediate cell layer and a superficial cell layer (See Fig. 1.1). It is separated from the underlying cervical stroma by a basement membrane and the epithelial-stromal junction is usually linear but sometimes slightly undulating with short projections of stroma at regular intervals called stromal papillae.

In haematoxylin and eosin stained histological sections basal layer epithelium consists of a single row of small cylindrical cells with relatively large ovoid nuclei and sparse eosinophilic cytoplasm. In normal cervical squamous epithelium the basal layer nuclei maintain a regular perpendicular orientation to the basement membrane. Growth and replacement of the squamous epithelium occurs from the basal layer and therefore nucleoli, numerous chromocentres and mitoses are identified in this layer.

The parabasal cell layer is composed of two or more layers of polyhedral cells with relatively large nuclei and distinct intercellular bridges. Mitoses may be found in this layer particularly in basal hyperplasia in response to chronic infection or trauma.

The intermediate cell layer is composed of polygonal cells with abundant glycogen rich, frequently vacuolated, cytoplasm and small nuclei.

The superficial cell layer is composed of similar cells to those in the intermediate cell layer except that the cells are flattened with even smaller nuclei and evident keratinisation.

Glycogenation of the intermediate and superficial layers is a sign of normal maturation under the influence of oestrogen. In the absence of oestrogen normal maturation does not occur and therefore after the menopause the squamous epithelium of the cervix does not mature beyond the parabasal layer and the epithelium is thin and atrophic.

Columnar Mucin Secreting Epithelium

The endocervical canal is lined by columnar epithelium composed of a single layer of tall slender cells with abundant cytoplasm and basal

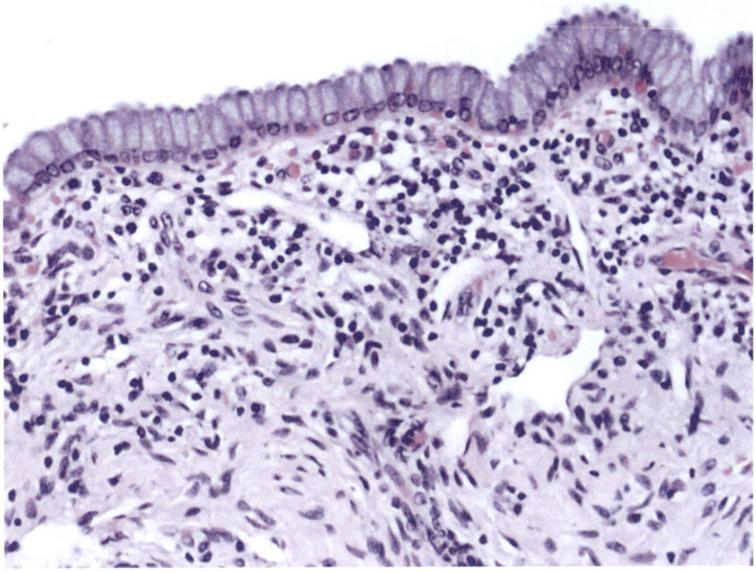

Fig. 1.2 Normal columnar glandular mucosa of the endocervix

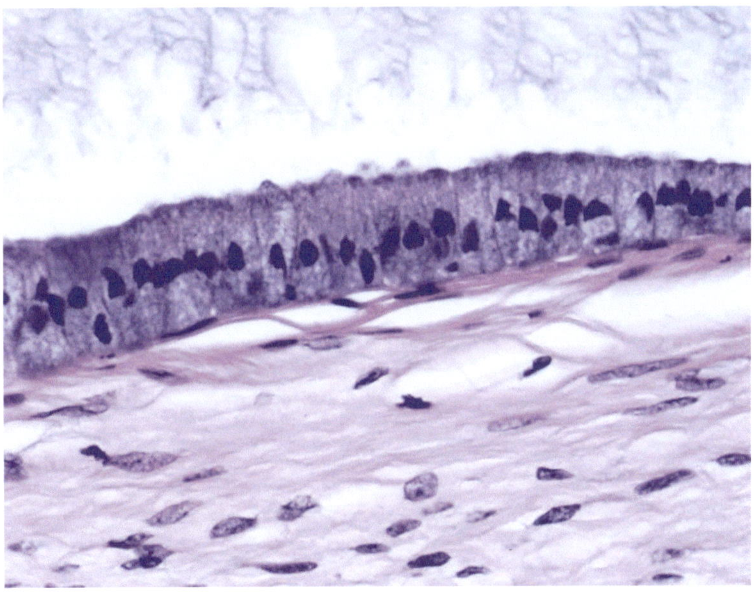

Fig. 1.3 Columnar epithelium of the endocervix with evidence of active secretion. Note the displaced nuclei and intracellular mucin accumulation

situated round or ovoid nuclei (See Fig. 1.2). The nuclei are usually situated in the basal part of the cell but may lie suprabasally or in the middle of the cell during active mucus secretion (See Fig. 1.3).

There are two types of columnar epithelial cell: non-ciliated secretory cells and ciliated cells.

The secretory cells predominate in the columnar epithelium and utilise both apocrine and merocrine secretion to produce both acid and neutral mucin, although the relative amounts vary with the menstrual cycle [3]. The ciliated cells are covered with tiny kinocilia that beat rhythmically towards the cervical canal and vagina. The distribution of the ciliated cells is not uniform in that they are found in highest concentration in the upper endocervical canal close to the endometrial junction and rarely seen close to the squamocolumnar junction (See Fig. 1.4).

The columnar epithelium does not form a single layer of cells lining the endocervical canal. Histological (two-dimensional) examination

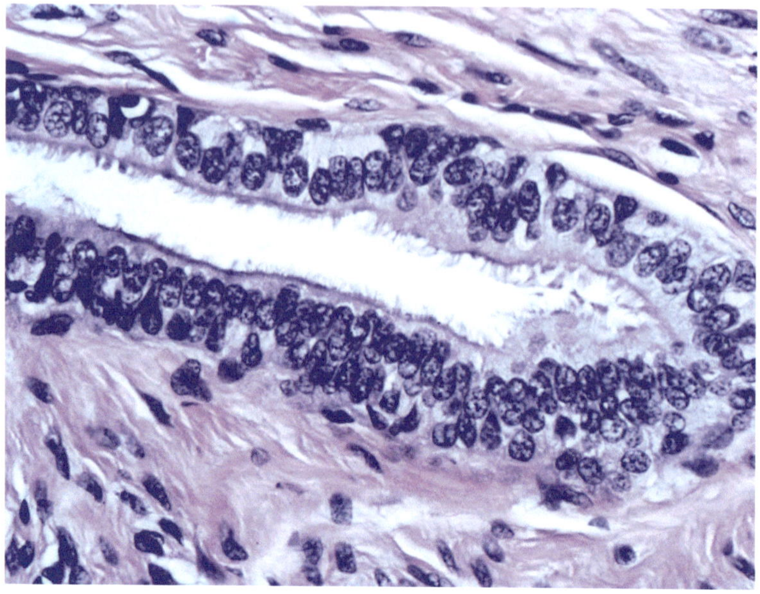

Fig. 1.4 Ciliated columnar cells lining an endocervical crypt in the upper endocervix

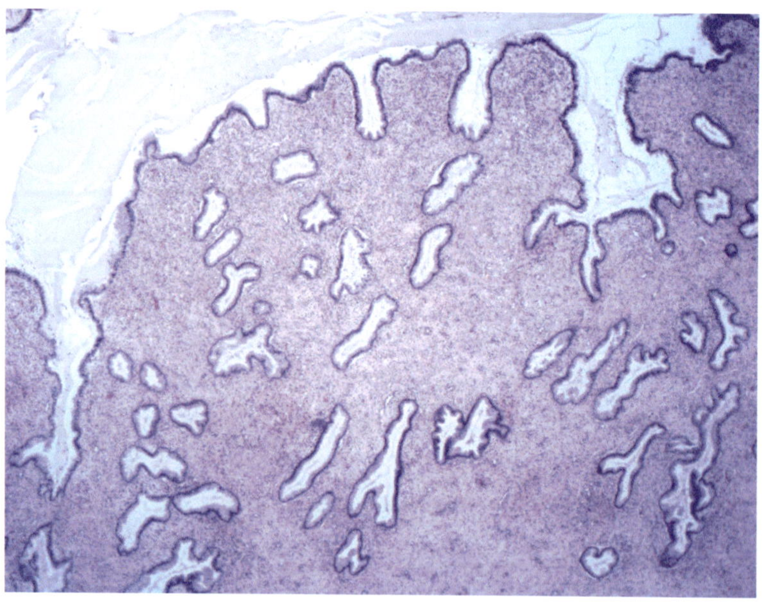

Fig. 1.5 Low power photomicrograph of the endocervix showing the complex crypt architecture

suggests that the endocervical canal is formed of numerous glands lined by columnar epithelium but elegant three-dimensional reconstruction has shown that these apparent glands are in fact a manifestation of an extensive cleft like system whereby there are numerous complex infoldings of endocervical epithelium on stroma to form endocervical folds and crypts [4, 5]. The crypts may extend to a depth of nearly 8 mm from the surface of the endocervical canal and these architectural features may be valuable in the diagnosis of invasive neoplastic lesions of the endocervix (see Chap. 5) (See Fig. 1.5) [6, 7].

Squamocolumnar Junction

The location of the junction between the columnar epithelium of the endocervix and the squamous epithelium of the ectocervix in

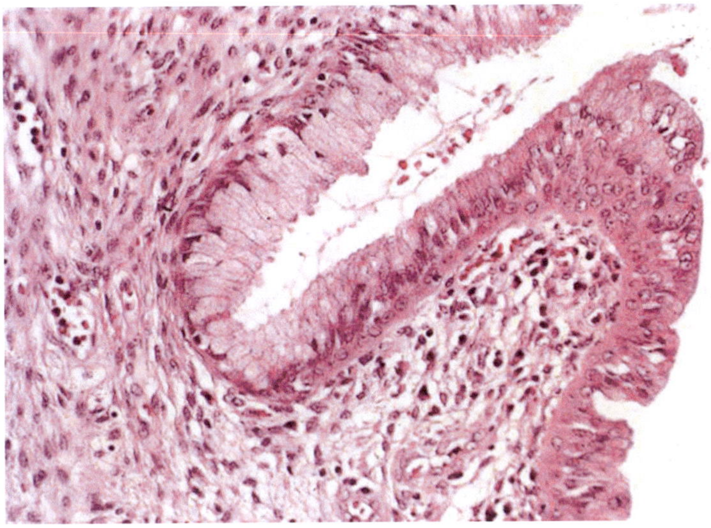

Fig. 1.6 Reserve cell hyperplasia. Initial displacement and replacement of columnar endocervical epithelium by small cuboidal cells

relation to the external os varies over a woman's lifetime and is dependent on hormonal influences, oral contraceptive use and physiological conditions such as pregnancy.

In childhood, the squamocolumnar junction is located at or very close to the external os. After puberty and during pregnancy the cervix swells and enlarges and the endocervical canal elongates under the influence of oestrogen. This leads to eversion of the columnar epithelium of the lower part of the endocervical canal onto the endocervix, a condition called ectropion or ectopy, which is clearly visible on naked eye examination as a prominent glistening red area.

Metaplastic Squamous Epithelium and the Transformation Zone

When the everted columnar epithelium in an ectropion is exposed to the acidic environment of the vagina, the buffer action of the mucus covering the columnar cells is destroyed and the columnar cells undergo metaplastic change and are transformed into squamous epithelium. Squamous metaplasia of the endocervix is a three step process proceeding from reserve cell hyperplasia to immature squamous metaplasia and mature squamous metaplasia.

The first sign of squamous metaplasia is the appearance and proliferation of sub columnar reserve cells, a unicellular layer of small cuboidal cells immediately beneath the normal endocervical columnar cells (See Fig. 1.6). The origin of the reserve cells is uncertain: opinion is divided as to whether they arise from primitive epithelial cells located between the columnar cells in the basement membrane or from sub epithelial stromal or mononuclear cells [8–12].

Progressive growth with stratification of reserve cells results in a multilayered epithelium showing some features of squamous differentiation and replacement of the columnar epithelium by immature squamous epithelium, a process known as immature squamous metaplasia. Immature metaplastic squamous epithelium lacks surface maturation and has inconspicuous intracytoplasmic glycogen in contrast to mature squamous epithelium (See Fig. 1.7).

Eventually the columnar epithelium is entirely replaced by mature squamous epithelium resembling native squamous epithelium and it overlies endocervical crypts (See Fig. 1.8). If endocervical crypt openings are completely occluded mucus accumulates in and expands the crypt to form mucous retention cysts called Nabothian cysts or follicles (See Fig. 1.9). The metaplastic process starts at the original squamocolumnar junction and moves toward the external os through the reproductive period. Thereby a new squamocolumnar junction is formed between the newly formed metaplastic squamous epithelium and the columnar epithelium remaining everted on the ectocervix. In the

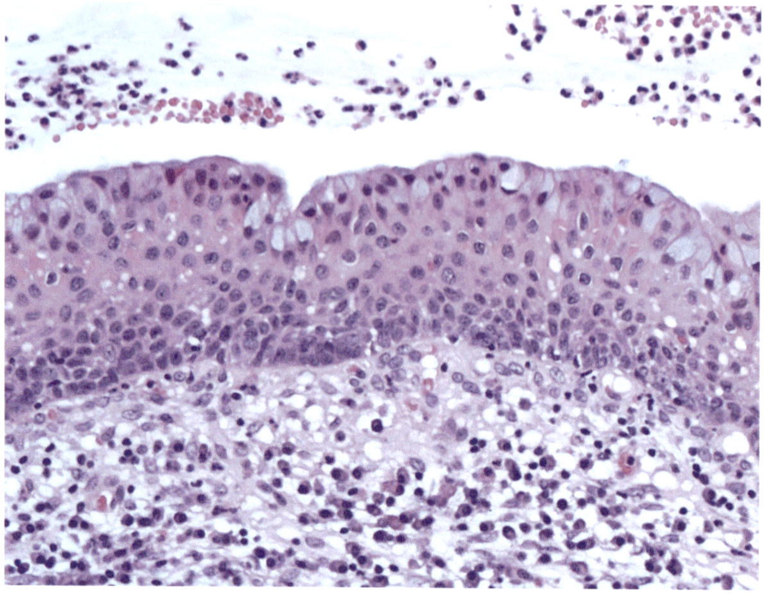

Fig. 1.7 Cervical transformation zone. The surface endocervical epithelium is partly replaced by immature metaplastic squamous epithelium

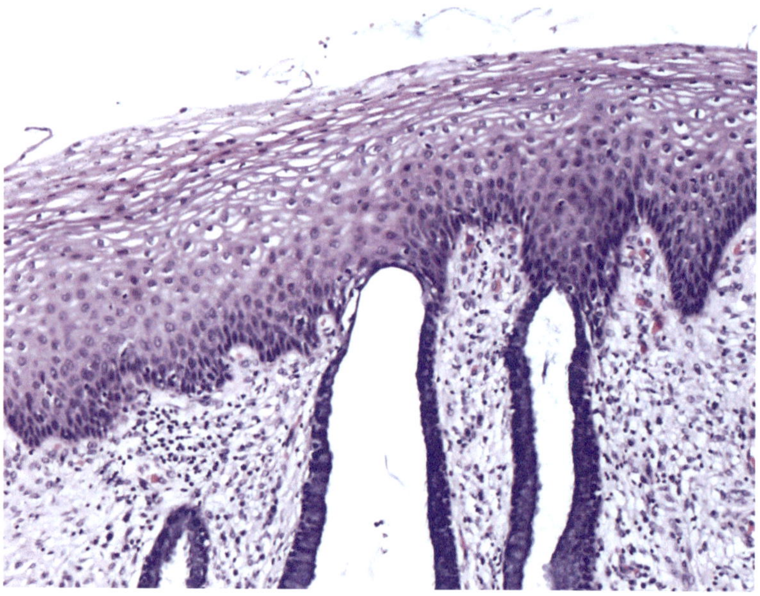

Fig. 1.8 Cervical transformation zone. The surface endocervical epithelium is completely replaced by mature metaplastic squamous epithelium which covers the crypt openings

perimenopausal age range the squamocolumnar junction progressively moves towards the external os and as the cervix shrinks after the onset of menopause due to lack of oestrogen the movement of the new squamocolumnar junction toward the external os is accelerated with the result that the new squamocolumnar junction is often not visible in postmenopausal women on colposcopic examination. Squamous metaplasia is an irreversible process but progresses at varying rates in different areas of the same cervix so that areas of differing maturity may be seen in the metaplastic squamous epithelium associated with residual islands of columnar epithelium. The metaplastic epithelium adjacent to the new squamocolumnar junction is immature whilst that near the original squamocolumnar junction is mature.

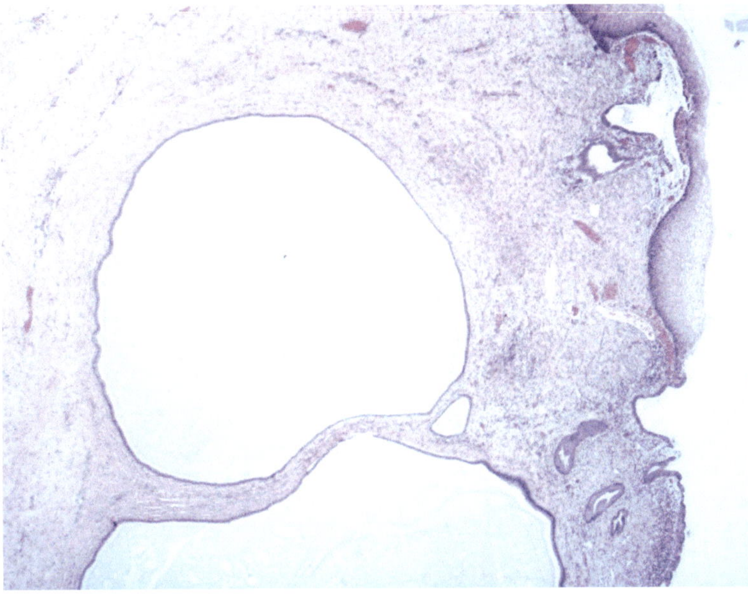

Fig. 1.9 Mucus retention cyst formation in the transformation zone as a result of complete occlusion of crypt openings by metaplastic squamous epithelium

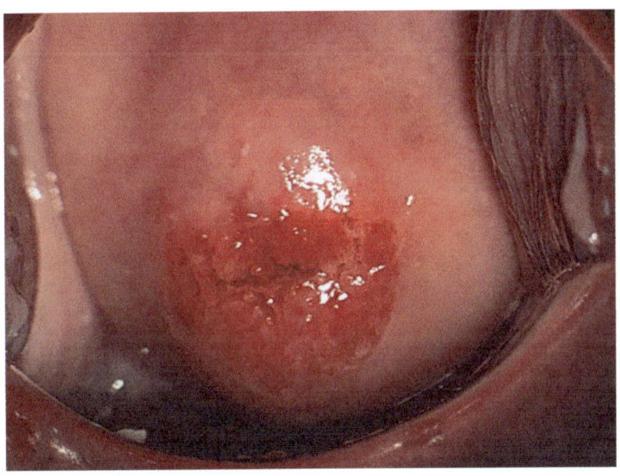

Fig. 1.10 Colposcopic appearance of the cervix in a woman in the reproductive age range showing the original and new squamocolumnar junctions

That part of the cervix where the columnar epithelium has been replaced or is being replaced by metaplastic squamous epithelium is referred to as the transformation zone and is delineated distally by the original squamocolumnar junction and proximally by the new squamocolumnar junction (See Fig. 1.10). It is in this area that oncogenic human papillomaviruses interact with the squamous and glandular epithelium and virtually all squamous neoplasms and the majority of glandular neoplasms of the cervix arise [13–17].

Cytology of Normal Endocervical Epithelium

Normal endocervical cells present in cervical cytology preparations as either cohesive groups or single dispersed cells. The cohesive groups when viewed end on have a characteristic honeycomb appearance with round nuclei, and when viewed in profile form palisades of columnar cells with basal situated ovoid nuclei resembling a "picket fence" (See Figs. 1.11 and 1.12). The individual cells within a cohesive group may show considerable variation in nuclear size but polarity is maintained and they lack other features of neoplasia (See Fig. 1.13). Single cells are recognised by their columnar shape with tall delicate cytoplasm and basal nuclei (See Fig. 1.14). The nuclei of endocervical cells have a fine chromatin pattern and one or more nucleoli may be identified close to the nuclear membrane. Ciliated cells may be identified, particularly in brush samples from the upper endocervical canal as noted above, and must be distinguished from the ciliated cells of tuboendometrioid metaplasia as described in Chap. 6 (See Fig. 1.15).

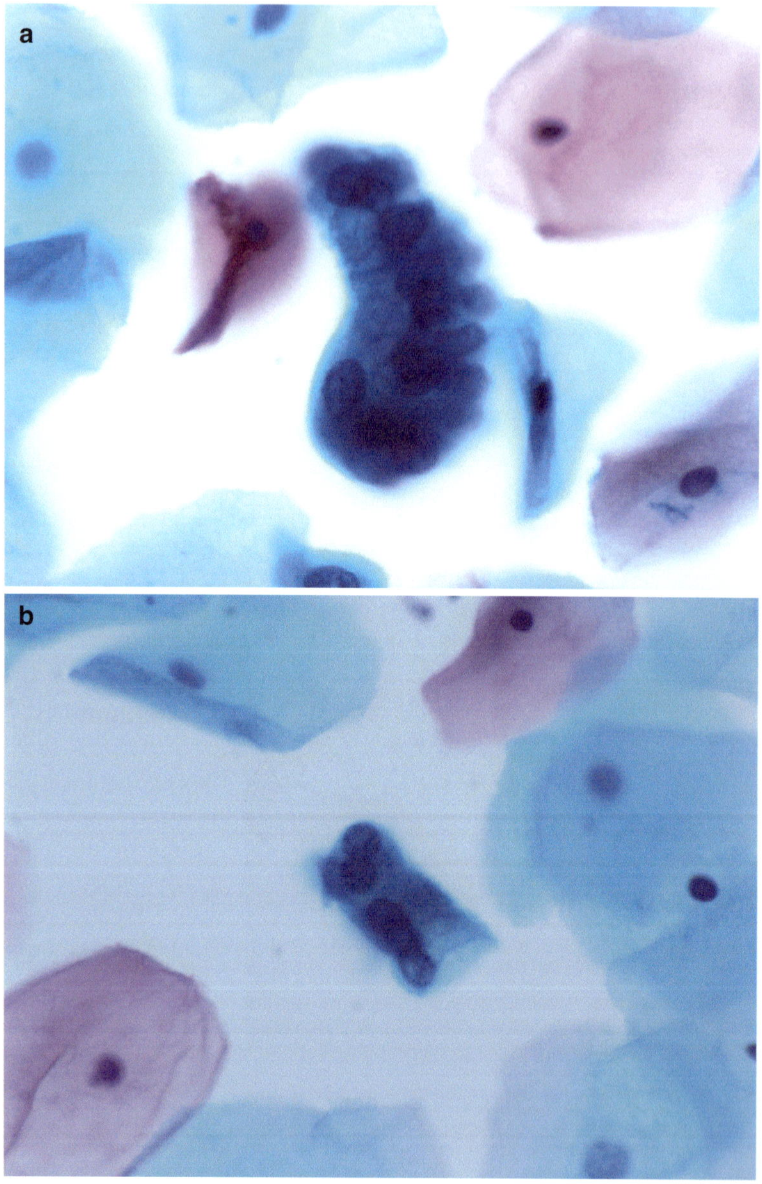

Fig. 1.11 (**a**, **b**) Normal endocervical cells in characteristic 'picket fence' configuration. Note that even in the slightly curved group the basal orientation of the nuclei is maintained (SurePath)

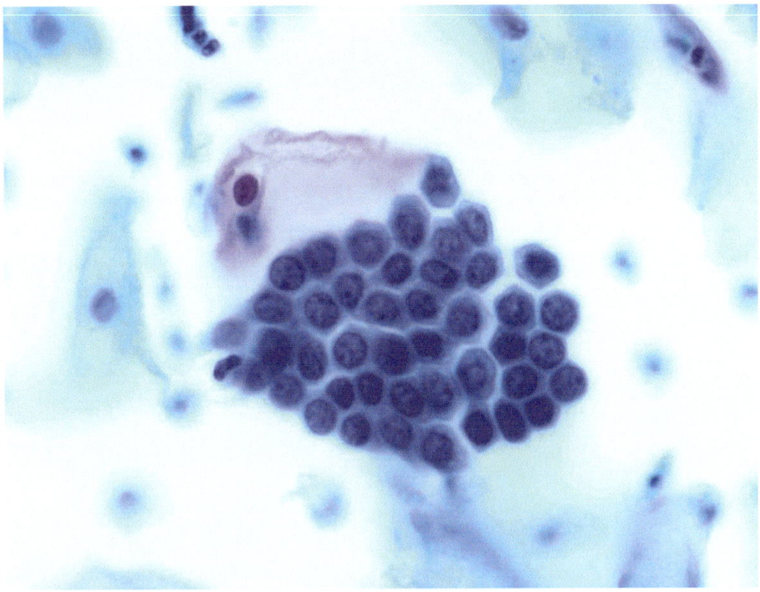

Fig. 1.12 A group of normal endocervical cells viewed end on in characteristic 'honey comb' configuration (SurePath)

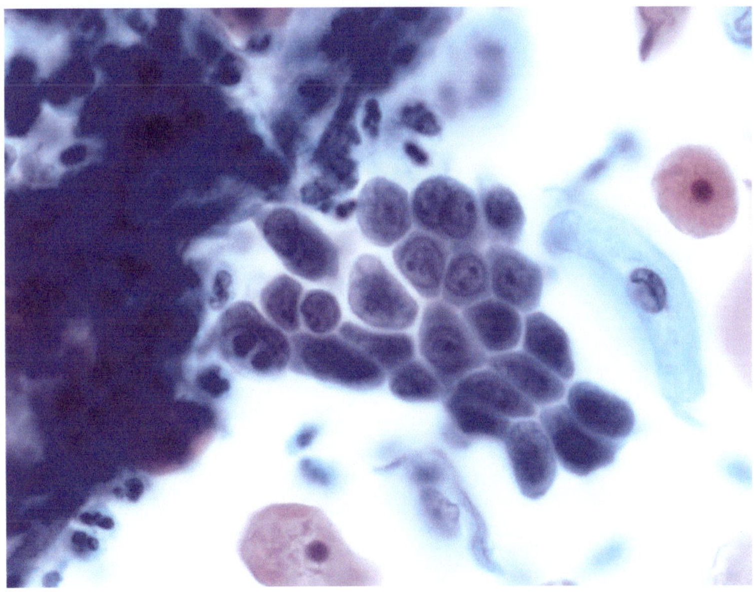

Fig. 1.13 A group of endocervical cells in an inflamed sample showing some variation in nuclear size but maintenance of orderly arrangement and no nuclear atypia (SurePath)

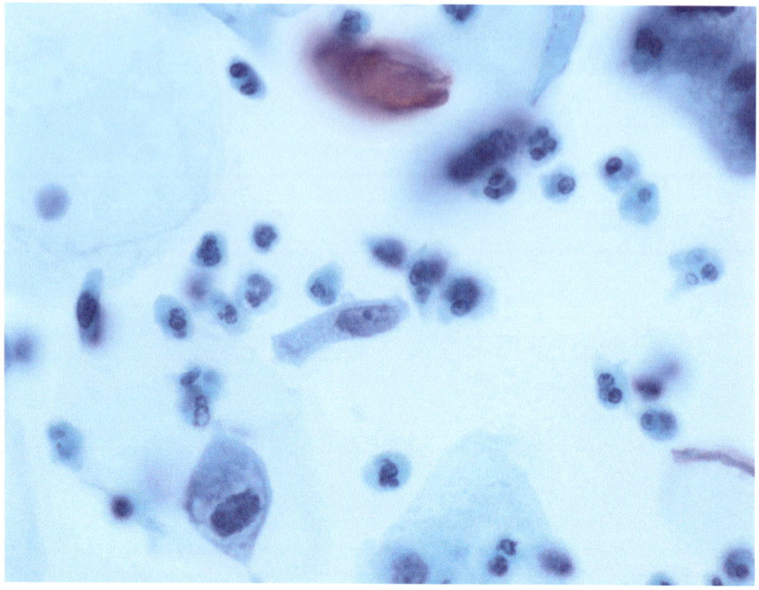

Fig. 1.14 A solitary normal dispersed endocervical cell in a LBC preparation (SurePath)

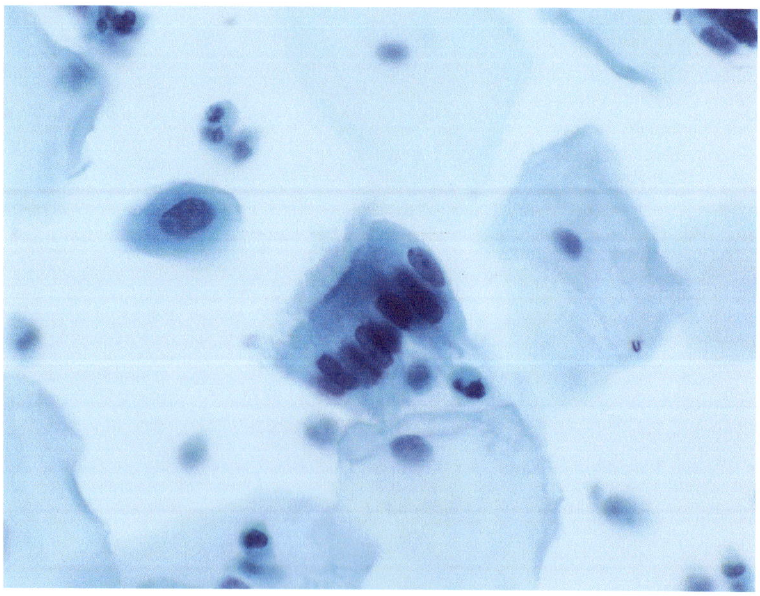

Fig. 1.15 An isolated strip of ciliated endocervical cells in a brush sample from high in the endocervical canal. Note the cilia, typical morphology of endocervical cells and bland nuclear features, which allows distinction from tuboendometrioid metaplasia (SurePath)

References

1. Hafez ES. Surface ultrastructure and functional histology of the uterine cervix. Reproduccion. 1981;5(4):243–9.
2. Hafez ES. Structural and ultrastructural parameters of the uterine cervix. Obstet Gynecol Surv. 1982;37(8):507–16.
3. Wakefield EA, Wells M. Histochemical study of endocervical glycoproteins throughout the normal menstrual cycle and adjacent to cervical intraepithelial neoplasia. Int J Gynecol Pathol. 1985;4(3):230–9.
4. Fluhmann CF. The nature and development of the so-called glands of the cervix uteri. Am J Obstet Gynecol. 1957;74(4):753–66.
5. Fluhmann CF. The glandular structures of the cervix uteri. Surg Gynecol Obstet. 1958;106(6):715–23.
6. Anderson MC, Hartley RB. Cervical crypt involvement by intraepithelial neoplasia. Obstet Gynecol. 1980;55(5):546–50.
7. Ostor AG, Pagano R, Davoren RA, et al. Adenocarcinoma in situ of the cervix. Int J Gynecol Pathol. 1984;3(2):179–90.

8. Fluhmann CF. The histogenesis of acquired erosions of the cervix uteri. Am J Obstet Gynecol. 1961;82:970–82.
9. Smedts F, Ramaekers F, Leube RE, et al. Expression of keratins 1, 6, 15, 16, and 20 in normal cervical epithelium, squamous metaplasia, cervical intraepithelial neoplasia, and cervical carcinoma. Am J Pathol. 1993;142(2):403–12.
10. Reid BL, Singer A, Coppleson M. The process of cervical regeneration after electrocauterization. I. Histological and colposcopic study. Aust NZ J Obstet Gynaecol. 1967;7(3):125–35.
11. Lawrence WD, Shingleton HM. Early physiologic squamous metaplasia of the cervix: light and electron microscopic observations. Am J Obstet Gynecol. 1980;137(6):661–71.
12. Maclean AB. Healing of cervical epithelium after laser treatment of cervical intraepithelial neoplasia. Br J Obstet Gynaecol. 1984;91(7):697–706.
13. Christopherson WM, Nealon N, Gray Sr LA. Noninvasive precursor lesions of adenocarcinoma and mixed adenosquamous carcinoma of the cervix uteri. Cancer. 1979;44(3):975–83.
14. Bertrand M, Lickrish GM, Colgan TJ. The anatomic distribution of cervical adenocarcinoma in situ: implications for treatment. Am J Obstet Gynecol. 1987;157(1):21–5.
15. Fu YS, Berek JS, Hilborne LH. Diagnostic problems of in situ and invasive adenocarcinomas of the uterine cervix. Appl Pathol. 1987;5(1):47–56.
16. Andersen ES, Arffmann E. Adenocarcinoma in situ of the uterine cervix: a clinico-pathologic study of 36 cases. Gynecol Oncol. 1989;35(1):1–7.
17. Colgan TJ, Lickrish GM. The topography and invasive potential of cervical adenocarcinoma in situ, with and without associated squamous dysplasia. Gynecol Oncol. 1990;36(2):246–9.

Benign Endocervical Glandular Lesions

2

W. Glenn McCluggage

Abstract

This chapter covers the many benign endocervical glandular lesions, some of which may mimic premalignant and malignant endocervical glandular lesions. Benign endocervical glandular lesions can be broadly divided into four groups, metaplasias and ectopias of endocervical glands, endocervical glandular "hyperplasias", reactive and inflammatory lesions and benign glandular neoplasms. The differential diagnosis with premalignant and malignant endocervical glandular lesions and the value of immunohistochemistry is discussed where appropriate.

Keywords

Cervix • Benign glandular lesions • Immunohistochemistry

Introduction

Within the cervix, there are many benign glandular lesions some of which are mimics of cervical glandular intraepithelial neoplasia (CGIN) or adenocarcinoma [1–3]. In general, these benign mimics are more common than premalignant and malignant endocervical glandular lesions. Most pose no particular diagnostic problem and the majority, but not all, are typically incidental microscopic findings which rarely produce a mass lesion. In evaluating a possible problematic benign cervical glandular lesion, the pathologist should always look for more typical areas; for example, unusual forms of microglandular hyperplasia may pose a diagnostic problem but are often associated with areas of more typical microglandular hyperplasia. It should be remembered that rarely CGIN involves a pre-existing benign endocervical glandular lesion and this may result in obvious diagnostic problems. Ancillary immunohistochemical studies are of some value in the distinction of benign mimics from CGIN and adenocarcinoma [2, 3]. However, there are pitfalls and, as in all aspects of pathology, the results of immunohistochemistry should always be correlated with the morphology.

Benign endocervical glandular lesions can broadly be categorised into four groups:

1. Metaplasias and ectopias of endocervical glands.
2. Endocervical glandular "hyperplasias".
3. Reactive and inflammatory lesions.
4. Benign glandular neoplasms.

W.G. McCluggage et al., *Cellular Pathology of Glandular Lesions and Uncommon Neoplasms of the Cervix*, DOI 10.1007/978-1-4471-2210-4_2, © Springer-Verlag London 2014

Metaplasias and Ectopias of Endocervical Glands

Tubal Metaplasia, Tuboendometrial Metaplasia (TEM) and Superficial Endometriosis

These comprise a spectrum of glandular lesions which are common within the cervix. There are two distinct types of cervical endometriosis, each with a different underlying pathogenesis. Superficial (primary) endometriosis is usually unassociated with pelvic endometriosis whereas deep (secondary) endometriosis (endometriosis involving the external surface of the cervix) is associated with pelvic endometriosis [4]. Deep endometriosis is discussed in the next section. Superficial endometriosis is often part of a spectrum including tubal metaplasia and TEM. In this spectrum of metaplastic glandular lesions, the glands may exhibit tubal, endometrioid or intermediate features. With tubal metaplasia and TEM, there is often slight increased cellularity and condensation of the stroma around the glands and when definite endometrioid type stroma is present, this constitutes superficial endometriosis. The term tubal metaplasia is sometimes used when the glands exhibit overt tubal differentiation, although the term TEM is preferred since there is often an overlap of tubal and endometrioid differentiation. Often these glandular lesions occur in combination and, as stated, they are best regarded as being part of a spectrum. Glands exhibiting tubal features with ciliation are a normal occurrence at the junction of the cervix and endometrium in the lower uterine segment/isthmus [5]. However, tubal or endometrioid type glands are an abnormal, but common, finding close to the transformation zone of the cervix [6–8]. They represent a metaplastic, usually reparative, phenomenon, often secondary to previous cervical biopsy, resection or ablation. Occasionally they are seen in the absence of such a history. Uncommonly, superficial endometriosis may occur secondary to implantation, possibly as a result of menstruation or prior endometrial curettage.

TEM may involve the surface glands or crypts and also sometimes dilated glands and Nabothian cysts. The morphology is usually, but not always, characterised by a heterogeneity of cell types. Ciliated and non-ciliated cells are present and there is often lymphocytic infiltration with intraepithelial lymphocytes, typically surrounded by a halo (Fig. 2.1). The non-ciliated cells may have apical snouts. There is nuclear stratification, mucin depletion, mild nuclear hyperchromasia and mild nuclear atypia; in occasional cases,

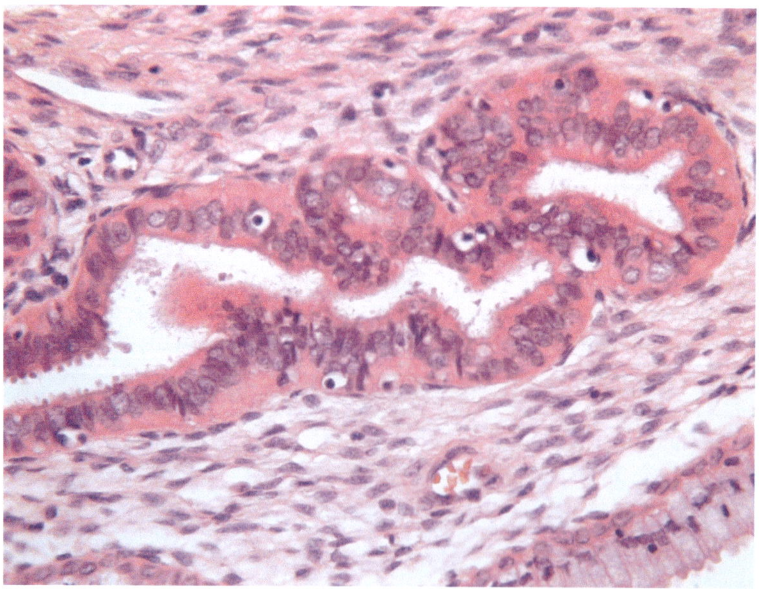

Fig. 2.1 Tuboendometrial metaplasia with ciliated and non-ciliated cells and lymphocytes surrounded by a halo

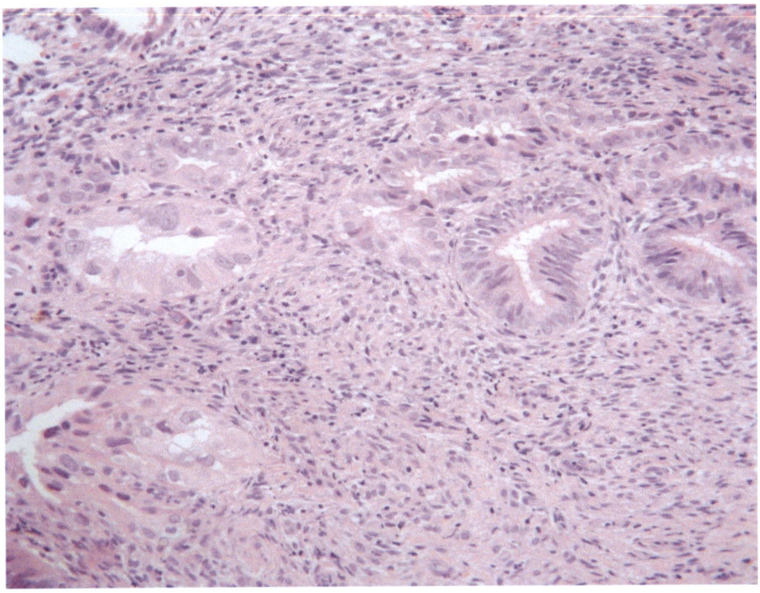

Fig. 2.2 In some cases of tuboendometrial metaplasia, there is quite marked nuclear atypia with an almost "symplastic-like" appearance

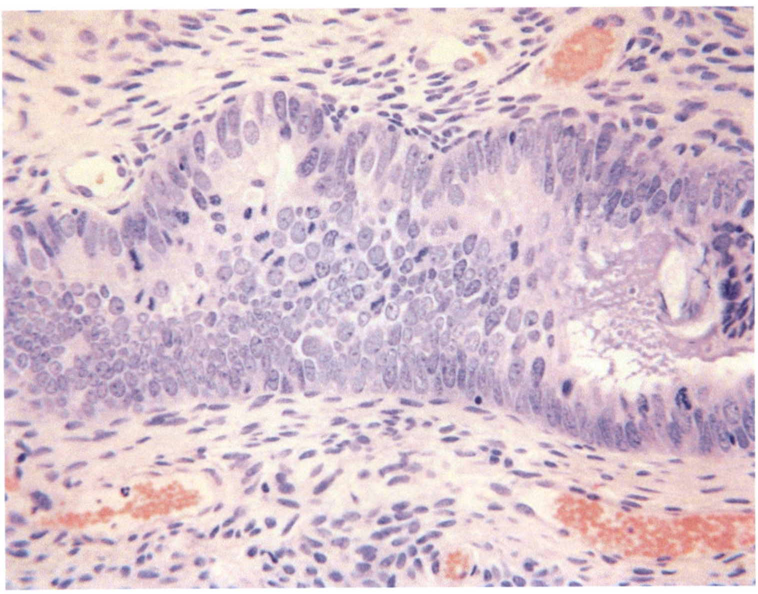

Fig. 2.3 In some cases of tuboendometrial metaplasia, mitoses are easily identified

some of the nuclei are quite atypical with an almost "symplastic-like" appearance but these are admixed with cells with bland nuclei (Fig. 2.2). Mitoses are sometimes present and occasionally are prominent, especially when the glands exhibit endometrioid differentiation (Fig. 2.3). Atypical mitoses are not seen. There may be a sharp demarcation between normal endocervical glands and glands involved by TEM or superficial endometriosis, both between adjacent glands and even within individual glands. The glands may be surrounded by true endometrioid stroma (superficial endometriosis), often with prominent engorgement of small vessels and extravasation of erythrocytes; these latter features are often a clue to the presence of endometrioid-type stroma which may otherwise be subtle (Fig. 2.4). There may be mild stromal condensation and hypercellularity surrounding the glands without overt endometrioid stromal differentiation (Fig. 2.5). CD10

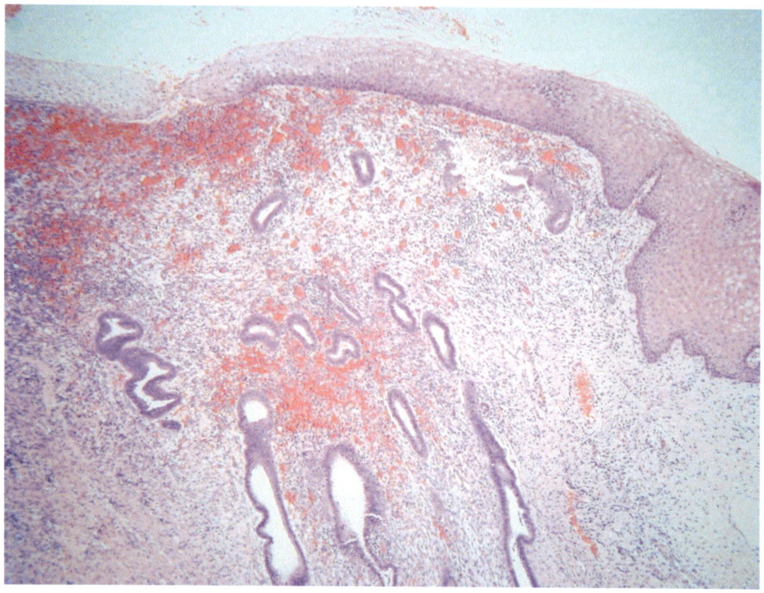

Fig. 2.4 Superficial endometriosis with endometrioid type glands and surrounding endometrioid type stroma

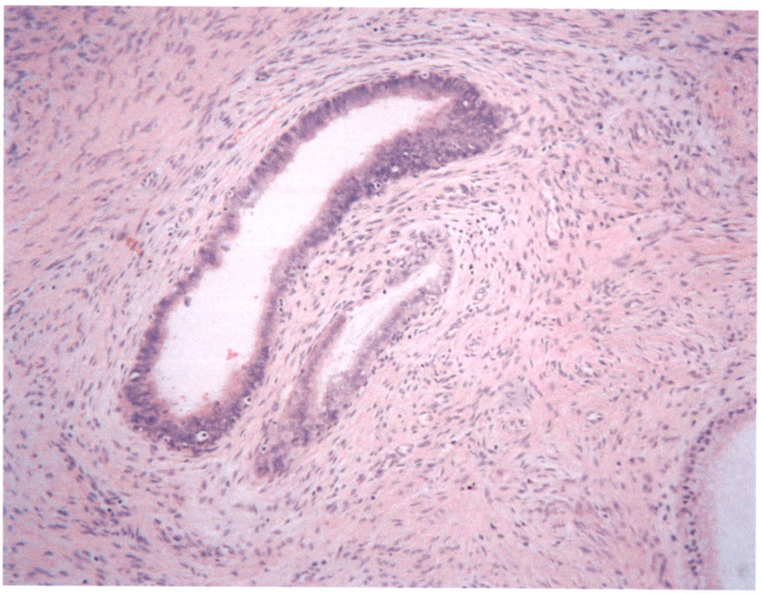

Fig. 2.5 In some cases of tuboendometrial metaplasia, there is stromal condensation and increased cellularity surrounding the glands

immunohistochemical staining may be useful in helping to confirm the presence of endometrioid-type stroma, although normal cervical stroma immediately surrounding endocervical glands can be positive [9, 10]. Usually the glands conform to the normal endocervical glandular architecture but occasional cases of TEM with a pseudoinfiltrative appearance have been described, including rare cases associated with in utero exposure to diethylstilbestrol [11].

Stromal endometriosis characterised by the presence of endometrioid-type stroma without glands occasionally occurs within the cervix. This is characterised by the presence of small superficial nodules or plaques of endometrioid-type stroma, sometimes with prominent engorgement of small vessels and extravasation of erythrocytes (Fig. 2.6).

In practice, this spectrum of lesions is the most likely within the cervix to be confused with CGIN. Features which may result in consideration

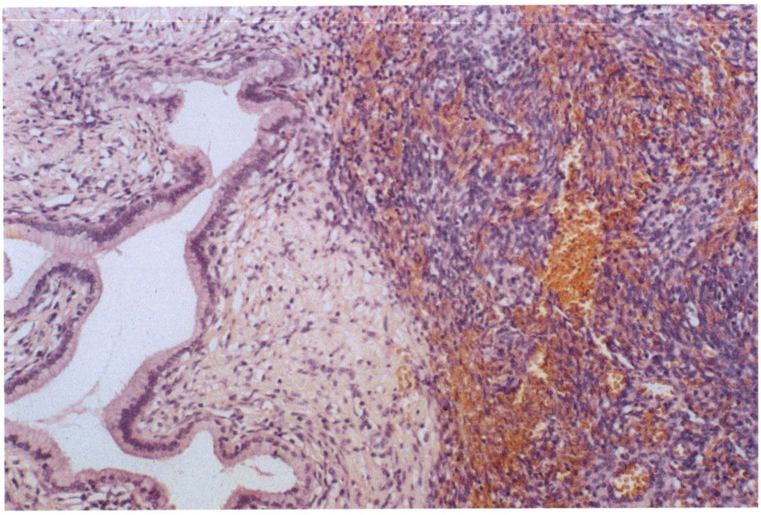

Fig. 2.6 Stromal endometriosis composed of aggregate of endometrial stromal cells without glands; there is engorgement of small vessels and extravasation of erythrocytes

of CGIN include the sometimes sharp demarcation from normal glands as well as nuclear stratification, nuclear atypia and hyperchromasia and mucin depletion. As discussed, mitoses are common, especially in cases exhibiting endometrioid differentiation, although abnormal mitotic figures are not a feature. Lymphocytes infiltrating the epithelium may mimic apoptotic bodies which are a feature of CGIN. Since TEM and superficial endometriosis are often a reparative phenomenon, there may be an associated stromal fibrotic or inflammatory reaction, rarely even mimicking an invasive adenocarcinoma.

Features useful in the distinction from CGIN include the presence of cilia in most examples of TEM and superficial endometriosis. However, cilia may not be prominent in those cases which exhibit overt endometrioid differentiation and a rare ciliated or tubal variant of CGIN exists [12]. Other points of distinction include the general absence of marked atypia in TEM and superficial endometriosis, except for occasional cases with "symplastic type" nuclei (see above) and the fact that there are, in general, fewer mitotic figures with no abnormal mitoses. There are few or no apoptotic bodies and the nuclei are less hyperchromatic than is the case in CGIN. Endometrioid-type stroma may be present.

Immunohistochemistry may be of value in distinguishing TEM and superficial endometriosis from CGIN (see Table 3.2- Chap. on 3). A useful panel of markers is MIB1, bcl2 and p16 [13–15]. Other antibodies which may be of value are CEA, vimentin and oestrogen receptor (ER). In general, TEM and superficial endometriosis exhibit a low MIB1 proliferation index of less than 30 % (in most cases, less than 10 %) whereas CGIN usually exhibits a much greater MIB1 proliferation index, in excess of 30 %. However, there is some overlap at the lower end of the CGIN and the upper end of the TEM and superficial endometriosis spectrum, especially in cases of endometriosis or TEM with prominent endometrioid differentiation. TEM and superficial endometriosis usually exhibit diffuse cytoplasmic positivity with bcl2 (Fig. 2.7) whereas CGIN is negative. p16 may be of value in that CGIN almost always exhibits diffuse positivity (usually a combination of nuclear and cytoplasmic staining). TEM and superficial endometriosis may be negative but are often positive, although usually with focal immunoreactivity (Fig. 2.8). Cytoplasmic CEA immunoreactivity is characteristic of a premalignant or malignant endocervical glandular lesion and favours CGIN over TEM or superficial endometriosis. However, in practice this marker is of limited value since luminal positivity may be present in benign glandular lesions and normal endocervical glands while some premalignant and malignant endocervical glandular lesions are negative; there is too much overlap in the CEA staining

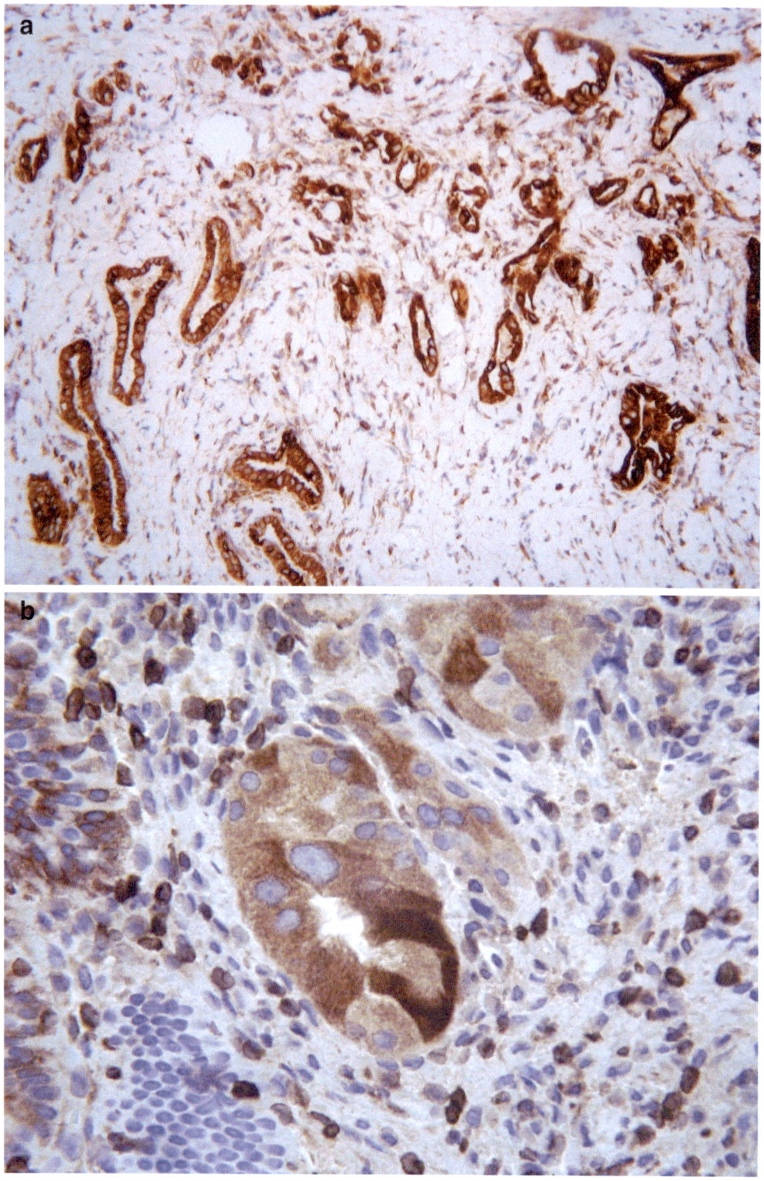

Fig. 2.7 Tuboendometrial metaplasia and tuboendometrial metaplasia with atypia exhibiting diffuse cytoplasmic staining with bcl2 (**a**, **b**)

patterns between benign and premalignant or malignant endocervical glandular lesions for this marker to be of value in an individual case. Vimentin may be of value in that CGIN is usually negative whereas TEM and endometriosis exhibit cytoplasmic positivity [16, 17]. ER may similarly be of use since TEM and superficial endometriosis are usually diffusely positive while CGIN is negative or focally positive. These markers may also be useful in cauterised endocervical glandular epithelium, for example the distinction between cauterised TEM or superficial endometriosis and cauterised CGIN.

Deep Endometriosis

Although not a metaplasia of endocervical glands, deep endometriosis is discussed here. This is associated with pelvic endometriosis and, as such, is usually secondary to retrograde menstruation. It involves the outer aspects of the cervical

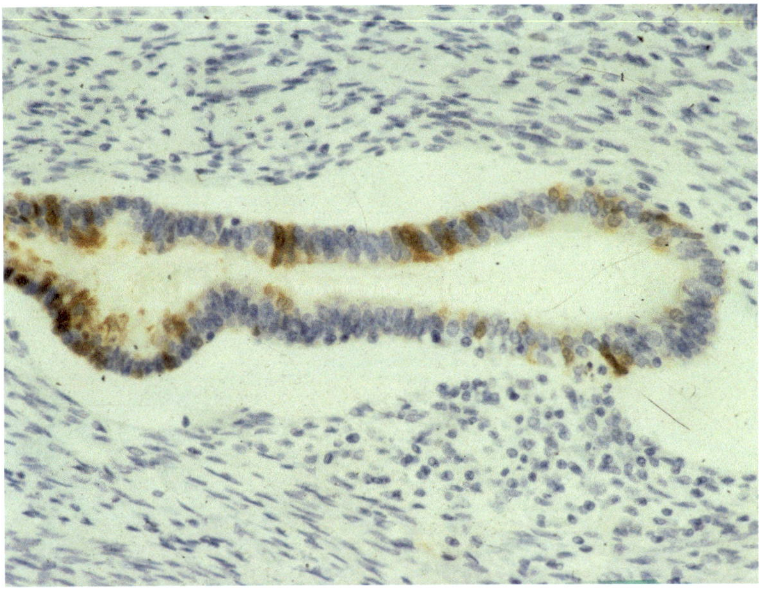

Fig. 2.8 Tuboendometrial metaplasia exhibiting focal staining with p16

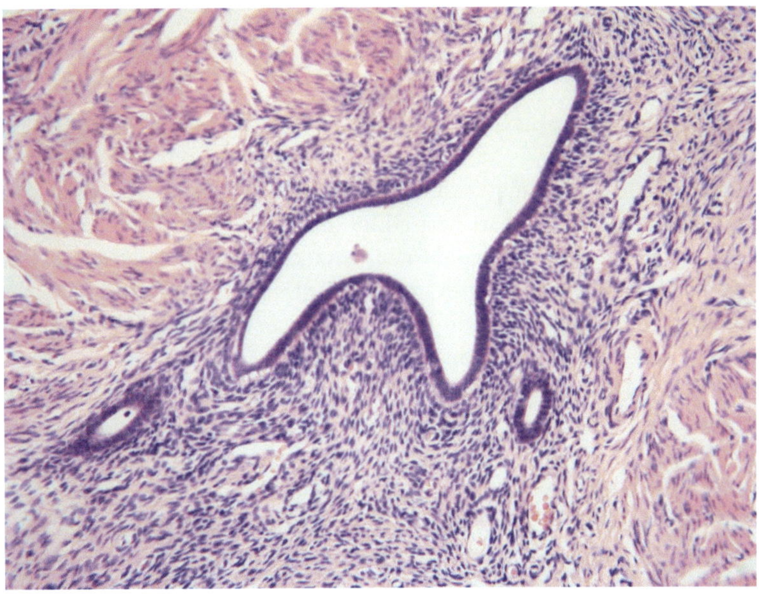

Fig. 2.9 Deep cervical endometriosis with endometrioid type glands and surrounding endometrioid type stroma in outer aspects of cervix

stroma and paracervical connective tissues (Fig. 2.9). The morphological features are similar to endometriosis in other locations with endometrioid type glands and surrounding stroma.

Atypical Oxyphilic Metaplasia

This is a rare incidental microscopic finding characterised by the presence of endocervical glands lined by cuboidal or polygonal cells with somewhat atypical hyperchromatic nuclei and abundant dense eosinophilic cytoplasm, sometimes with apical snouts, the cytoplasmic appearances being the characteristic morphological feature of this lesion (Fig. 2.10) [18]. The nuclei may be multilobated and usually the changes are focal involving only a few glands or even a single gland. There is no mitotic activity. The features somewhat resemble apocrine metaplasia within

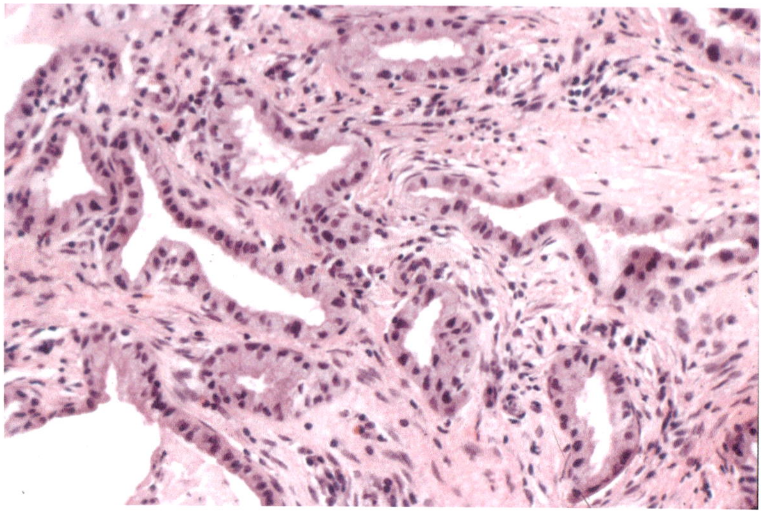

Fig. 2.10 Atypical oxyphilic metaplasia characterized by endocervical glands lined by cells with abundant eosinophilic cytoplasm and atypical hyperchromatic nuclei

the breast. Radiation atypia may have a very similar appearance and a history of prior pelvic irradiation should be excluded.

Intestinal Metaplasia

Endocervical glands may exhibit intestinal differentiation which is characterised by the presence of goblet cells and rarely neuroendocrine or Paneth cells. Almost all examples of intestinal metaplasia involving non-invasive endocervical glands represent an intestinal variant of CGIN [19] (discussed in Chap. 3, Premalignant Glandular Lesions of the Cervix). While rare examples of "benign" intestinal metaplasia occur within the cervix, for example in association with lobular endocervical glandular hyperplasia [20], this is extremely rare and true intestinal differentiation is almost always indicative of a premalignant or malignant lesion. In one reported case of "benign" cervical intestinal metaplasia, there was also gastric/pyloric metaplasia within the cervix and intestinal metaplasia within the endometrium [20], suggesting an occasional association between intestinal metaplasia at various sites within the female genital tract.

There have been occasional reported cases of intestinal-type epithelium lining the cervix secondary to spread from a primary appendiceal mucinous neoplasm [21]. In such cases, similar intestinal-type epithelium may line the endometrium and/or fallopian tube.

Simple Gastric (Pyloric) Metaplasia

Most examples of so-called gastric or pyloric metaplasia involving endocervical glands represent lobular endocervical glandular hyperplasia (LEGH) (See section on "Lobular endocervical glandular hyperplasia"). However, rarely endocervical glands without architectural features of LEGH exhibit immunoreactivity for HIK1083 [22, 23], a marker of pyloric gland mucins. In one study, Zhao et al. showed that the surface epithelium or crypt epithelium of non-neoplastic endocervical glands with a normal architecture were positive for pyloric gland mucin in 0.7 % of cases using this marker [23]. Such cases may be best designated as simple gastric (pyloric) metaplasia. Morphologically, this is extremely subtle and is characterized by pre-existing endocervical glands lined by columnar cells with abundant pale eosinophilic cytoplasm, in contrast to the rather basophilic cytoplasm of normal endocervical glands. The significance of this is unknown but it may represent an early phase of LEGH. In the rare scenario of this being diagnosed in a biopsy specimen, the coexistence of prototypical LEGH is a concern and radiological examination is advised

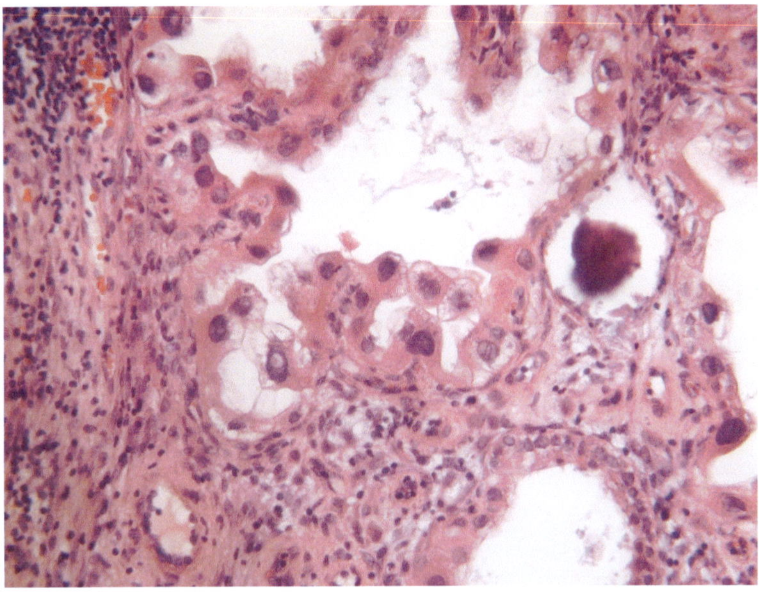

Fig. 2.11 Arias-Stella reaction involving endocervical glands with atypical nuclei and hobnail cells

to look for the presence or absence of features suggestive of LEGH.

Arias-Stella Reaction

The Arias-Stella reaction (Arias-Stella effect) uncommonly involves endocervical glands, usually in association with pregnancy or, more rarely, hormonal preparations [24]. This is usually a focal finding involving the surface or crypt epithelium or sometimes the glands of an endocervical polyp. The histological features are well known and are similar to those seen within the endometrium, comprising cells with enlarged somewhat pleomorphic and hyperchromatic nuclei with hobnail features, intraglandular papillary tufts and abundant clear vacuolated or eosinophilic cytoplasm (Fig. 2.11). Intranuclear pseudoinclusions, a cribriform architecture and occasional mitotic figures may be seen. Rarely, the Arias-Stella reaction may be mistaken for a premalignant or malignant lesion, most commonly a clear cell carcinoma. However, the history of pregnancy should result in a correct diagnosis. Useful in the distinction from clear cell carcinoma (this is only likely to be problematic on a small biopsy) is the absence of a mass lesion and of a desmoplastic response and infiltrative growth pattern and the fact that the Arias-Stella reaction is usually a focal finding involving a few glands. There is generally more atypia and mitotic activity in clear cell carcinoma, although some clear cell carcinomas may be cytologically bland with few mitotic figures. Stromal hyalinisation is characteristic of clear cell carcinomas.

Endocervicosis

This rare condition may be viewed as the mucinous counterpart of endometriosis and can be associated with endometriosis and/or endosalpingiosis (collectively known as Mullerianosis). The most common sites of involvement are the outer aspects of the cervix (usually the anterior wall), the vagina, the bladder, the peritoneum and the pelvic lymph nodes [25, 26]. In the cervix, endocervicosis may be associated with a prior caesarean section and occasionally results in the formation of a mass lesion. The histological features are of glands lined by cytologically bland, or at the most mildly atypical, mucinous epithelium (Fig. 2.12). Mitotic figures are rare or absent. Some of the glands may be dilated and there can be minor foci of ciliated or endometrioid type glands. Helpful in the distinction from a mucinous variant of minimal deviation adenocarcinoma (adenoma malignum) is the fact

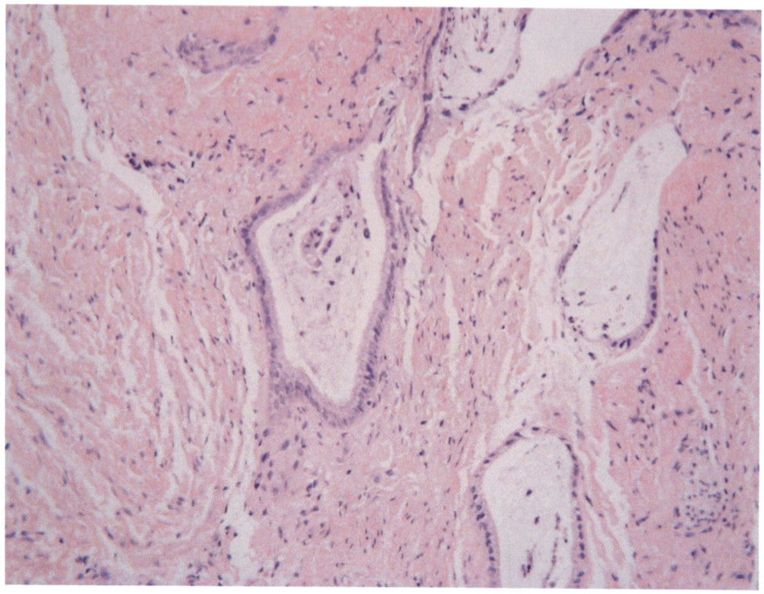

Fig. 2.12 Endocervicosis characterized by bland mucinous glands within outer cervical stroma

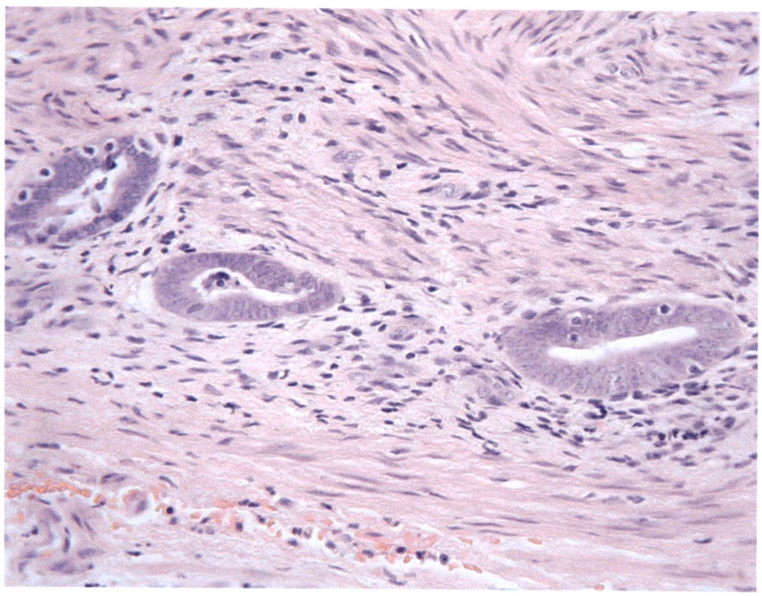

Fig. 2.13 Endosalpingiosis characterized by ciliated tubal type glands in outer aspects of cervical stroma

that endocervicosis involves the outer aspects of the cervix and paracervical connective tissue with a zone of uninvolved tissue between the lesion and the native endocervical glands. There is minimal nuclear atypia and no desmoplastic stromal response, although there may be a focal stromal reaction to mucin extravasation. There is no vascular invasion, although perineural infiltration has been described [25]. Endocervicosis is a benign lesion but a single vaginal case with malignant transformation has been reported [27].

Endosalpingiosis/Florid Cystic Endosalpingiosis

Endosalpingiosis is usually an incidental microscopic finding and is characterised by the presence of benign glands lined by ciliated tubal type epithelium (Fig. 2.13). When occurring in the cervix, it involves the outer aspects of the stroma and the surrounding tissues. Rarely there is marked glandular dilatation resulting in the formation of multiple cysts,

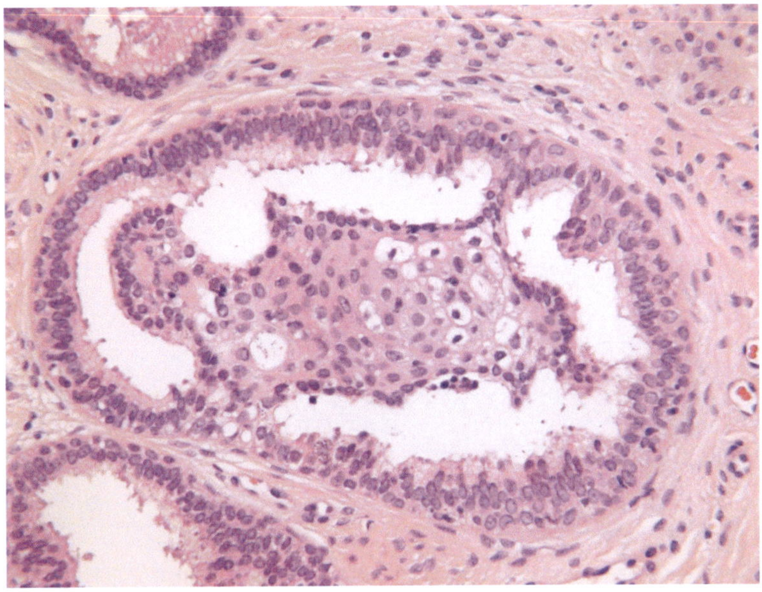

Fig. 2.14 Ectopic prostatic tissue in cervix characterized by squamous and glandular elements, the latter lined by a double cell layer

predominantly involving the serosa of the uterus, cervix, adnexae and intestine; this is referred to as florid cystic endosalpingiosis and in rare cases there is transmural involvement of the cervix [28]. While the bland cytological features usually result in a benign diagnosis, an adenocarcinoma, for example a minimal deviation adenocarcinoma of endometrioid type or an endocervical adenocarcinoma with cystic features, may be considered. Distinction from TEM is based on the location of the tubal type glands, TEM being situated superficially within the cervix while endosalpingiosis predominantly involves the outer aspect and surrounding tissues.

Ectopic Prostatic Tissue

So-called ectopic prostatic tissue is uncommon within the cervix and is usually an incidental microscopic finding, although in very rare cases a mass lesion is formed [29–31]. There is debate whether this represents a developmental anomaly or a metaplasia of endocervical glands. The "prostatic" tissue may be present superficially or deep within the cervical stroma and is usually located predominantly in the ectocervix rather than at the transformation zone, although sometimes the transformation zone is involved; the typical ectocervical location is evidence that this represents a developmental anomaly rather than a metaplasia of endocervical glands.

The basic morphological appearance is of rounded epithelial elements of both glandular and squamous type; tubules lined by bland epithelium are typically present around the periphery of the squamous elements and, in some cases, the glandular elements, at least focally, form a double cell layer (Fig. 2.14). Cribriform and papillary patterns are common. Although the glandular element of ectopic prostatic tissue is typically positive with prostate specific antigen and prostatic acid phosphatase (Fig. 2.15), this is not always the case. Occasional examples are negative with one or both markers and often positive staining is focal rather than diffuse. Prostatic acid phosphatase is more likely to be positive than prostate specific antigen [31]. p63 and other basal markers highlight the presence of a basal cell layer within the glandular or tubular elements.

An uncommon vaginal polyp, referred to as vaginal tubulosquamous polyp, is morphologically similar to cervical ectopic prostatic tissue and may exhibit positive immunohistochemical staining with prostatic markers [31, 32]. It is thought that cervical ectopic prostatic tissue and vaginal tubulosquamous polyp are derived from paraurethral Skene's glands which are the female equivalent of prostatic glands in the male [31, 32]. Uncommon findings in

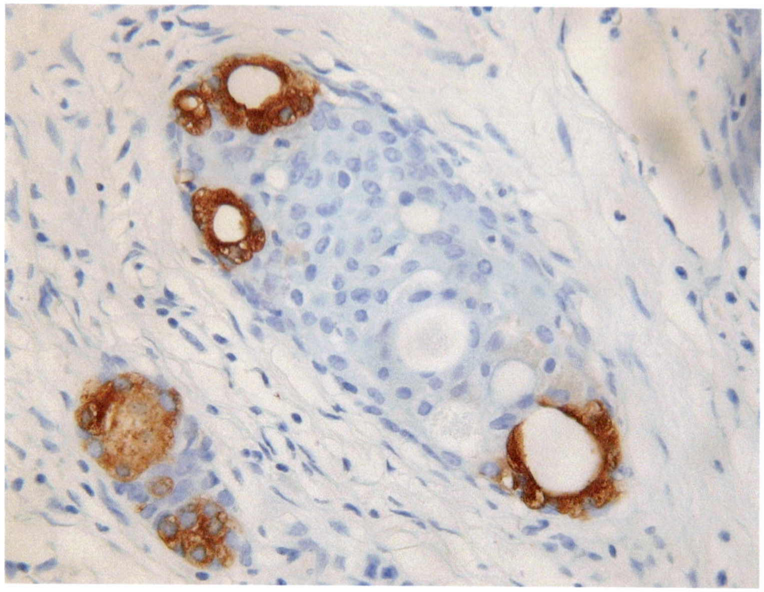

Fig. 2.15 Ectopic prostatic tissue in cervix is focally positive with prostatic acid phosphatase

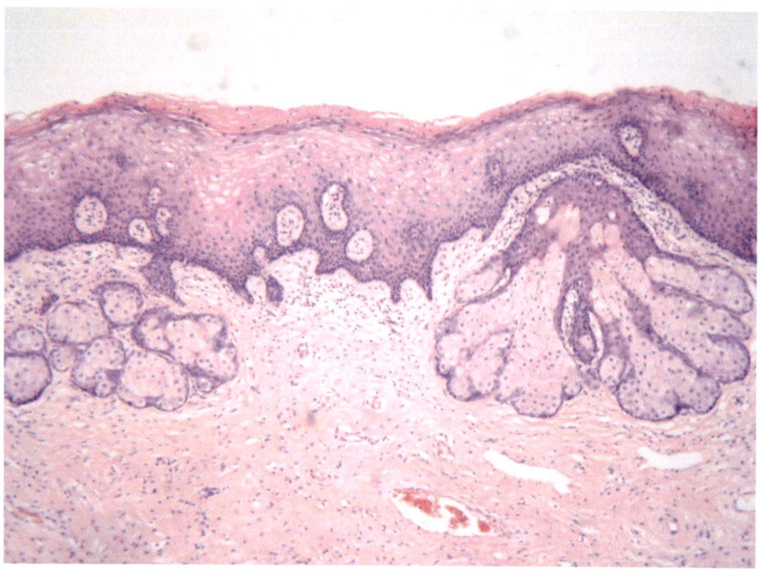

Fig. 2.16 Ectopic sebaceous glands within superficial cervical stroma

these lesions include the presence of sebaceous glands, basaloid formations resembling hair follicle structures and a microglandular proliferation resembling nephrogenic adenoma [31]. Occasionally, similar microscopic lesions are seen in the vulva [31, 33]. It has been proposed that these benign lesions in the cervix, vagina and vulva, which may exhibit immunoreactivity with prostatic markers, are derived from eutopic or misplaced Skene's glands [31].

Sebaceous Glands and Hair Follicle Structures

So-called ectopic sebaceous glands are a rare incidental microscopic finding within the cervix (Fig. 2.16); they may also be found in the vagina [34–38]. They are usually attached to or situated just beneath the ectocervical squamous epithelium and are possibly more common in association with uterine prolapse. The overlying squamous epithelium may be keratinised and occasionally hair follicle structures are also present, sometimes forming pilosebaceous units in association with sebaceous glands; rarely sweat gland-like structures are present [38]. It has been debated whether ectopic ectodermal structures (sebaceous glands, hair follicles and sweat glands) in the cervix and vagina are a result of congenital misplacement or an acquired metaplastic change [34–38]; the latter theory is preferred whereby the ectodermal structures are a response to prolonged irritation or chronic injury [38].

Endocervical Glandular Hyperplasias

It is arbitrary as to what constitutes an endocervical glandular hyperplasia, since normal endocervical glands may vary considerably in prominence, depending amongst other things on the menopausal status and parity of the patient and whether exogenous hormones are being taken. There is little point in rendering a diagnosis of non-specific endocervical glandular hyperplasia and this terminology is not recommended. However, there are several lesions, including some where the term hyperplasia is used, which should be recognised by the pathologist.

Tunnel Clusters

Tunnel clusters are a relatively common, usually incidental, microscopic finding within the cervix, although uncommonly they are visible grossly. Rarely, they are associated with a mucoid vaginal discharge. They were first described by Fluhmann in 1961 [39] and are divided into type A (non-cystic) and type B (cystic) variants; type B is much more common [40, 41]. Tunnel clusters are usually superficially located within the cervix but occasionally extend quite deeply. There is some degree of overlap between type A and B with occasional cases exhibiting an admixture of patterns. There is an association with parity and it has been suggested that tunnel clusters represent involution of pregnancy associated "hyperplastic" endocervical glands [40, 41].

The more common type B tunnel clusters have a characteristic low power appearance with well demarcated clusters of closely packed, dilated endocervical glands with a lobular architecture (Fig. 2.17). The clusters may be multifocal. On high power, the glands are lined by flattened epithelium with minimal intracytoplasmic mucin. There is little or no nuclear atypia or mitotic activity. Sometimes, there is mucin extravasation with an associated stromal reaction in the form of histiocytes and other inflammatory cells.

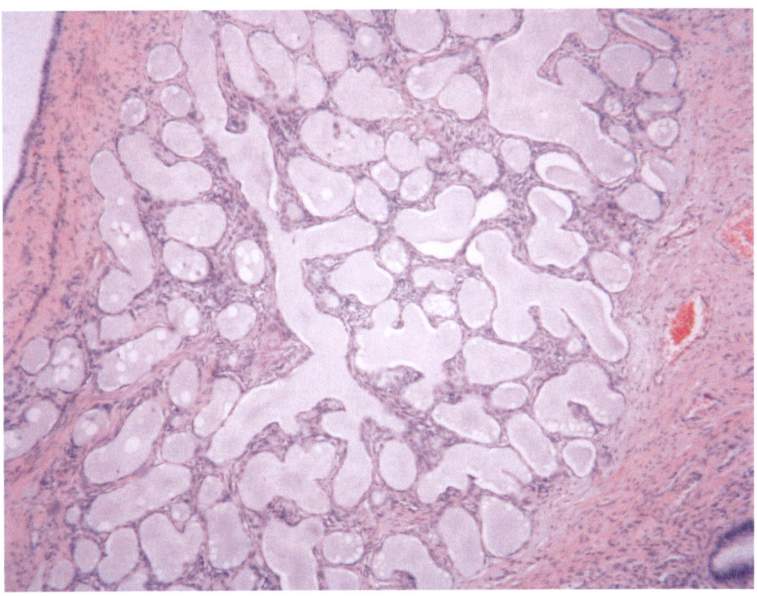

Fig. 2.17 Type B tunnel clusters characterized by lobular arrangement of glands with cystic dilatation

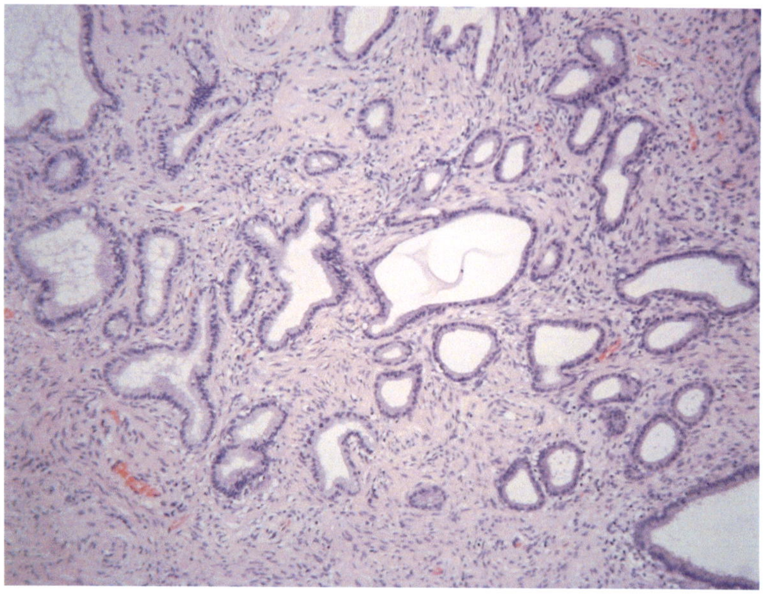

Fig. 2.18 Type A tunnel clusters consisting of non-dilated glands

Although the histological features of type B tunnel clusters are characteristic they may rarely be mistaken for adenoma malignum or an adenocarcinoma with cystic features, either a microcystic variant of usual endocervical type adenocarcinoma [42] or a cystic variant of clear cell carcinoma. However, the absence of a mass lesion and of nuclear atypia and stromal desmoplasia are in favour of a benign lesion; in fact, it is more likely to misdiagnose a cystic variant of adenocarcinoma as tunnel clusters.

Type A tunnel clusters are characterized by a lobular proliferation of predominantly small-calibre, nondilated, closely packed glands which may be arranged around a central endocervical cleft (Fig. 2.18). Most are well circumscribed but occasionally there is a slightly irregular border with a pseudoinfiltrative appearance which can result in consideration of an adenocarcinoma. The glands are lined by columnar or low cuboidal cells containing intracytoplasmic mucin. Occasional cases exhibit mild cytologic atypia and there can be a degree of hypercellularity of the stroma surrounding the glands but there is no desmoplasia [40]. These features, together with the pseudoinfiltrative appearance, may result in consideration of adenocarcinoma.

It has been shown that some type A tunnel clusters, in contrast to normal endocervical glands and type B tunnel clusters, contain neutral mucins and exhibit positive immunohistochemical staining with antibodies against gastric/pyloric mucins, such as HIK1083 and MUC6. Along with lobular endocervical glandular hyperplasia, type A tunnel clusters may be part of a spectrum of benign endocervical glandular lesions exhibiting gastric differentiation; in fact, some type A tunnel clusters may represent an early or incipient form of lobular endocervical glandular hyperplasia (see section on "Lobular endocervical glandular hyperplasia") [22, 43, 44].

Lobular Endocervical Glandular Hyperplasia (LEGH)

LEGH is an uncommon cervical lesion [45, 46]. While this is most commonly an incidental microscopic finding, sometimes there is a mass lesion which may be "picked up" on radiological examination. Some patients present with watery vaginal discharge and occasional patients have Peutz Jeghers syndrome. LEGH is usually situated in the upper part of the endocervical canal close to the internal os rather than at the transformation zone. Morphologically, this constitutes a well demarcated lesion which is usually confined to the inner half of the cervix. It is characterised by the presence of small glands arranged in a lobular fashion surrounding larger glands or duct-like structures; the ducts and lobular elements are lined by low columnar cells with pale eosinophilic cytoplasm and basally located small bland nuclei (Fig. 2.19a). Sometimes there is mild nuclear atypia and/or occasional mitotic activity. Intraglandular bridging or a cribriform architecture may be seen focally. Occasionally, there is a focal diffuse architecture rather than the normal lobular pattern. Rarely, there is focal intestinal metaplasia with goblet cells, especially within the centrally located glands (Fig. 2.19b). Hormone receptors (ER and PR) are negative (Fig. 2.19c), in contrast to normal endocervical glands and most other benign cervical glandular lesions [22, 45–47]. Cytokeratin (CK) 7 and 20 are positive and negative respectively and CEA is positive only in the apical aspect of the columnar cells, in contrast with the cytoplasmic immunoreactivity in most adenocarcinomas.

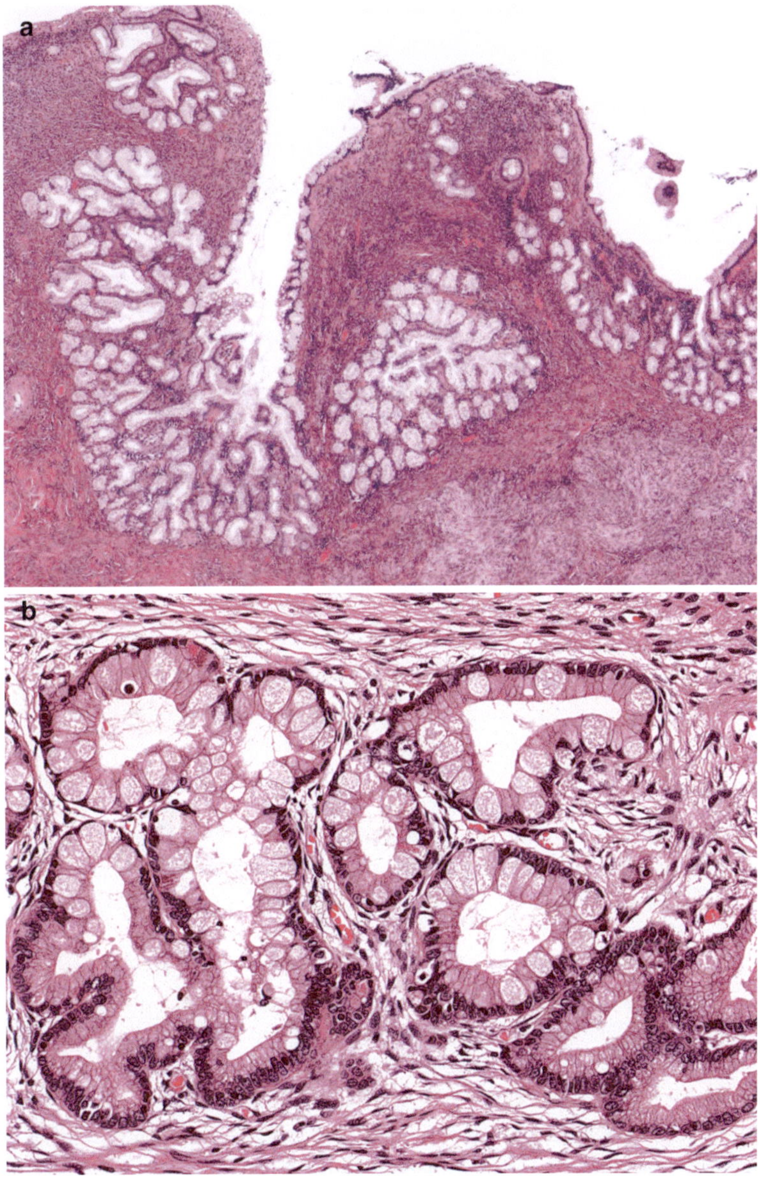

Fig. 2.19 Lobular endocervical glandular hyperplasia characterized by central duct-like structure and surrounding lobules (**a**). Rarely there is focal intestinal metaplasia with goblet cells (**b**). ER is negative but positive in the surrounding stromal cells (**c**). There is positive staining with HIK1083 (**d**)

Fig. 2.19 (continued)

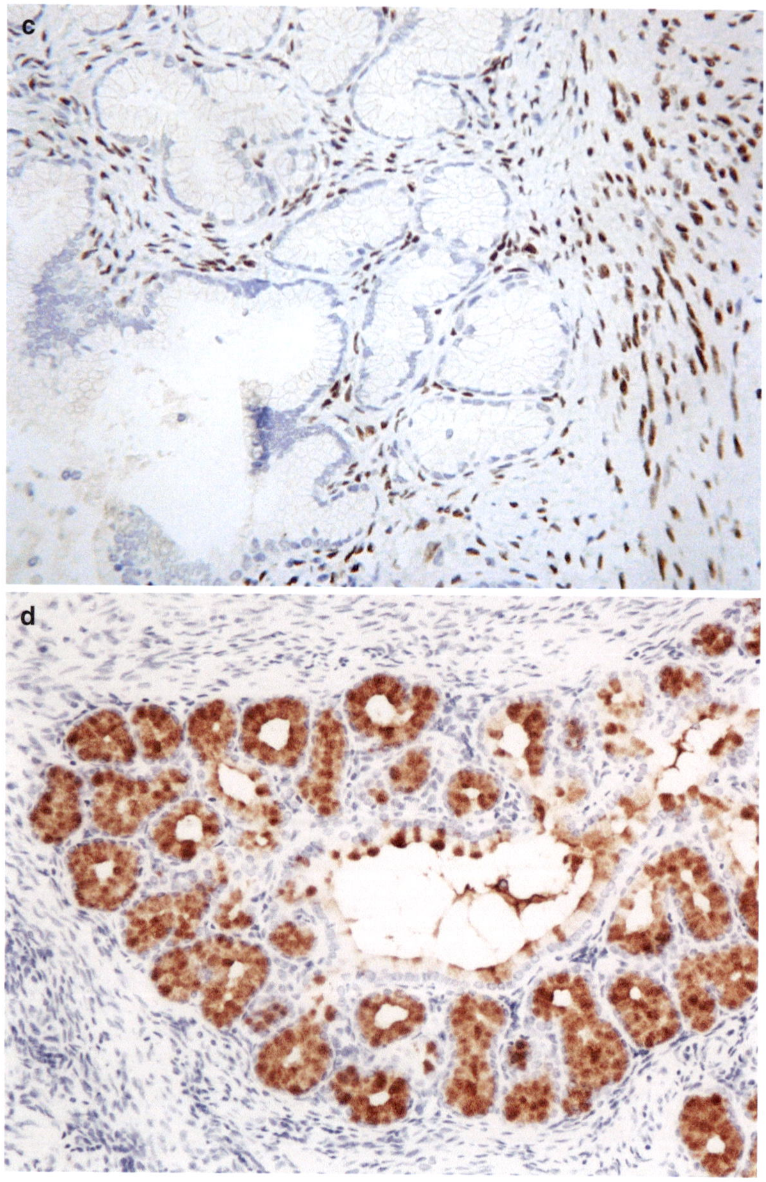

There may be scattered chromogranin A and/or synaptophysin-positive neuroendocrine cells

LEGH, along with type A tunnel clusters, has been proposed to be part of a spectrum of benign cervical glandular lesions exhibiting gastric/pyloric differentiation [22]. These various glandular lesions contain neutral mucins and stain red with combined Alcian-blue/PAS while normal endocervical glands stain a purple-violet colour due to their admixture of acid and neutral mucins [48]. These gastric lesions are also positive with HIK1083 (Fig. 2.19d) and MUC6, markers of pyloric gland mucins [49–51]. Comparing these two markers, HIK1083 is more specific but less sensitive while MUC6 is more sensitive but less specific; staining with both markers, especially HIK1083, is often focal. There are also a variety of premalignant and malignant cervical glandular lesions exhibiting gastric differentiation (Table 2.1).

Although extremely uncommon, atypical variants of LEGH have been described which are characterised by cytological abnormalities (mild nuclear atypia and mitotic activity) and/or

Table 2.1 Endocervical glandular lesions exhibiting gastric differentiation

Benign	Lobular endocervical glandular hyperplasia (complex pyloric/gastric metaplasia)
	Simple gastric/pyloric metaplasia
	Tunnel cluster (type A)
Possible in situ/premalignant	Atypical lobular endocervical glandular hyperplasia
	Adenocarcinoma in situ of gastric type
Malignant	Gastric type adenocarcinoma[a]
	Minimal deviation adenocarcinoma (adenoma malignum)[a]
Specific clinical or clinicopathologic conditions	Synchronous mucinous metaplasia and neoplasia of the female genital tract (SMMN-FGT)
	Peutz-Jeghers syndrome

[a]These comprise a spectrum of cervical gastric type adenocarcinomas with some neoplasms having an admixture of both tumour types and others exhibiting overlapping morphological features

architectural abnormalities, mainly in the form of short papillary projections, and it has been proposed that these represent a precursor of cervical adenocarcinomas exhibiting gastric differentiation [52–54]. In one study, comparative genomic hybridization revealed recurrent chromosomal imbalances, in the form of gains of chromosome 3q and a loss of 1p (aberrations which are common in minimal deviation adenocarcinoma and other cervical mucinous adenocarcinomas), in 3 of 14 LEGHs analyzed (21 %) [54]. LEGHs with chromosomal imbalances exhibited a degree of cellular atypia in the hyperplastic glandular epithelium. Dual-colour fluorescence in situ hybridization confirmed a gain of chromosome 3 fragment in these cervical glandular lesions. This study demonstrated a molecular-genetic link between LEGH and cervical mucinous adenocarcinomas, including adenoma malignum, supporting the hypothesis that a proportion of LEGHs (atypical LEGH) are precancerous precursors of gastric type adenocarcinomas. Gastric type mucinous glandular lesions in the cervix may be associated with synchronous mucinous lesions, including metaplasias and neoplasms, elsewhere within the female genital tract, for example the endometrium, fallopian tube and ovary; in some cases, it may be problematic to ascertain whether these represent synchronous independent mucinous lesions or metastatic disease from one site to another [55–57].

The morphological features of LEGH may result in consideration of an adenocarcinoma, especially adenoma malignum (mucinous variant of minimal deviation adenocarcinoma) and in occasional examples of the latter neoplasm there are areas resembling LEGH, providing evidence that LEGH may, in some cases, represent a precursor lesion of adenoma malignum. The distinction from adenoma malignum is facilitated by the usual absence of an obvious tumour mass in LEGH, its location high in the endocervical canal, its more superficial location, lobular architecture, absence of irregular stromal infiltration and a desmoplastic stromal reaction, no evidence of focal nuclear atypia and no evidence of vascular or perineural infiltration. It has been suggested that a combination of ER and smooth muscle actin (SMA) staining may assist in the distinction [47]. In LEGH and other benign glandular lesions, the stroma surrounding the glands is ER positive and largely SMA negative while in adenoma malignum and other adenocarcinomas, the stroma is SMA positive and there is a decrease in staining with ER as a result of the desmoplasia [47].

While LEGH per se is a benign condition, occasionally an adenocarcinoma can be associated with this (see Chap. 4, section on "Mucinous variant of minimal deviation adenocarcinoma"). Those adenocarcinomas which are associated with LEGH are of gastric type, including adenoma malignum. Therefore, some gynaecologists or patients may prefer hysterectomy in cases of LEGH diagnosed on loop excision to confirm that there is no co-existing adenocarcinoma. Loop excision with close surveillance, especially where fertility preservation is an issue, is also an option. Currently, the exact risk of coexistence or future development of adenocarcinoma is unknown, although this is likely to be low. However, in the presence of a clinically significant mass and/or massive watery vaginal discharge, the patient should be managed with caution.

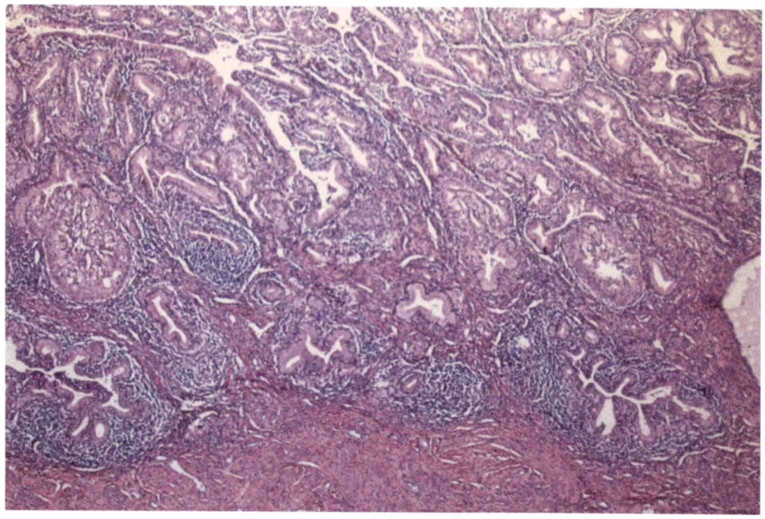

Fig. 2.20 Diffuse laminar endocervical glandular hyperplasia consisting of proliferation of endocervical glands with an associated inflammatory infiltrate; a straight line can be drawn under the proliferation

Diffuse Laminar Endocervical Glandular Hyperplasia (DLEGH)

This rare lesion is an incidental microscopic finding within the cervix and usually occurs within the reproductive years [58]. It is characterised by a band-like proliferation of endocervical glands which is sharply demarcated from the underlying stroma such that a straight line can almost be drawn under the proliferation (Fig. 2.20). DLEGH is usually confined to the inner third of the cervix and is characterised by the presence of moderately sized, evenly spaced, closely packed glands. There may be mild nuclear atypia and an inflammatory or oedematous stromal reaction. Adenoma malignum (mucinous variant of minimal deviation adenocarcinoma) may be considered in the differential. Features that assist in this distinction are that in DLEGH, there is no mass lesion, irregular stromal infiltration, desmoplastic stromal response or focal malignant cytological features.

Deep Glands and Nabothian Cysts

Occasionally normal endocervical glands and dilated glands (Nabothian cysts) are located deep within the cervical stroma, sometimes extending close to the paracervical connective tissues (Fig. 2.21) [59, 60]. The Nabothian cysts may be visible macroscopically. The glands and cysts are lined by bland mucinous epithelium which may be focally or extensively attenuated. Sometimes there is focal tubal differentiation with cilia. When the features are florid, deep glands and cysts may be confused with adenoma malignum but the overall appearances differ from the latter and misdiagnosis is unlikely. There is no evidence of focal cytologic atypia and there is an absence of a desmoplastic stromal reaction, vascular and perineural invasion.

Microglandular Hyperplasia (MGH)

This is a very common finding within the cervix and was previously referred to as microglandular adenosis. It is usually an incidental microscopic finding but occasionally, when florid, results in the formation of a grossly visible lesion and clinically appears as an erosion or a polyp or there may even be clinical suspicion of malignancy. Rarely, there is vaginal discharge or bleeding. MGH typically, but not always, occurs in women in the reproductive years (<5 % in postmenopausal patients) and there is usually a history of hormone usage or pregnancy, although this is not invariable; for example, in one study only 58 % of women had a recent history of hormone usage or pregnancy [61]. Most cases probably arise as a

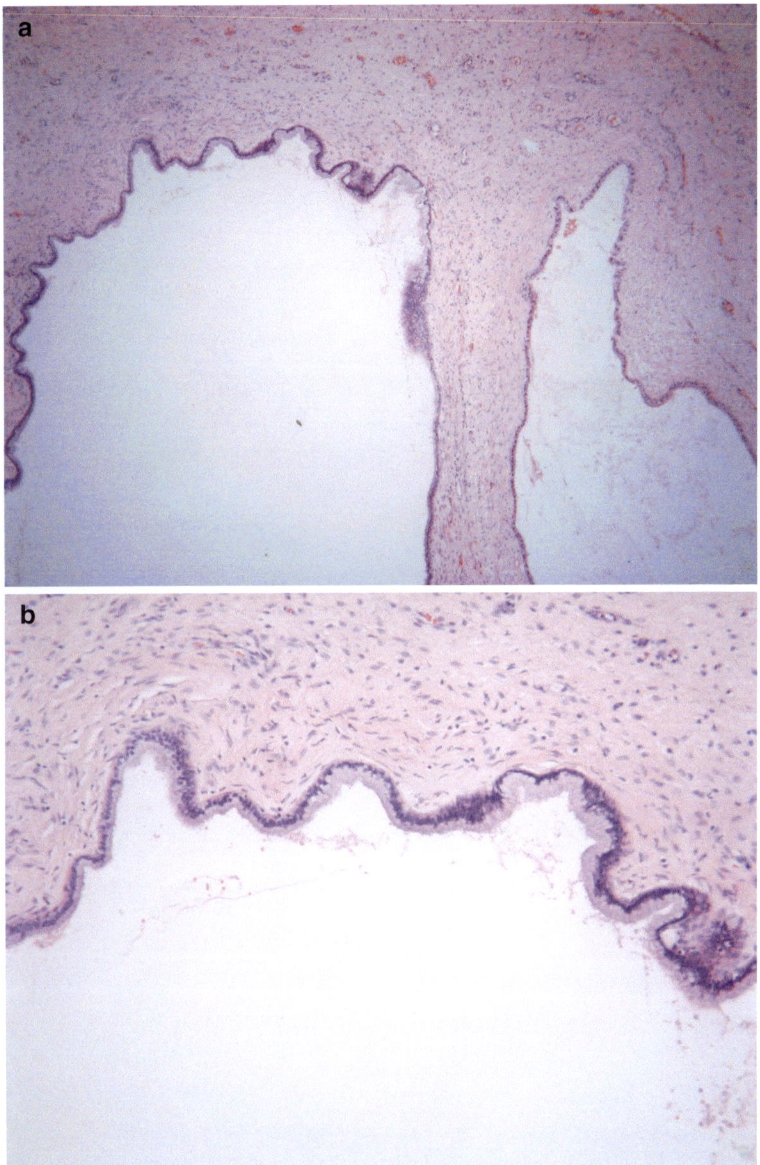

Fig. 2.21 Deep Nabothian cysts within cervical stroma (**a**). On high power, the deep Nabothian cysts are lined by bland mucinous epithelium (**b**)

result of exogenous or endogenous progestogen effect.

MGH involves the endocervical glands at the transformation zone or more proximally. It is often multifocal and may be particularly florid within endocervical polyps, especially involving the surface. The typical morphology is of microglandular architecture with cytoplasmic vacuolation, resulting in a "lace-like" pattern (Fig. 2.22a). There is often associated reserve cell hyperplasia and immature squamous metaplasia. The glands are lined by low columnar, cuboidal or flattened cells which exhibit little in the way of nuclear atypia or mitotic activity. Some of the glands may be dilated. There is characteristically a brisk inflammatory cell infiltrate, including neutrophils and plasma cells (Fig. 2.22b). Cytoplasmic vacuolation is the most common characteristic feature and this may be seen in early forms before the microglandular architecture is apparent. In some cases, the reserve cell hyperplasia and/or immature squamous metaplasia is the predominant feature. Cervical MGH exhibits a low MIB1 proliferation

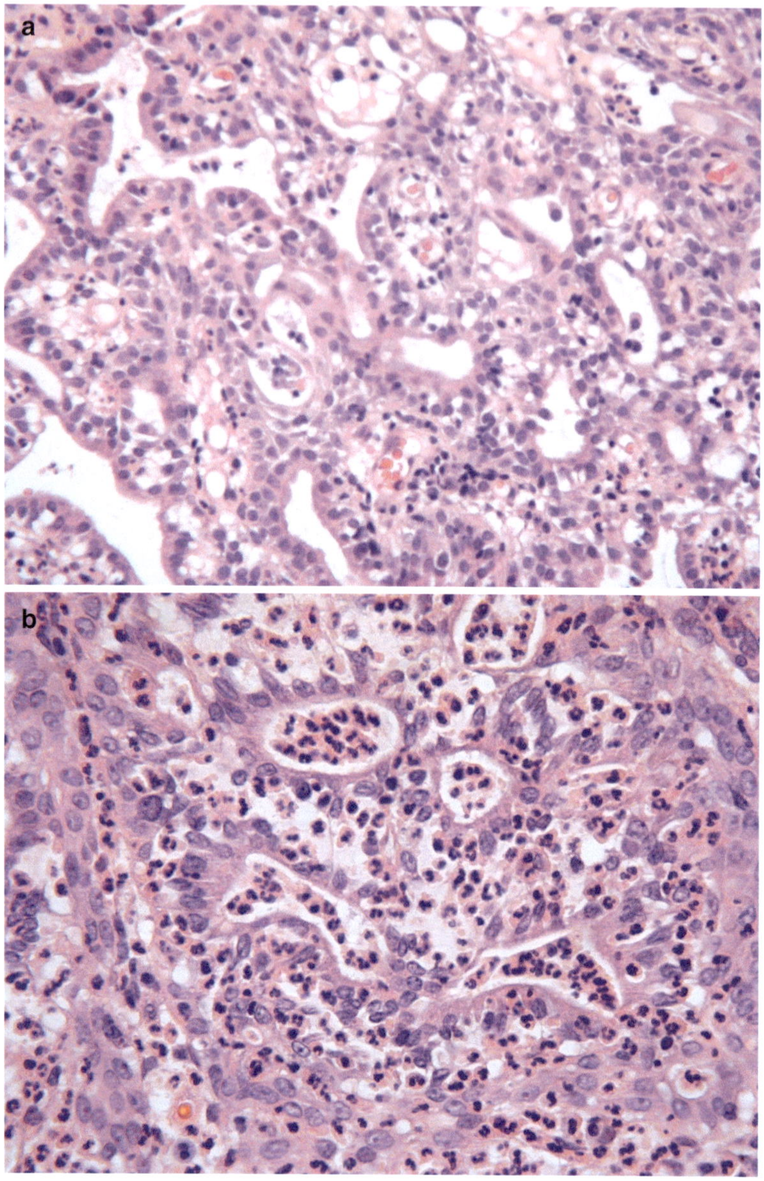

Fig. 2.22 Microglandular hyperplasia consisting of closely packed small glands with cytoplasmic vacuolation (**a**). In some cases of microglandular hyperplasia, there is prominent polymorph infiltration (**b**)

index and is negative with p16 and bcl2; CEA is usually negative [13, 62].

A variety of atypical features may occasionally be seen which can result in consideration of a malignant process [63]. In evaluating such cases, the presence of more typical areas of MGH is often a clue to the correct diagnosis. These atypical features include the presence of solid formations, signet ring cells, marked stromal hyalinisation creating an impression of infiltration, corded, papillary, reticular or trabecular architecture, myxoid stroma, hobnail cells and mild to moderate nuclear atypia (Fig. 2.23). These features, especially when florid, may potentially result in confusion with a clear cell carcinoma or a microglandular variant of adenocarcinoma (especially a microglandular variant of endometrial adenocarcinoma of endometrioid or mucinous type). The stromal hyalinisation, in particular, may result in consideration of clear cell carcinoma, since eosinophilic stromal hyalinisation is characteristic of this neoplasm.

Distinction from a carcinoma is only likely to be a problem in a small biopsy specimen and the identification of areas of typical MGH, if present, is in favour of this diagnosis.

The distinction in a small biopsy specimen between cervical MGH and a microglandular variant of adenocarcinoma of the endometrium may be particularly problematic and caution should be exercised before rendering a diagnosis of cervical MGH in an endometrial biopsy in a postmenopausal woman. Some endometrial adenocarcinomas of endometrioid or mucinous type exhibit a microglandular growth pattern, especially towards the surface [64–66]. This surface component is likely to be sampled by endometrial biopsy and may closely mimic cervical MGH (or endometrial papillary syncytial metaplasia). Cytoplasmic vacuolation is characteristic of MGH, as this is not usually found in microglandular adenocarcinomas [66]. Areas of adenocarcinoma without a microglandular architecture are obviously of value in

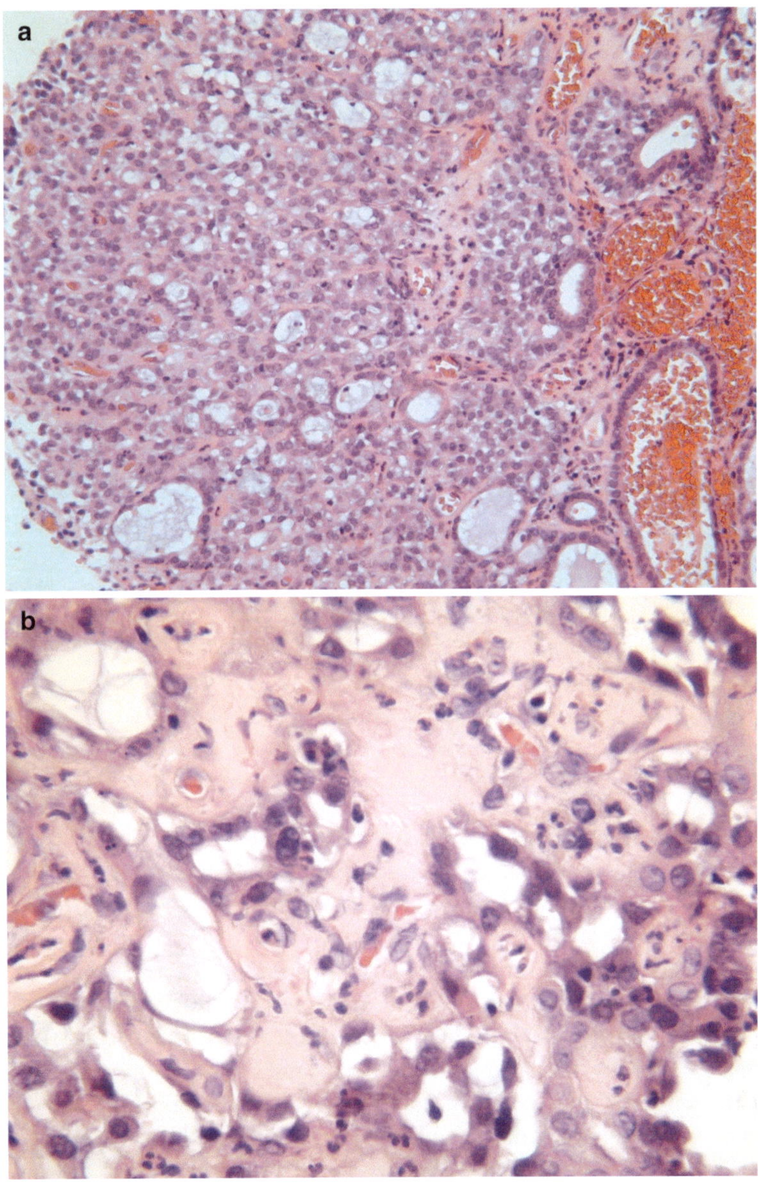

Fig. 2.23 Atypical features in microglandular hyperplasia with solid formations (**a**), stromal hyalinization (**b**), signet ring cells (**c**) and a papillary architecture (**d**)

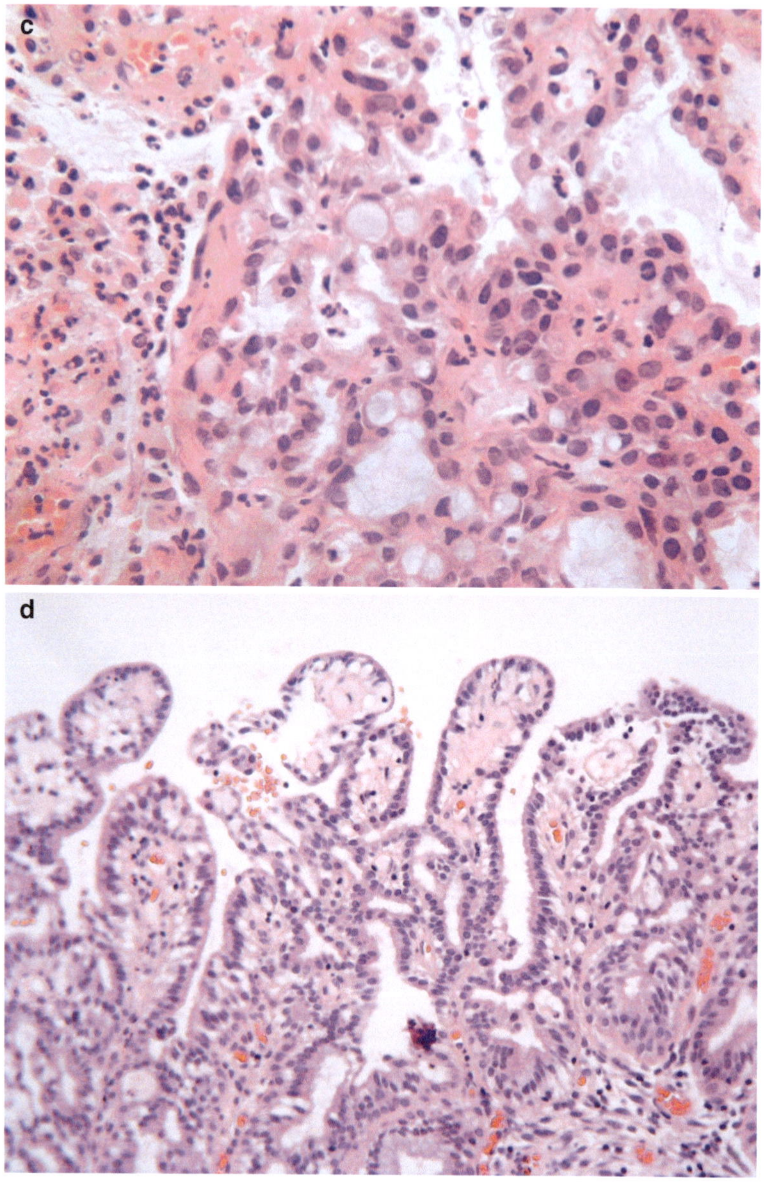

Fig. 2.23 (continued)

diagnosis. There is considerable immunophenotypic overlap such that in an individual case, markers may not assist [67]. However, vimentin may be useful in that many microglandular adenocarcinomas of the endometrium are positive whereas cervical MGH is usually negative [66]. However, some microglandular adenocarcinomas, especially those which exhibit mucinous differentiation, are vimentin negative. One study which investigated a number of markers found that p16 was more likely to be positive in microglandular adenocarcinoma of the endometrium than cervical MGH and that this was the most useful marker in the differential diagnosis [65].

Mesonephric Remnants and Mesonephric Gland Hyperplasia

Mesonephric remnants are not uncommonly seen within the cervix (approximately 10 % of cervices) [68]. They are usually situated deep within

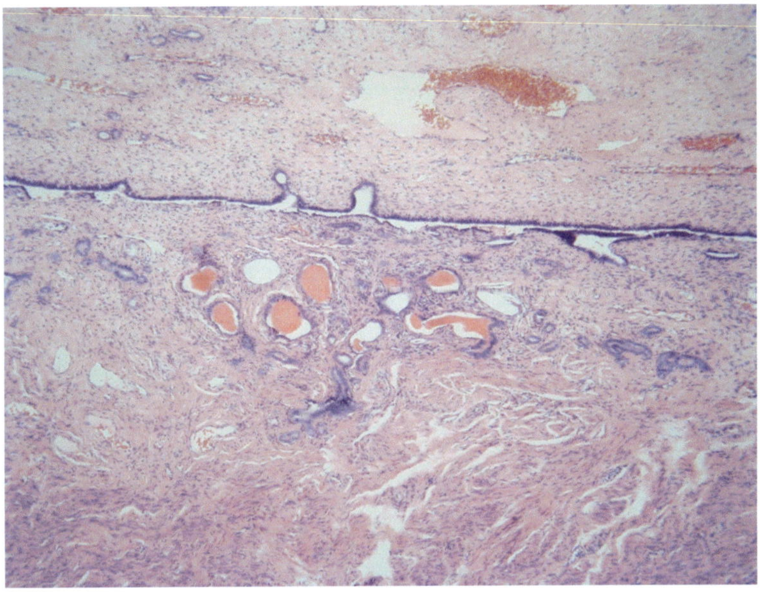

Fig. 2.24 Mesonephric remnants consisting of central duct and surrounding small tubules containing eosinophilic luminal colloid-like material; a linear arrangement is often a feature

the cervical stroma in the lateral walls; they also occur extremely rarely within the vagina. Mesonephric remnants and hyperplasia may involve the ectocervix, transformation zone or endocervix and may also extend proximally to involve the lower uterine segment. The distinction between "normal" and "hyperplastic" mesonephric remnants is arbitrary and a 6 mm cut-off has been suggested [68]. On low power examination, mesonephric remnants typically have a somewhat linear arrangement, the linear arrays being arranged parallel to the mucosal surface beneath normal endocervical glands or squamous epithelium (Fig. 2.24). Sometimes, there is a rather infiltrative low power appearance with the glands appearing to "melt-through" the stroma. There may be mild increased cellularity surrounding the glands. The remnants usually have at least focally a lobular arrangement, being composed of central duct-like structures and surrounding small tubules, although ducts are not present in all cases. Occasionally, some of the tubules are dilated. The ducts and tubules are lined by cuboidal cells with vesicular nuclei and scant cytoplasm; occasionally there is cytoplasmic clearing. There is little nuclear stratification (occasionally there is mild stratification and bridging), pleomorphism or mitotic activity and no intracytoplasmic mucin. The presence of PAS positive eosinophilic secretions (often referred to as colloid-like) within some of the ductal and tubular lumina is characteristic.

Lobular, diffuse and ductal variants of mesonephric hyperplasia have been described and sometimes there are admixtures [68]. In lobular variants, the architecture is similar to that seen in "normal" mesonephric remnants. Diffuse mesonephric hyperplasia consists mainly of small tubules without a lobular architecture (Fig. 2.25) while the uncommon ductal variant is composed of larger duct-like structures without tubules (Fig. 2.26). The ducts usually have a somewhat linear arrangement and small papillary infoldings may be present. When there is florid mesonephric hyperplasia, the ducts and tubules may involve much of the cervix and be admixed amongst normal endocervical glands. There may rarely even be extension into the lower uterine segment and/or paracervical connective tissues.

Distinction from other benign endocervical glandular lesions is chiefly based on the location and the characteristic morphological appearances but immunohistochemistry may assist in problematic cases. Markers which may be positive in mesonephric glands include CD10 (characteristic apical luminal positivity), epithelial membrane antigen (EMA), androgen receptor, calretinin, vimentin, PAX2 and PAX8 [69–73]. ER, PR and

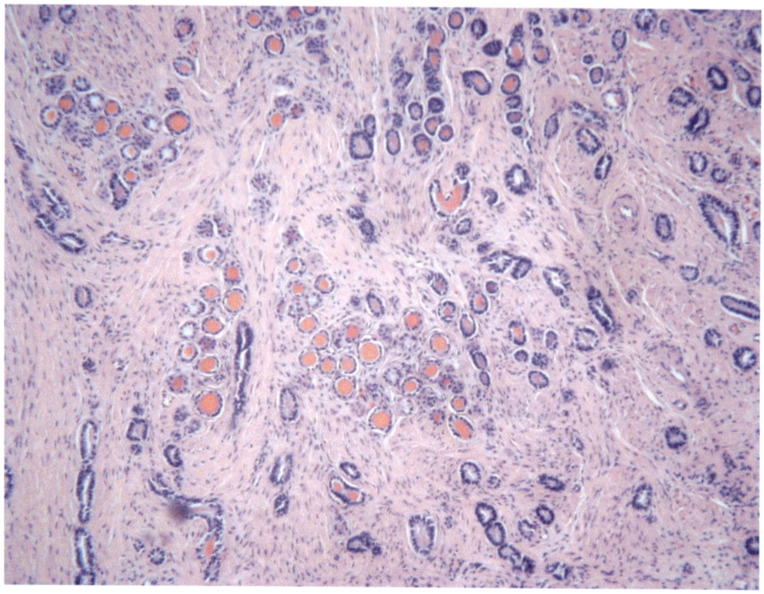

Fig. 2.25 Diffuse mesonephric hyperplasia with small tubules containing eosinophilic luminal colloid-like material throughout cervical stroma

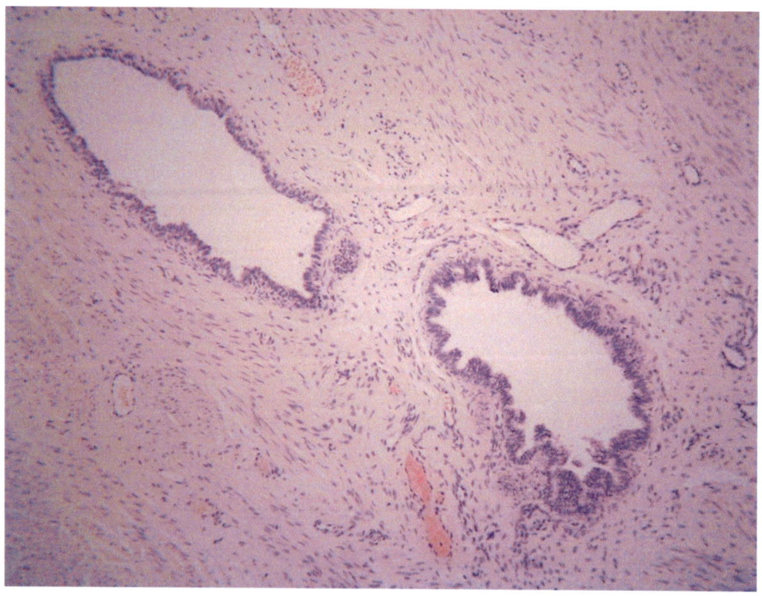

Fig. 2.26 Ductal mesonephric remnants composed of duct-like structures with small papillary infoldings

CEA are usually negative. The combination of positive staining with CD10 and vimentin and totally negative staining with ER and PR is characteristic and allows distinction from other benign endocervical glandular lesions. CD10 positivity is uncommon in other benign endocervical glandular lesions but may be seen in malignant endocervical glandular lesions [69]. p16 may be focally positive in mesonephric glands [73]. Purely ductal mesonephric hyperplasia may rarely be confused with CGIN but is characteristically situated deep to normal endocervical glands. Some of the aforementioned immunohistochemical markers may assist in this distinction, although CGIN, like mesonephric remnants, is usually ER and PR negative. It may be extremely difficult to distinguish between florid diffuse mesonephric hyperplasia and a mesonephric adenocarcinoma [72, 74]. Mesonephric hyperplasia is almost always an

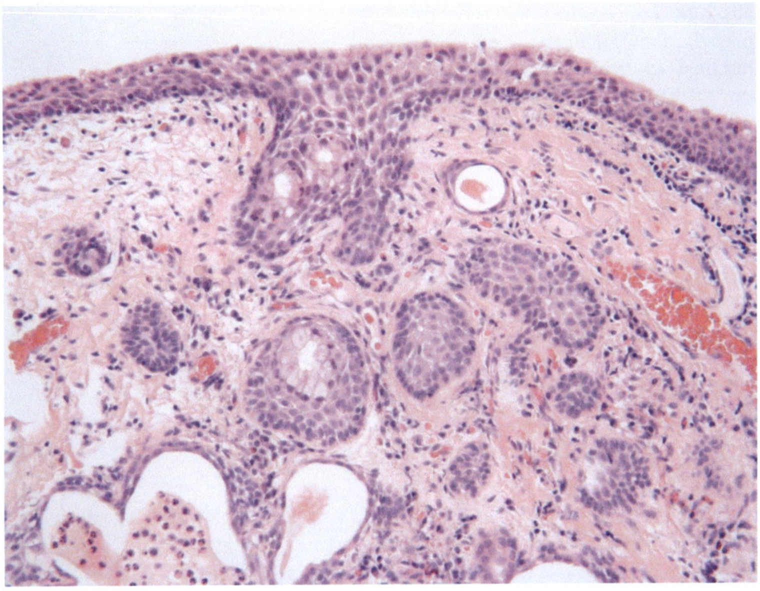

Fig. 2.27 Adenoid basal hyperplasia consisting of small buds of cells with a basaloid appearance attached to the surface squamous epithelium

incidental microscopic finding while most, but not all, mesonephric adenocarcinomas form an obvious tumour mass. Although some areas may be cytologically bland, almost all mesonephric adenocarcinomas contain foci which are obviously cytologically malignant with significant glandular crowding, nuclear atypia and mitotic activity, destructive stromal invasion and sometimes lymphovascular permeation. It should be noted that mesonephric hyperplasia and adenocarcinoma may coexist and the boundary between these may not be clear in individual cases.

Adenoid Basal Hyperplasia

This is a not uncommon incidental microscopic finding which has not been extensively described in the literature. It is most common in postmenopausal women, but may also occur in the reproductive age group, and consequently is most commonly seen in hysterectomy specimens.

Morphologically, adenoid basal hyperplasia is characterised by multiple small buds of cells with a basaloid appearance emanating from the overlying normal squamous or glandular epithelium and involving the superficial cervical stroma (Fig. 2.27) [75]. Some of the buds are attached to the surface while others appear to lie free within the stroma. Sometimes small glandular lumina are formed or there may be focal squamous differentiation. There is little or no nuclear atypia or mitotic activity and no stromal reaction. This lesion has also been termed postmenopausal basaloid proliferation [76].

The main differential is likely to be adenoid basal carcinoma and it has been suggested that adenoid basal hyperplasia represents an early form of adenoid basal carcinoma [75], although there is no firm evidence for this. Adenoid basal hyperplasia is distinguished from adenoid basal carcinoma by its tiny size, superficial location and contact with the overlying epithelium, although in some cases the distinction between the two can be difficult and somewhat arbitrary. There is usually no associated premalignant or malignant squamous lesion in adenoid basal hyperplasia, these being commonly seen in association with adenoid basal carcinoma.

Reactive and Inflammatory Lesions

Endocervical Polyps

Endocervical polyps are non-neoplastic inflammatory-related lesions and are thus discussed here. They are common lesions which

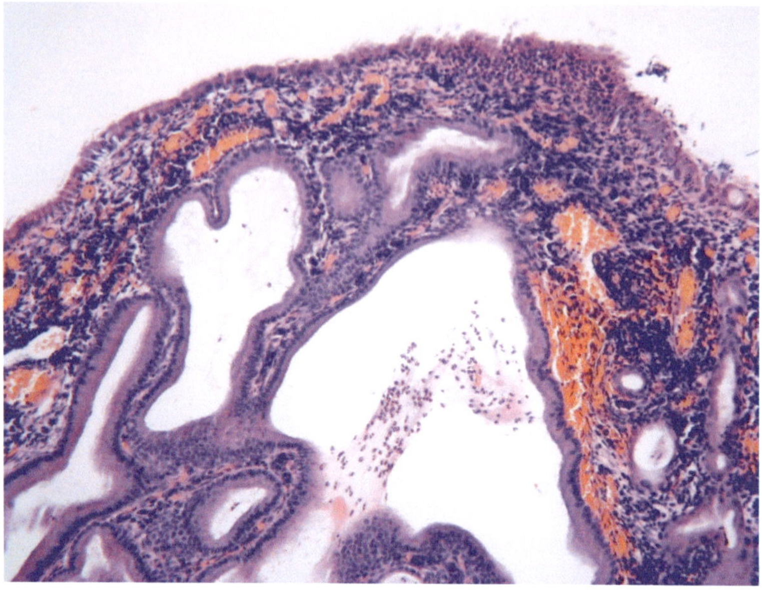

Fig. 2.28 Endocervical polyp lined by columnar mucinous epithelium which invaginates into the underlying stroma

occur over a wide age range. They are single or more uncommonly multiple and are most common in the reproductive years. They may be an incidental finding at a smear test or on colposcopic examination or be associated with symptoms such as abnormal vaginal bleeding or discharge. They can also result in an abnormal cervical smear since the glandular epithelial cells can exhibit a degree of atypia.

Morphologically these have a polypoid appearance and are lined by typical endocervical columnar mucinous epithelium. The columnar epithelium invaginates into the underlying stroma to form glands (Fig. 2.28). The surface epithelium or glands may exhibit focal tubal or tuboendometrial metaplasia and there is often mature or immature squamous metaplasia which may be florid and involve much of the surface or expansively fill the underlying glands. The stroma is typically inflamed with a mixture of acute and chronic inflammatory cells and is often oedematous. The inflammatory cells are often most conspicuous just deep to the surface. Occasionally, a few smooth muscle fibres are present within the stroma. There may be surface erosion and not uncommonly the surface glandular or squamous epithelium exhibits a degree of reactive nuclear atypia. This may be particularly marked involving the glandular epithelium but characteristically there is a low nuclear to cytoplasmic ratio. The reactive glandular epithelium sometimes has a hobnail appearance with enlarged nuclei with prominent nucleoli and sometimes there is multinucleation or multilobated nuclei are present (Fig. 2.29). The cytoplasm is typically abundant and eosinophilic and contains neutrophils. These "reactive" glandular changes are similar morphologically to those which involve the epithelium of some ovarian endometriotic cysts. In some endocervical polyps, there is a focal club-like (phyllodes-like) architecture with intraglandular stromal protrusions and increased cellularity around glands. These features may result in consideration of a lesion in the adenofibroma/adenosarcoma category but in such cases, follow-up is usually uneventful [77]. Occasionally, there is a focal "overgrowth" of loose oedematous stroma without glands which results in consideration of a benign mesenchymal lesion; however, this is part of the spectrum of endocervical polyps.

In some cases, microglandular hyperplasia is present, especially on the surface of the polyp, and when florid, this may result in a "busy" appearance. Cervical polyps in pregnancy may exhibit the Arias Stella reaction and/or there may be stromal decidualisation (Fig. 2.30). Uncommonly, there is focal involvement of an

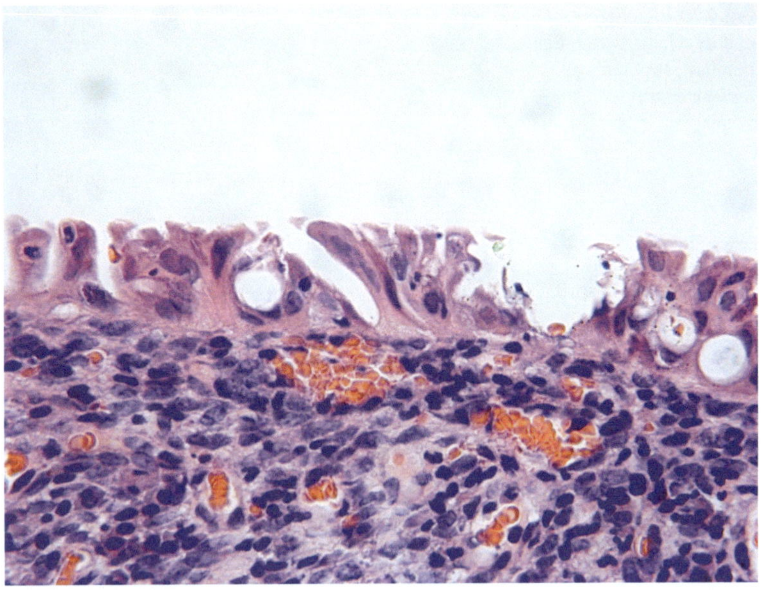

Fig. 2.29 Atypical cells on surface of endocervical polyp with a hobnail appearance

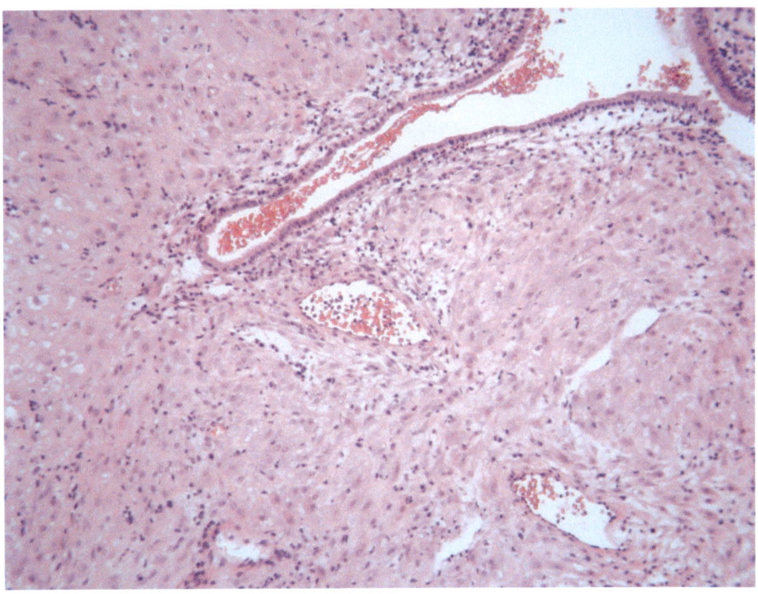

Fig. 2.30 Cervical polyp in pregnancy exhibiting extensive stromal decidualisation

endocervical polyp by CIN, CGIN or an invasive carcinoma [78]. Although the premalignant or malignant lesion may be confined to the polyp, there is also more commonly involvement of the cervix outside the confines of the polyp.

Rare cervical polyps containing benign adipose tissue, cartilage or glial tissue, which may be of foetal origin, have been reported [79, 80]. Fibroepithelial polyps rarely occur within the cervix; these do not contain a glandular component but rather are lined entirely by squamous epithelium. Similar to their much more common counterparts within the vulva and vagina, atypical stromal fibroblasts may be present.

Inflammatory Atypia

In association with inflammation, the endocervical epithelium may exhibit a degree of

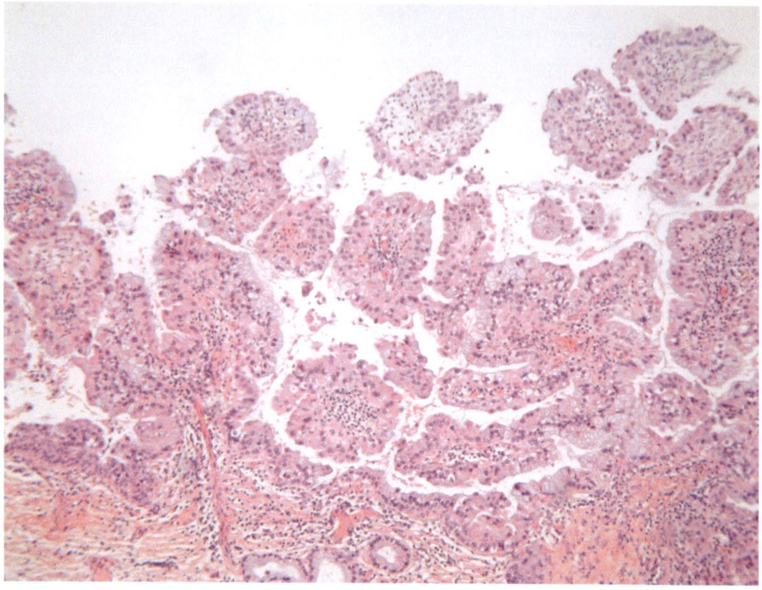

Fig. 2.31 Papillary endocervicitis with inflamed papillary structures and associated mild nuclear atypia

nuclear atypia. This is especially common on the surface of benign endocervical polyps, as discussed in the last section. Although there may be quite significant atypia, individual cells are usually involved and there is typically both nuclear and cytoplasmic enlargement with the maintenance of a low nuclear to cytoplasmic ratio. As discussed in the last section, the atypical cells may contain abundant eosinophilic cytoplasm and have a hobnail appearance being morphologically somewhat similar to the reactive atypia commonly seen within endometriotic cysts of the ovary. If fragments of inflamed endocervical glandular tissue are present in an endometrial biopsy, an erroneous diagnosis of endometritis may be made.

Papillary Endocervicitis

When the endocervix becomes inflamed, the surface epithelium commonly assumes a papillary architecture; this is referred to as papillary endocervicitis (Fig. 2.31) [1]. When florid, a gross lesion or "erosion" may be seen. With papillary endocervicitis, there may be associated reactive nuclear atypia. In most cases, there are no issues in diagnosis but when the papillary architecture is florid with associated nuclear atypia, there is some potential for confusion with a villoglandular adenocarcinoma or a papillary cervical adenocarcinoma of usual type. However, any atypia is mild, sometimes with multinucleate cells, and there is little in the way of mitotic activity. In problematic cases, p16 may be of use since this is negative in papillary endocervicitis but diffusely positive in most adenocarcinomas with a papillary architecture.

Follicular Cervicitis

This refers to inflammation of the cervix, usually the endocervix, containing lymphoid follicles, often with germinal centres. There is often associated plasmacytic and neutrophilic infiltration. Some cases may be secondary to Chlamydia infection [81].

Radiation-Associated Change/Atypia

Obviously in establishing a diagnosis of radiation-associated changes, the history is paramount. Prior radiation therapy (or chemoradiation), which may have been recent or many years previously, can result in quite marked atypia of the endocervical glands [1, 82]. However, as with

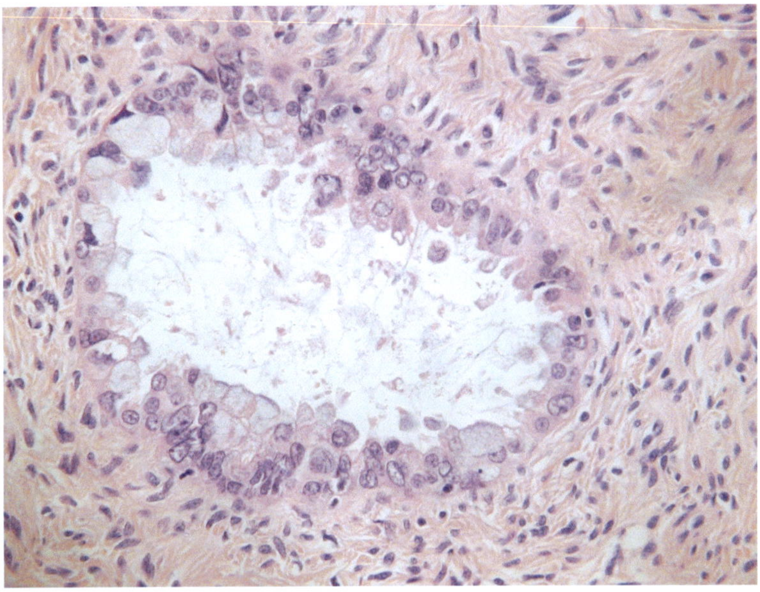

Fig. 2.32 Radiation atypia characterized by endocervical glands lined by cells exhibiting a degree of nuclear atypia

many other reactive glandular conditions in the cervix, a low nuclear to cytoplasmic ratio is usually maintained and the cells often have abundant eosinophilic cytoplasm; the morphological features are similar to those seen in atypical oxyphilic metaplasia involving the endocervical glands [18]. The nuclear enlargement may be quite marked and bizarre nuclear forms can be seen, sometimes with multinucleation and prominent eosinophilic nucleoli (Fig. 2.32). The nuclei are hyperchromatic and, in some cases, have a "smudged" appearance. There are few mitotic figures. Cytoplasmic vacuolation may be present. Often the atypical nuclei are present individually or in small clusters with intervening normal endocervical nuclei. The features may be mistaken for CGIN, an adenocarcinoma, especially of serous type, or serous endometrial intraepithelial carcinoma (serous EIC). However, the normal glandular architecture is typically maintained with no glandular crowding, there is a low nuclear to cytoplasmic ratio and the atypical cells are admixed with normal cells. There are also commonly stromal changes, such as hyaline thickening of blood vessels and atypical fibroblasts. p16 may be positive, usually with focal immunoreactivity, in some cases of radiation affected endocervical glands [83]. p53 usually exhibits "wild-type" staining (focal, weak, heterogenous) in radiation affected endocervical glands while most cases of serous adenocarcinoma or serous EIC exhibit diffuse nuclear immunoreactivity.

Changes Secondary to Mucin Extravasation

A variety of benign endocervical glandular lesions (or normal endocervical glands) may be associated with a stromal inflammatory, oedematous or mild fibroblastic reaction secondary to rupture of glands [25, 26]. The inflammatory cell infiltrate often includes foamy histiocytes and multinucleate giant cells (Fig. 2.33). The benign nature of the underlying glandular lesion is usually obvious but mucin extravasation with a stromal reaction may occur in association with a variety of benign endocervical glandular lesions which in themselves may be diagnostically challenging. In such cases, the presence of a stromal reaction to mucin extravasation may result in further diagnostic confusion.

Cytomegalovirus Infection

Cytomegalovirus (CMV) may affect the cervix and in most cases the characteristic cytoplasmic

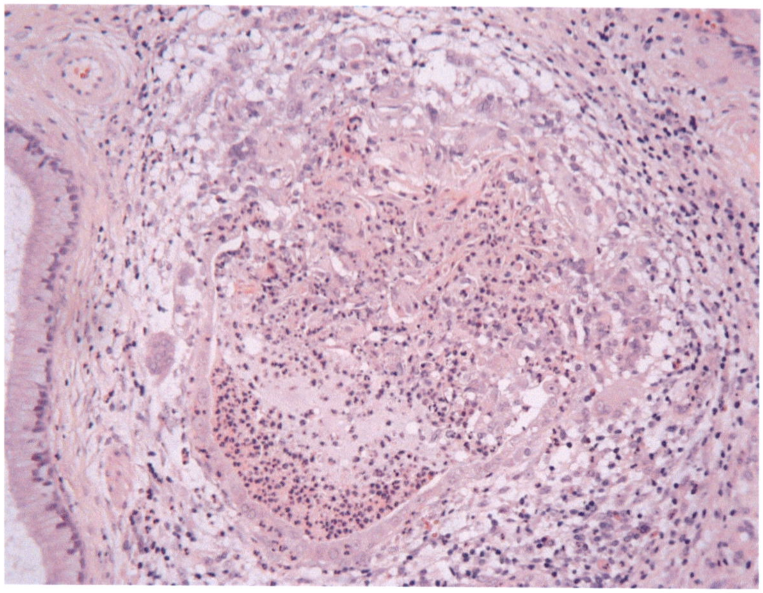

Fig. 2.33 Ruptured endocervical gland with mucin extravasation and a histiocytic and giant cell reaction

inclusions are predominanty found within endocervical glands (Fig. 2.34a); endothelial and stromal cells more uncommonly contain inclusions [84]. Usually only scattered individual endocervical cells are affected and there may be associated mild nuclear atypia [84]. There may be inflammation, including lymphoid follicles, and fibrin thrombi can be present within vessels. Occasional cases are associated with a "lymphoma-like" lesion (see Chap. 5, section on "Lymphoma-like lesion"). Although some patients are immunosuppressed, most cases of CMV infection within the cervix are an incidental microscopic finding in patients who are not immunocompromised. Diagnosis is straightforward, using anti-CMV antibodies (Fig. 2.34b), once the characteristic inclusions are seen.

Cautery Artefact

Iatrogenic cautery may result in nuclear changes involving the endocervical glands (and also cervical squamous epithelium) which can mimic CGIN. This is most commonly seen in large loop excisions of the transformation zone (LLETZs) and the alterations are most marked at the edge of the specimen, although when severe the entire tissue may be affected. The degree of artefact depends somewhat on the instrumentation and technique used [85]. Typically, the nuclei exhibit streaming artefact with elongation and extrusion of nuclear material, resulting in a "crushed" appearance (Fig. 2.35). The cervical stroma is characteristically homogenized and darkly stained and there may be signet ring alteration of the stroma [86]. In the distinction from CGIN, immunohistochemistry may be useful in that although the glands are artefacted, they usually maintain their characteristic staining patterns; cauterized normal endocervical glands are MIB1, p16 and bcl2 negative. Benign cervical glandular lesions, especially TEM, may also be affected by cautery artefact but again maintain their characteristic staining patterns, TEM being bcl2 positive, p16 negative or focally positive and there is a low MIB1 proliferation index.

Multinucleate Endocervical Cells

The occurrence of multinucleate endocervical cells or endocervical cells with multilobated nuclei is a not uncommon incidental finding, usually close to the transformation zone (Fig. 2.36). Usually only isolated individual cells

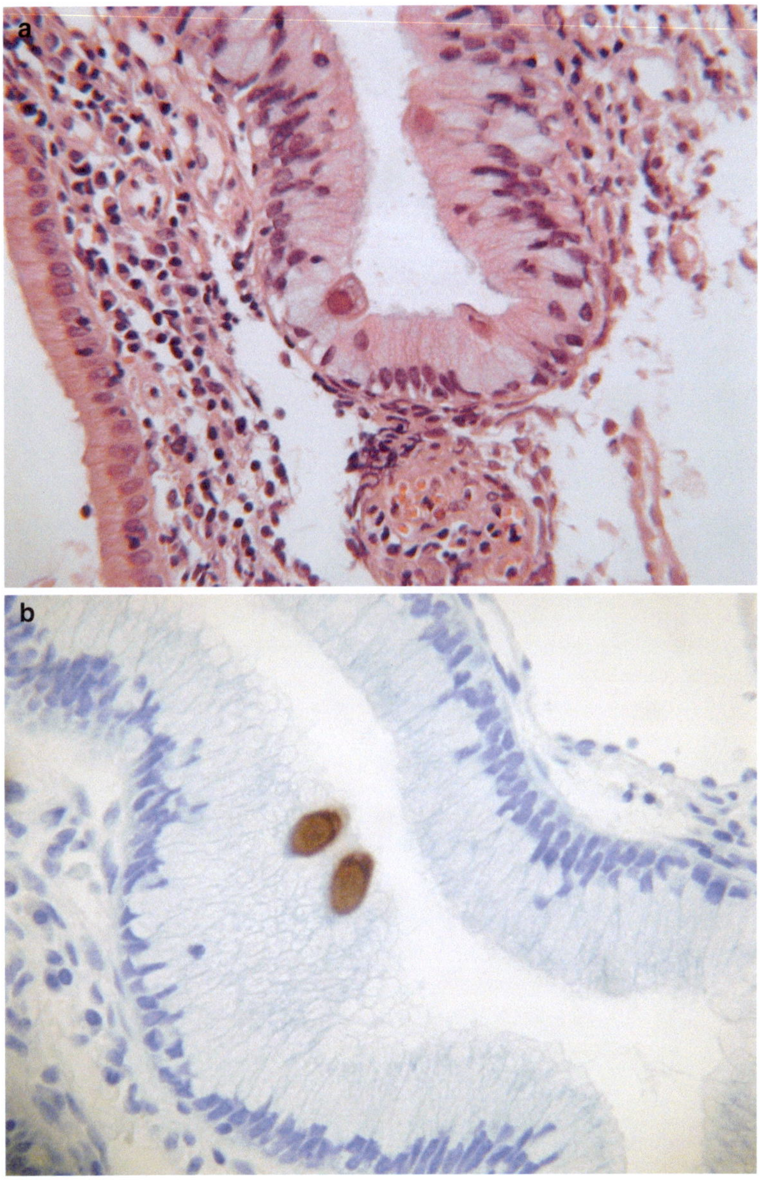

Fig. 2.34 Cytomegalovirus inclusions involving endocervical glands. There is positive immunohistochemical staining of the inclusions with ant-CMV antibodies

exhibit this phenomenon but occasionally many cells are affected. Commonly there is associated inflammation and the changes are likely to be secondary to this. In spite of the multinucleation and multilobation, there is no significant atypia and little or no mitotic activity. The multinucleate cells are not a manifestation of HPV or herpes simplex virus infection; these both generally affect cervical squamous rather than glandular epithelium.

Endocervical Glandular Changes Secondary to Recent Endometrial Curettage or Biopsy

It is not uncommon to see changes in the endocervix in cases where a hysterectomy has been performed a short time following an endometrial curettage or biopsy, especially a curettage [87]. In most cases, there are no diagnostic difficulties but when the features are florid, problems may

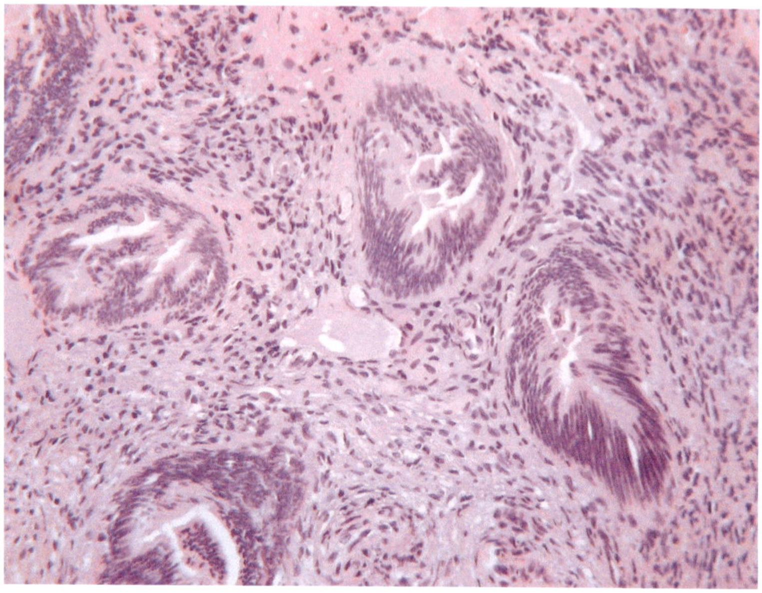

Fig. 2.35 Cautery artifact involving endocervical glands with marked nuclear streaming and homogenization of the tissues

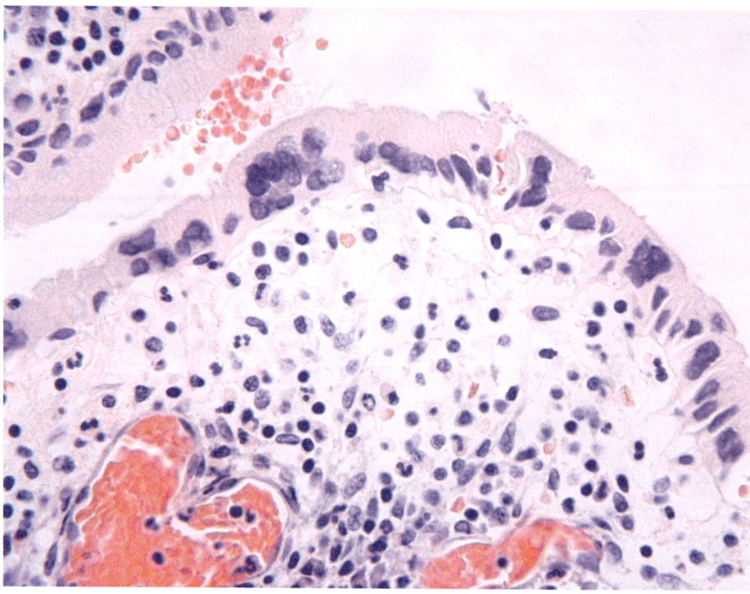

Fig. 2.36 Multinucleate endocervical cells

ensue. If the hysterectomy was performed for endometrial carcinoma, overdiagnosis of cervical glandular or even stromal involvement by tumour can occur. The changes have been referred to as atypical reactive proliferation of the endocervix [87]. The histological features, not all of which are present in every case, include nuclear stratification and multilayering with a micropapillary architecture, squamoid change, hobnail cells, cytoplasmic clearing and mild cytological atypia (Fig. 2.37a). There is often associated surface erosion, fibrin deposition and an inflammatory cell infiltrate. There can be fibrosis of the subepithelial stroma with entrapment of epithelial cells which can result in overdiagnosis of cervical stromal involvement by tumour. In some cases, there is a florid granulation tissue-like appearance (Fig. 2.37b). Awareness of this phenomenon and knowledge of the recnet biopsy procedure are important in avoiding misinterpretation.

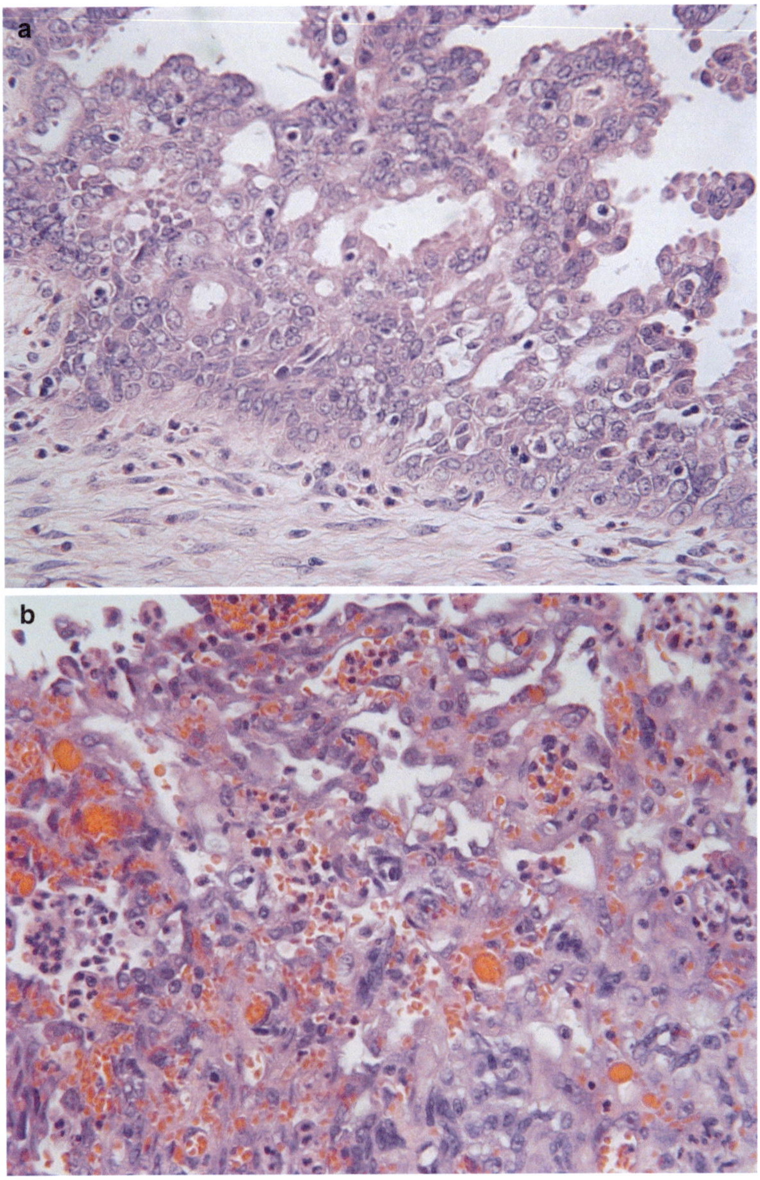

Fig. 2.37 Atypical reactive proliferation of endocervix with short micropapillary processes (**a**). Atypical reactive proliferation with florid granulation tissue-like appearance (**b**)

Benign Glandular Neoplasms

Endocervical Adenomyoma

Adenomyomas of endocervical type are uncommon lesions usually occurring in women of reproductive or postmenopausal age. They vary in size and are most commonly polypoid and project from the mucosal surface of the cervix. Rare examples are intramural or exophytic. They are grossly well circumscribed, usually grey-white to tan and may contain small cysts. Histologically, they are composed of bland mucinous glands of endocervical type, often with a somewhat lobular arrangement, embedded in a stroma containing abundant smooth muscle (Fig. 2.38a) [88]. Some of the glands may be dilated. There may be focal mild nuclear atypia and minor foci of tubal or endometrioid type epithelium but there is no stromal desmoplasia (Fig. 2.38b). These are benign lesions but occasionally persist or recur following local excision.

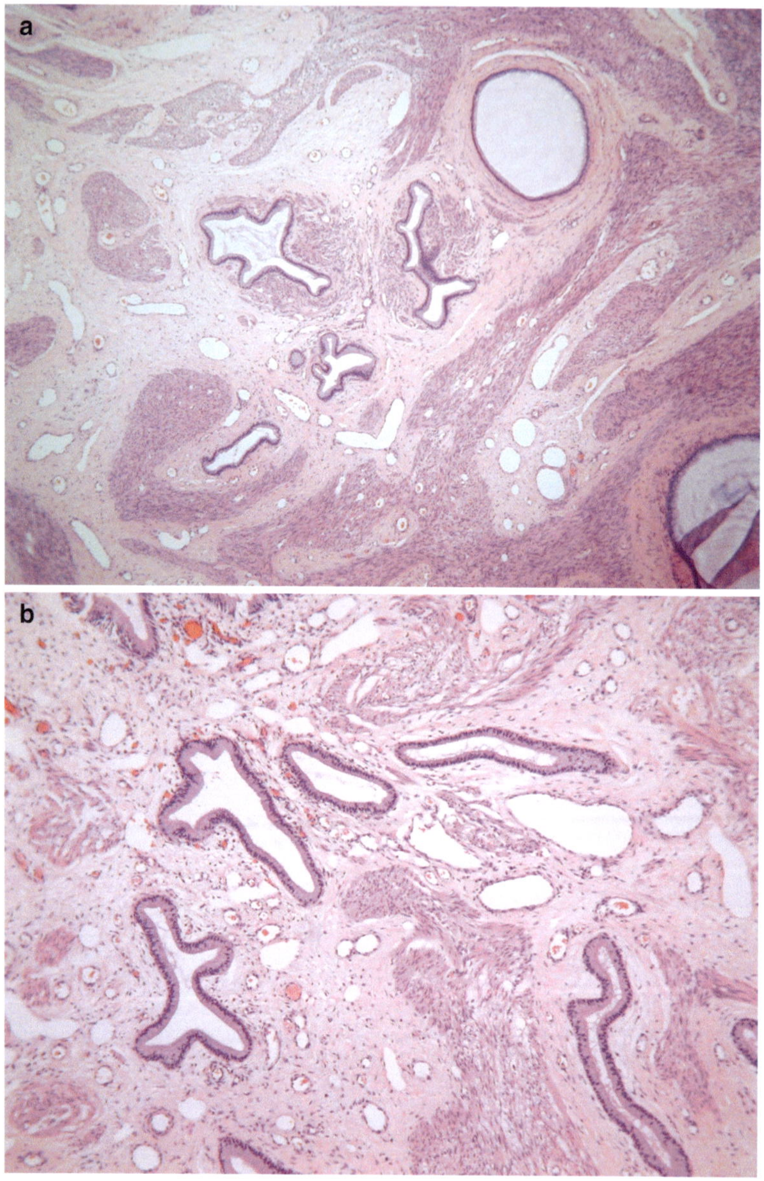

Fig. 2.38 Endocervical adenomyoma consisting of mucinous glands in an abundant myomatous stroma (**a**). High power view of endocervical adenomyoma showing bland mucinous glands in a myomatous stroma with no stromal reaction (**b**)

The main differential diagnoses are adenoma malignum (mucinous variant of minimal deviation adenocarcinoma) and lobular endocervical glandular hyperplasia. The circumscription of the lesion together with absence of irregular stromal infiltration, a desmoplastic stromal response and focal significant nuclear atypia and the presence of abundant smooth muscle assists in excluding adenoma malignum. Lobular endocervical glandular hyperplasia may be considered since in endocervical adenomyoma the glands can have a somewhat lobular arrangement. However, lobular endocervical glandular hyperplasia is not polypoid, is usually an incidental microscopic finding and lacks a smooth muscle component. Usual endocervical polyps may contain a minor population of smooth muscle fibres within the stroma but this should not result in diagnostic confusion.

Endometrioid type adenomyomas of usual type and atypical polypoid adenomyomas, similar to those seen more commonly within the uterine corpus, rarely occur in the cervix [89].

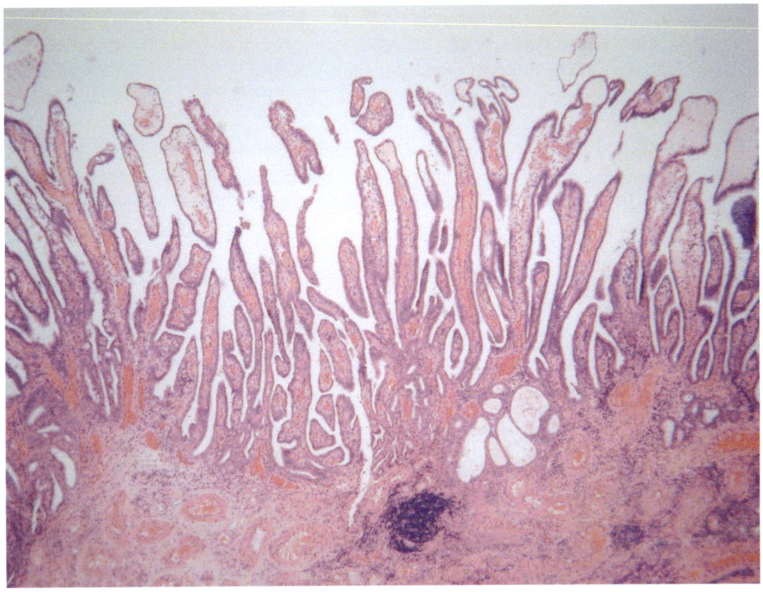

Fig. 2.39 Mullerian papilloma in the form of a surface lesion composed of slender papillae lined by bland cells

Villous Adenoma

Villous adenomas have rarely been reported within the cervix [90, 91]. All of the reported cases have been associated with an invasive adenocarcinoma, casting doubt on the existence of villous adenoma as a true entity within the cervix. The diagnosis should be made with great caution and only on a resection specimen with clear margins. This is because a villous pattern may be seen on the surface of cervical papillary adenocarcinomas, either of usual endocervical type or of villoglandular type, and these malignancies may be cytologically bland and confined to the surface without infiltration of the underlying stroma. The diagnosis of villous adenoma should be reserved for lesions where there is a pronounced villous architecture, the nuclear features are entirely bland and the lesion is confined to the surface without stromal infiltration; the lesion should be sampled in its entirety.

Cervical Adenofibroma

Adenofibroma is a benign variant of mixed Mullerian tumour which rarely occurs in the cervix. It is discussed in the Chap. on 5.

Mullerian Papilloma

This rare lesion was previously thought to be of mesonephric derivation but is now considered to be of Mullerian origin. It occurs almost exclusively in children, usually between age 2 and 5, and is most common in the vagina [92] but has occasionally been reported in the cervix [93, 94]. Presentation is usually with vaginal bleeding and a friable polypoid mass. Mullerian papilloma is composed of slender, sometimes branching, papillae lined by a single layer of bland cuboidal, columnar or flattened epithelial cells (Fig. 2.39). Occasionally there is focal squamous metaplasia and the papillae are typically oedematous and contain inflammatory cells. Rarely, psammoma bodies or osseous metaplasia is present. These are benign lesions, although occasionally they recur following local excision. A single vaginal case has been reported with "borderline" change in a recurrence [95]. The differential diagnosis may include papillary endocervicitis, villous adenoma and villoglandular adenocarcinoma.

References

1. Young RH, Clement PB. Pseudoneoplastic glandular lesions of the uterine cervix. Semin Diagn Pathol. 1991;8:234–49.

2. McCluggage WG. Glandular lesions of the uterine cervix. Curr Diagn Pathol. 2000;6:1–12.
3. McCluggage WG. Endocervical glandular lesions: controversial aspects and ancillary techniques. J Clin Pathol. 2003;56:164–73.
4. Baker PM, Clement PB, Bell DA, Young RH. Superficial endometriosis of the uterine cervix: a report of 20 cases of a process that may be confused with endocervical glandular dysplasia or adenocarcinoma in situ. Int J Gynecol Pathol. 1999;18: 198–205.
5. Hoogduin KJ, Hopman AN, Ramaekers FC, McCluggage WG, Smedts F. BCL2 and keratin 5 define the uterine-cervix-isthmus junction, a transition between endocervical and tubal-like epithelium. Int J Gynecol Pathol. 2013;32:122–30.
6. Oliva E, Clement PB, Young RH. Tubal and tubo-endometrioid metaplasia of the uterine cervix. Unemphasized features that may cause problems in differential diagnosis: a report of 25 cases. Am J Clin Pathol. 1995;103:618–23.
7. Ismail SM. Cone biopsy causes cervical endometriosis and tubo-endometrioid metaplasia. Histopathology. 1991;18:107–14.
8. Al-Nafussi AI, Rahilly M. The prevalence of tubo-endometrial metaplasia and adenomatoid proliferation. Histopathology. 1993;22:177–9.
9. McCluggage WG, Oliva E, Herrington CS, McBride H, Young RH. CD10 and calretinin staining of endocervical glandular lesions, endocervical stroma and endometrioid adenocarcinomas of the uterine corpus: CD10 positivity is characteristic of, but not specific for, mesonephric lesions and is not specific for endometrial stroma. Histopathology. 2003;43:144–50.
10. Sumathi VP, McCluggage WG. CD10 is useful in demonstrating endometrial stroma at ectopic sites and in confirming a diagnosis of endometriosis. J Clin Pathol. 2002;55:391–2.
11. Vang R, Vinh TN, Burks RT, et al. Pseudoinfiltrative tubal metaplasia of the endocervix: a potential form of in utero diethylstilbestrol exposure-related adenosis simulating minimal deviation adenocarcinoma. Int J Gynecol Pathol. 2005;24:391–8.
12. Schlesinger C, Silverberg SG. Endocervical adenocarcinoma in situ of tubal type and its relation to atypical tubal metaplasia. Int J Gynecol Pathol. 1999;18: 1–4.
13. Cameron RI, Maxwell P, Jenkins D, McCluggage WG. Immunohistochemical staining with MIB1, bcl2 and p16 assists in the distinction of cervical glandular intraepithelial neoplasia from tubo-endometrial metaplasia, endometriosis and microglandular hyperplasia. Histopathology. 2002;41:313–21.
14. McCluggage WG, Maxwell P, McBride HA, Hamilton PW, Bharucha H. Monoclonal antibodies Ki-67 and MIB1 in the distinction of tuboendometrial metaplasia from endocervical adenocarcinoma and adenocarcinoma in situ in formalin-fixed material. Int J Gynecol Pathol. 1995;14:209–16.
15. McCluggage G, McBride H, Maxwell P, Bharucha H. Immunohistochemical detection of p53 and bcl-2 proteins in neoplastic and non-neoplastic endocervical glandular lesions. Int J Gynecol Pathol. 1997;16: 22–7.
16. Marques T, Andrade LA, Vassallo J. Endocervical tubal metaplasia and adenocarcinoma in situ: role of immunohistochemistry for carcinoembryonic antigen and vimentin in differential diagnosis. Histopathology. 1996;28:549–50.
17. Stewart CJ, Little L. Diagnostic value and implications of vimentin expression in normal, reactive and neoplastic endocervical epithelium. Pathology. 2010; 42:217–33.
18. Jones MA, Young RH. Atypical oxyphilic metaplasia of the endocervical epithelium: a report of six cases. Int J Gynecol Pathol. 1997;16:99–102.
19. McCluggage WG, Shah R, Connolly LE, McBride HA. Intestinal-type cervical adenocarcinoma in situ and adenocarcinoma exhibit a partial immunophenotype with consistent expression of CDX2. Int J Gynecol Pathol. 2008;27:92–100.
20. Nicolae A, Goyenaga P, McCluggage WG, Preda O, Nogales FF. Endometrial intestinal metaplasia: a report of two cases, including one associated with cervical intestinal and pyloric metaplasia. Int J Gynecol Pathol. 2011;30:492–6.
21. Moore WF, Bentley RC, Kim KR, Olatidoye B, Gray SR, Robboy SJ. Goblet-cell mucinous epithelium lining the endometrium and endocervix: evidence of metastasis from an appendiceal primary tumor through the use of cytokeratin-7 and –20 immunostains. Int J Gynecol Pathol. 1998;17:363–7.
22. Mikami Y, McCluggage WG. Endocervical glandular lesions exhibiting gastric differentiation: an emerging spectrum of benign, premalignant and malignant lesions. Adv Anat Pathol. 2013;20:227–37.
23. Zhao S, Hayasaka T, Osakabe M, et al. Mucin expression in nonneoplastic and neoplastic glandular epithelia of the uterine cervix. Int J Gynecol Pathol. 2003;22:393–7.
24. Nucci MR, Young RH. Arias-Stella reaction of the endocervix: a report of 18 cases with emphasis on its varied histology and differential diagnosis. Am J Surg Pathol. 2004;28:608–12.
25. Young RH, Clement PB. Endocervicosis involving the uterine cervix: a report of four cases of a benign process that may be confused with deeply invasive endocervical adenocarcinoma. Int J Gynecol Pathol. 2000;19:322–8.
26. Clement PB, Young RH. Endocervicosis of the urinary bladder: a report of six cases of a benign Mullerian lesion that may mimic adenocarcinoma. Am J Surg Pathol. 1992;16:533–42.
27. McCluggage WG, Price JH, Dobbs SP. Primary adenocarcinoma of the vagina arising in endocervicosis. Int J Gynecol Pathol. 2001;20:399–402.
28. Clement PB, Young RH. Florid cystic endosalpingiosis with tumor-like manifestations: a report of four cases including the first reported cases of transmural

endosalpingiosis of the uterus. Am J Surg Pathol. 1999;23:166–75.
29. Nucci MR, Ferry JA, Young RH. Ectopic prostatic tissue in the uterine cervix: a report of four cases and review of ectopic prostatic tissue. Am J Surg Pathol. 2000;24:1224–30.
30. McCluggage WG, Ganesan R, Hirschowitz L, Miller K, Rollason TP. Ectopic prostatic tissue in the uterine cervix and vagina: report of a series with a detailed immunohistochemical analysis. Am J Surg Pathol. 2006,30:209–15.
31. Kelly P, McBride HA, Kennedy K, Connolly LE, McCluggage WG. Misplaced Skene's glands: glandular elements in the lower female genital tract that are variably immunoreactive with prostate markers and that encompass vaginal tubulosquamous polyp and cervical ectopic prostatic tissue. Int J Gynecol Pathol. 2011;30:605–12.
32. McCluggage WG, Young RH. Tubulo-squamous polyp: a report of ten cases of a distinctive hitherto uncharacterized vaginal polyp. Am J Surg Pathol. 2007;31:1013–9.
33. Kazakov DV, Stewart CJ, Kacerovska D, et al. Prostatic-type tissue in the lower female genital tract: a morphologic spectrum, including vaginal tubulosquamous polyp, adenomyomatous hyperplasia of paraurethral Skene glands (female prostate), and ectopic lesion in the vulva. Am J Surg Pathol. 2010;34: 950–5.
34. Kazakov DV, Hejda V, Kacerovska D, Michal M. Hyperplasia of ectopic sebaceous glands in the uterine cervix: case report. Int J Gynecol Pathol. 2010;29: 605–8.
35. Robledo MC, Vazquez JJ, Contreras-Mejuto F, et al. Sebaceous glands and hair follicles in the cervix uteri. Histopathology. 1992;21:278–80.
36. Kazakov DV, Mukensnabl P, Kacerovska D, Michal M. Mantle structures in the uterine cervix. Int J Gynecol Pathol. 2009;28:568–9.
37. Belousova IE, Kazakov DV, Michal M. Ectopic sebaceous glands in the vagina. Int J Gynecol Pathol. 2005;24:193–5.
38. Brady AJ, McCluggage WG. Ectodermal structures within the uterine cervix and vagina: report of a series of cases. Int J Gynecol Pathol. 2013;32:602–5.
39. Fluhmann CF. Focal hyperplasias (tunnel clusters) of the cervix uteri. Obstet Gynecol. 1961;17: 206–14.
40. Jones MA, Young RH. Endocervical type A (noncystic) tunnel clusters with cytologic atypia. A report of 14 cases. Am J Surg Pathol. 1996;20:1312–8.
41. Segal GH, Hart WR. Cystic endocervical tunnel clusters. A clinicopathologic study of 29 cases of so-called adenomatous hyperplasia. Am J Surg Pathol. 1990;14:895–903.
42. Tambouret R, Bell DA, Young RH. Microcystic endocervical adenocarcinomas: a report of eight cases. Am J Surg Pathol. 2000;24:369–74.
43. Kondo T, Hashi A, Murata SI, et al. Gastric mucin is expressed in a subset of endocervical tunnel clusters: type A tunnel clusters of gastric phenotype. Histopathology. 2007;50:843–50.
44. McCluggage WG. New developments in endocervical glandular lesions. Histopathology. 2013;62: 138–60.
45. Nucci MR, Clement PB, Young RH. Lobular endocervical glandular hyperplasia, not otherwise specified: a clinicopathologic analysis of thirteen cases of a distinctive pseudoneoplastic lesion and comparison with fourteen cases of adenoma malignum. Am J Surg Pathol. 1999;23:886–91.
46. Mikami Y, Hata S, Melamed J, et al. Lobular endocervical glandular hyperplasia is a metaplastic process with a pyloric gland phenotype. Histopathology. 2001;39:364–72.
47. Mikami Y, Kiyokawa T, Moriya T, Sasano H. Immunophenotypic alteration of the stromal component in minimal deviation adenocarcinoma ('adenoma malignum') and endocervical glandular hyperplasia: a study using oestrogen receptor and alpha-smooth muscle actin double immunostaining. Histopathology. 2005;46:130–6.
48. Hayashi I, Tsuda H, Shimoda T. Reappraisal of orthodox histochemistry for the diagnosis of minimal deviation adenocarcinoma of the cervix. Am J Surg Pathol. 2000;24:559–62.
49. Ichimura T, Koizumi T, Tateiwa H, et al. Immunohistochemical expression of gastric mucin and p53 in minimal deviation adenocarcinoma of the uterine cervix. Int J Gynecol Pathol. 2001;20:220–6.
50. Toki T, Shiozawa T, Hosaka N, Ishii K, Nikaido T, Fujii S. Minimal deviation adenocarcinoma of the uterine cervix has abnormal expression of sex steroid receptors, CA125, and gastric mucin. Int J Gynecol Pathol. 1997;16:111–6.
51. Utsugi K, Hirai Y, Takeshima N, et al. Utility of the monoclonal antibody HIK1083 in the diagnosis of adenoma malignum of the uterine cervix. Gynecol Oncol. 1999;75:345–8.
52. Mikami Y, Kiyokawa T, Hata S, Fujiwara K, Moriya T, Sasano H, et al. Gastrointestinal immunophenotype in adenocarcinomas of the uterine cervix and related glandular lesions: a possible link between lobular endocervical glandular hyperplasia/pyloric gland metaplasia and 'adenoma malignum'. Mod Pathol. 2004;17:962–72.
53. Nara M, Hashi A, Murata S, et al. Lobular endocervical glandular hyperplasia as a presumed precursor of cervical adenocarcinoma independent of human papillomavirus infection. Gynecol Oncol. 2007;106: 289–98.
54. Kawauchi S, Ksuda T, Liu XO, et al. Is lobular endocervical glandular hyperplasia a cancerous precursor of minimal deviation adenocarcinoma?: a comparative molecular-genetic and immunohistochemical study. Am J Surg Pathol. 2008;32:1807–15.
55. Mikami Y, Kiyokawa T, Sasajima Y, et al. Reapprasial of synchronous and multifocal mucinous lesions of the female genital tract: a close association with gastric metaplasia. Histopathology. 2009;54:184–91.

56. Seidman JD. Mucinous lesions of the fallopian tube. Am J Surg Pathol. 1994;18:1205–12.
57. Young RH, Scully RE. Mucinous tumors of the ovary associated with mucinous adenocarcinomas of the cervix. A clinicopathologic analysis of 16 cases. Int J Gynecol Pathol. 1988;7:99–111.
58. Jones MA, Young RH, Scully RE. Diffuse laminar endocervical glandular hyperplasia. A benign lesion often confused with adenoma malignum (minimal deviation adenocarcinoma). Am J Surg Pathol. 1991; 15:1123–9.
59. Daya D, Young RH. Florid deep glands of the uterine cervix. Another mimic of adenoma malignum. Am J Clin Pathol. 1995;103:614–7.
60. Clement PB, Young RH. Deep nabothian cysts of the uterine cervix. A possible source of confusion with minimal-deviation adenocarcinoma (adenoma malignum). Int J Gynecol Pathol. 1989;8:340–8.
61. Greeley C, Schroeder S, Silverberg SG. Microglandular hyperplasia of the cervix: a true "pill" lesion? Int J Gynecol Pathol. 1995;14:50–4.
62. Speers WC, Picaso LG, Silverberg SG. Immunohistochemical localization of carcinoembryonic antigen in microglandular hyperplasia and adenocarcinoma of the endocervix. Am J Clin Pathol. 1983;79:105–7.
63. Young RH, Scully RE. Atypical forms of microglandular hyperplasia of the cervix simulating carcinoma. A report of five cases and review of the literature. Am J Surg Pathol. 1989;13:50–6.
64. Jacques SM, Qureshi F, Lawrence WD. Surface epithelial changes in endometrial adenocarcinoma: diagnostic pitfalls in curettage specimens. Int J Gynecol Pathol. 1995;14:191–7.
65. Chekmareva M, Ellenson LH, Pirog EC. Immunohistochemical differences between mucinous and microglandular adenocarcinomas of the endometrium and benign endocervical epithelium. Int J Gynecol Pathol. 2008;27:547–54.
66. Qui W, Mittal K. Comparison of morphologic and immunohistochemical features of cervical microglandular hyperplasia with low-grade mucinous adenocarcinoma of the endometrium. Int J Gynecol Pathol. 2003;22:261–5.
67. McCluggage WG. A critical appraisal of the value of immunohistochemistry in diagnosis of uterine neoplasms. Adv Anat Pathol. 2004;11:162–71.
68. Seidman JD, Tavassoli FA. Mesonephric hyperplasia of the uterine cervix: a clinicopathologic study of 51 cases. Int J Gynecol Pathol. 1995;14:293–9.
69. Ordi J, Ramagosa C, Tavassoli FA. CD10 expression in epithelial tissues and tumors of the gynecologic tract. Am J Surg Pathol. 2003;27:178–86.
70. Devouassoux-Shisheboran M, Silver SA, Tavassoli FA. Wolffian adnexal tumor, so-called female adnexal tumor of probable Wolffian origin (FATWO): immunohistochemical evidence in support of a Wolffian origin. Hum Pathol. 1999;30:856–63.
71. Rabban JT, McAlhany S, Lerwill MF, Grenert JP, Zaloudek CJ. PAX2 distinguishes benign mesonephric and mullerian glandular lesions of the cervix from endocervical adenocarcinoma, including minimal deviation adenocarcinoma. Am J Surg Pathol. 2010; 34:137–46.
72. Kenny SL, McBride HA, Jamison J, McCluggage WG. Mesonephric adenocarcinomas of the uterine cervix and corpus: HPV negative neoplasms which are commonly PAX8, CA125 and HMGA2 positive and which may be immunoreactive with TTF1 and Hepatocyte Nuclear Factor 1 Beta. Am J Surg Pathol. 2012;36:799–807.
73. Truskinovsky AM, Stelow EB, Jessurun J, et al. Staining for p16 of cervical mesonephric remnants and hyperplasia: A potential diagnostic pitfall. Mod Pathol. 2006;19:199A.
74. Clement PB, Young RH, Keh P, Ostor AG, Scully RE. Malignant mesonephric neoplasms of the uterine cervix. A report of eight cases, including four with a malignant spindle cell component. Am J Surg Pathol. 1995;19:1158–71.
75. Brainard JA, Hart WR. Adenoid basal epitheliomas of the uterine cervix. A reevaluation of distinctive cervical basaloid lesions currently classified as adenoid basal carcinoma and adenoid basal hyperplasia. Am J Surg Pathol. 1998;22:965–75.
76. Al-Nafussi A. Histopathological challenges in assessing invasion in squamous and glandular neoplasia of the cervix. Curr Diagn Pathol. 2006;12:364–93.
77. Howitt BE, Quade BJ, Nucci MR. Atypical uterine polyps sub-diagnostic of Mullerian adenosarcoma: a clinicopathologic analysis of 28 cases with long term follow-up. Mod Pathol. 2012;25 Suppl 2:1159.
78. Heatley MK. Squamous intraepithelial lesions arising in benign endocervical polyps: a report of 9 cases with correlation to the pap smears, HPV analysis, and immunoprofile. Int J Gynecol Pathol. 2009;28:567.
79. Ilhan R, Yavuz E, Iplikci A, et al. Hamartomatous endocervical polyp with heterologous mesenchymal tissue. Pathol Int. 2001;51:305–7.
80. Siddon A, Hui P. Glial heterotopia of the uterine cervix: DNA genotyping confirmation of its fetal origin. Int J Gynecol Pathol. 2010;29:394–7.
81. Kiviat NB, Paavonen JA, Wolner-Hanssen P, et al. Histopathology of endocervical infection caused by Chlamydia trachomatis, herpes simplex virus, Trichomonas vaginalis, and Neisseria gonorrhoeae. Hum Pathol. 1990;21:831–7.
82. Lesack D, Wahab I, Gilks CB. Radiation-induced atypia of endocervical epithelium: A histologic, immunohistochemical and cytometric study. Int J Gynecol Pathol. 1996;15:42–7.
83. El-Bahrawy M. Expression of p16 in post-radiotherapy cervical biopsies. Histopathology. 2011;58:1174–6.
84. McGalie CE, McBride HA, McCluggage WG. Cytomegalovirus infection of the cervix: morphological observations in five cases of a possibly under-recognised condition. J Clin Pathol. 2004;57:691–4.
85. Nagar HA, Dobbs SP, McClelland HR, et al. The large loop excision transformation zone cut or blend artefact study: a randomized control trial. Int J Gynecol Cancer. 2004;14:1108–11.

86. McKenna M, McCluggage WG. Signet ring cells of stromal derivation in the uterine cervix secondary to cauterisation: report of a previously undescribed phenomenon. J Clin Pathol. 2008;61:648–51.
87. Scott M, Lyness RW, McCluggage WG. Atypical reactive proliferation of endocervix: a common lesion associated with endometrial carcinoma and likely related to prior endometrial sampling. Mod Pathol. 2006;19:470–4.
88. Gilks CB, Young RH, Clement PB, Hart WR, Scully RE. Adenomyomas of the uterine cervix of endocervical type: a report of ten cases of a benign cervical tumor that may be confused with adenoma malignum [corrected]. Mod Pathol. 1996;9:220–4.
89. Gilks CB, Clement PB, Hart WR, Young RH. Uterine adenomyomas excluding atypical polypoid adenomyomas and adenomyomas of endocervical type: a clinicopathologic study of 30 cases of an underemphasized lesion that may cause diagnostic problems with brief consideration of adenomyomas of other female genital tract sites. Int J Gynecol Pathol. 2000;19:195–205.
90. Michael H, Sutton G, Hull MT, et al. Villous adenoma of the uterine cervix associated with invasive adenocarcinoma: A histologic, ultrastructural and immunohistochemical study. Int J Gynecol Pathol. 1986;5:163–9.
91. Alvaro T, Nogales F. Villous adenoma and invasive adenocarcinoma of the cervix. Int J Gynecol Pathol. 1988;7:96.
92. McCluggage WG, Nirmala V, Radhakurami K. Intramural mullerian papilloma of the vagina. Int J Gynecol Pathol. 1999;18:94–5.
93. Lane BR, Ross JH, Wart WR, et al. Mullerian papilloma of the cervix in a child with multiple renal cysts. Urology. 2005;65:388.
94. Smith YR, Quint EH, Hinton EL. Recurrent benign mullerian papilloma of the cervix. J Pediatr Adolesc Gynecol. 1998;11:29–31.
95. Dobbs SP, Shaw PA, Brown LJ, Ireland D. Borderline malignant change in recurrent müllerian papilloma of the vagina. J Clin Pathol. 1998;51:875–7.

Premalignant Glandular Lesions of the Cervix

3

W. Glenn McCluggage

Abstract

Premalignant endocervical glandular lesions are increasing in incidence. The various terminologies applied to these lesions (adenocarcinoma in situ or cervical glandular intraepithelial neoplasia), which are the precursors of usual type cervical adenocarcinoma, are discussed. These lesions are usually associated with high risk human papillomavirus (HPV) infection. The morphological features are discussed, as is the immunophenotype, differential diagnosis and management.

Keywords

Cervical glandular intraepithelial neoplasia • Adenocarcinoma in situ • Stratified mucin producing intraepithelial lesion

Introduction

Friedel and MacKay first described a premalignant endocervical glandular lesion which they termed adenocarcinoma in situ (AIS) in 1953 [1]. Premalignant (and malignant) endocervical glandular lesions are much more uncommon than their squamous counterparts in the cervix but are increasing in incidence [2]. Part of this is a relative increase, compared to squamous carcinoma, because of a reduction in the latter in developed countries secondary to organised cervical screening programmes. However, there is also evidence that there is a real increase in the prevalence of premalignant and malignant endocervical glandular lesions; while some of this may be due to better recognition of these lesions by pathologists, it is also probable that some of this increase is due to an increased prevalence of human papillomavirus (HPV) infection and/or a change in the distribution of HPV types [2]. A study from Sweden found that the incidence of cervical adenocarcinoma increased from 1.59/100,000 person years in the 1950s and 1960s to 2.36 in the early 1990s [3]. The corresponding figures for cervical AIS were 0.04 and 1.37 reflecting an even greater increase [3]. Another study found the risk of cervical adenocarcinoma to be 14 times greater in women born in the early 1960s compared to those born before 1935 [4]. According to the Surveillance Epidemiology and End Results (SEER) database, the age-adjusted incidence rate of cervical adenocarcinoma per 100,000 women increased from

W.G. McCluggage et al., *Cellular Pathology of Glandular Lesions and Uncommon Neoplasms of the Cervix*,
DOI 10.1007/978-1-4471-2210-4_3,

1.34 in the 1970s to 1.73 in the 1990s [4]. The ratio of patients with adenocarcinoma versus squamous carcinoma doubled in this period with the incidence of adenocarcinoma increasing to 26 % of all cervical carcinomas [4].

Terminology of Premalignant Endocervical Glandular Lesions

Cervical glandular intraepithelial neoplasia (CGIN) is the term in widespread use in the United Kingdom for endocervical glandular lesions which are the precursor of usual type cervical adenocarcinoma (referred to as mucinous adenocarcinoma of endocervical type by the World Health Organization (WHO)) [5, 6]. CGIN is divided into low grade and high grade. In WHO terminology, low grade CGIN corresponds to glandular dysplasia and high grade CGIN to AIS [5, 6] (Table 3.1). The CGIN terminology is recommended since, like the CIN classification scheme used for premalignant squamous lesions, this suggests there is a continuum of premalignant endocervical glandular lesions. However, the different terminologies in use make it difficult to directly compare various studies and the CGIN classification is not widely used outside the United Kingdom. Previously some authors divided premalignant endocervical glandular lesions into low grade CGIN, high grade CGIN and AIS or used a three tier grading system for CGIN [7–9]; however, high grade CGIN and AIS are now regarded as the same lesion and a two tier classification is recommended, although many authorities recognise only a single category of premalignant endocervical glandular lesion (high grade CGIN or AIS) (see below). The WHO definition of AIS is a lesion in which normally situated endocervical glands are partly or wholly replaced by cytologically malignant epithelium [6]. The WHO definition of glandular dysplasia is a glandular lesion characterised by significant nuclear abnormalities that are more striking than in glandular atypia but falling short of the criteria for AIS [6]. Most examples of CGIN (AIS) are of the so-called usual or endocervical type, although several morphological subtypes have been described (see below).

Table 3.1 Comparison of WHO and United Kingdom Systems for Classification of Premalignant Endocervical Glandular Lesions

WHO	United Kingdom
Glandular dysplasia	Low grade CGIN
Adenocarcinoma in-situ	High grade CGIN

CGIN cervical glandular intraepithelial neoplasia

Aetiology and Pathogenesis of Premalignant Endocervical Glandular Lesions

Most, but not all, premalignant (and malignant) endocervical glandular lesions are associated with high risk HPV, most commonly types 16 and 18 [10–12]; HPV 18 is proportionally much more common than in CIN and is probably more prevalent than HPV 16 in premalignant and malignant endocervical glandular lesions [10–12]. In a significant percentage and probably a majority of cases, premalignant endocervical glandular lesions coexist with CIN since both are, for the most part, HPV-related lesions; in some, but not all, cases the same HPV type is found in the premalignant squamous and glandular lesion, although this is not always the case [13]. Many cases of CGIN are identified as an incidental finding in a patient with CIN and, in general, CGIN occurs in a similar age group to CIN. There is a suggestion that premalignant and malignant endocervical glandular lesions may be associated with the use of hormonal agents but this is not proven [14, 15].

More uncommon morphological variants of cervical adenocarcinoma, including clear cell, mesonephric, gastric type and adenoma malignum, are usually not HPV-related and do not arise from CGIN [10, 11]. It has been suggested that the benign endocervical glandular lesion, lobular endocervical glandular hyperplasia (see Chap. on 2) may be a precursor of adenoma malignum and gastric type cervical adenocarcinoma [16–18].

Clinical Features of Premalignant Endocervical Glandular Lesions

Most women with a premalignant endocervical glandular lesion are asymptomatic and the lesion is discovered following an abnormal cervical smear. The smear result may have suggested a glandular or squamous abnormality or the premalignant glandular lesion may be an incidental finding in a patient with a premalignant or malignant squamous lesion. The age range is similar to that of patients with CIN, both the median and mean age being in the fourth decade (10–15 years younger than the corresponding median and mean ages of patients with cervical adenocarcinoma).

Premalignant endocervical glandular lesions are more likely to be seen in an excisional rather than a punch biopsy since they are often not visible colposcopically and excision biopsy of the transformation zone is usually undertaken if a premalignant glandular lesion is strongly suspected on a cervical smear.

Evidence for Low Grade CGIN Being a Premalignant Lesion

It seems logical to assume that there is a precursor lesion to high grade CGIN. However, low grade CGIN is much more uncommon than high grade and it is unusual to identify low grade CGIN in pure form without a high grade lesion. Some authorities doubt the existence of low grade CGIN (glandular dysplasia) and do not diagnose this since the morphological features are not clearly defined, the diagnosis is poorly reproducible, the natural history is not known and there are no clear management guidelines. Points of evidence in favour of low grade CGIN being a precursor of high grade include the observation that in some studies low grade CGIN has occurred in a younger age group than high grade, the fact that low grade CGIN may be seen adjacent to high grade and the presence of similar HPV types in some studies [19–23]. On the other hand, it is unclear what criteria were used to diagnose low grade CGIN in these studies, low grade CGIN is uncommonly seen in pure form and in many cases there is an abrupt transition between normal glandular epithelium and a high grade glandular lesion.

A reasonable approach is to accept that low grade CGIN is a precursor of high grade but it is uncommonly seen in the absence of a high grade lesion and it should not be diagnosed unless the morphological features are unequivocally those of a premalignant lesion, although of lesser severity than high grade CGIN; diffuse p16 immunoreactivity would be a prerequisite to the diagnosis. If diagnosing low grade CGIN in pure form, it is recommended to state on the pathology report that management should be as for high grade CGIN. An alternative, and equally acceptable, viewpoint is that low grade CGIN (glandular dysplasia) is not diagnosed but rather that cases which are equivocal for high grade CGIN be subject to immunohistochemical analysis. If p16 is negative or focally positive and there is a low MIB1 proliferation index, the lesion should be regarded as benign but if p16 is diffusely positive and there is an elevated MIB1 proliferation index, it is classified as high grade CGIN [24].

Morphological Features of CGIN

Most examples of CGIN are of so-called usual or endocervical type but several subtypes have been described, including intestinal, endometrioid and tubal (discussed below). Clear cell and serous variants have also been postulated to exist but these are likely to merely represent growth patterns at the periphery of primary clear cell and serous carcinomas of the cervix rather than true precursor lesions.

Usual or Endocervical Type CGIN

This is the most common type of CGIN, although the term usual or endocervical type is not generally used in the pathology report. CGIN usually occurs at or close to the transformation zone and there is coexistent CIN in a high proportion of cases. It was previously considered that both skip

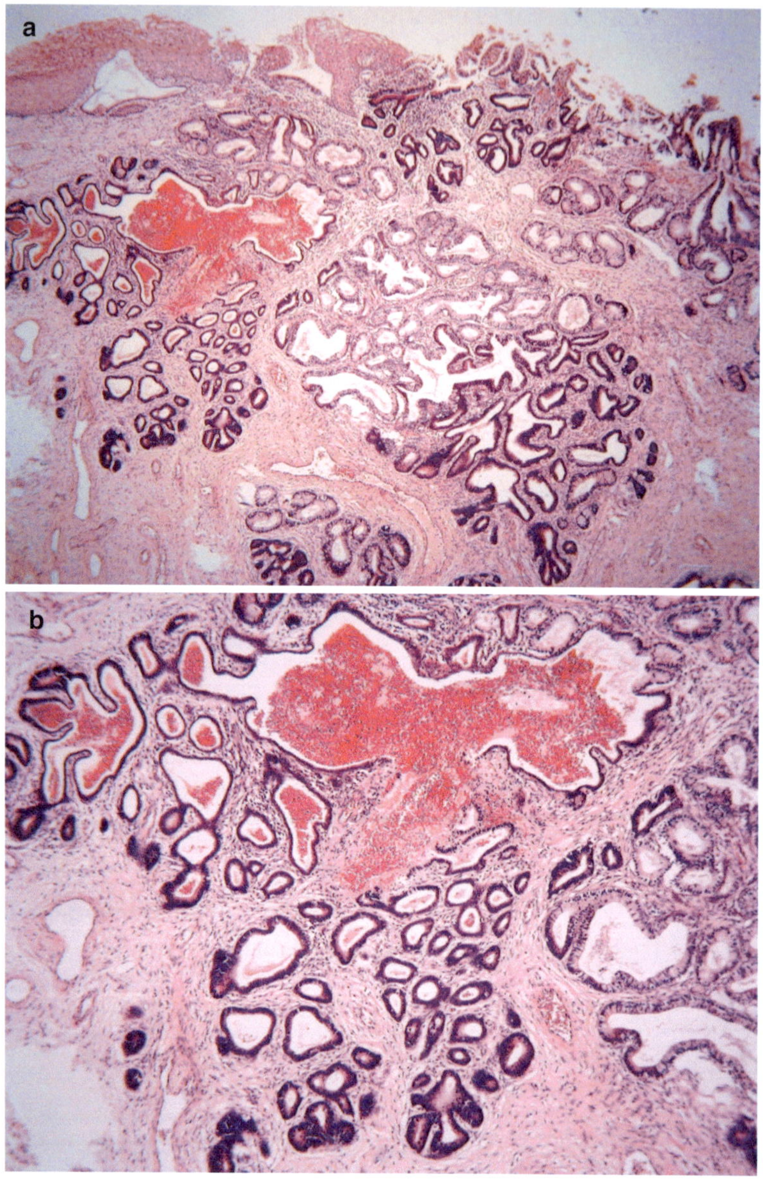

Fig. 3.1 Low power view of high grade CGIN showing accentuation of the normal lobular endocervical glandular architecture (**a**). Higher power of same lesion (**b**)

lesions and extension high up the endocervical canal were common in CGIN but, although these sometimes occur, both are relatively uncommon [25, 26]; tangentional sectioning may result in an impression of skip lesions. However, there have been occasional reports of CGIN with extension to the endometrium [27, 28]. Some of these cases have been misdiagnosed as a primary adenocarcinoma of the uterine corpus or have resulted in ovarian metastasis, sometimes even in the absence of obvious invasion within the cervix [27]. Those cases with ovarian metastases have not generally been associated with an adverse outcome and the ovarian disease is likely secondary to transuterine and transtubal spread [27].

CGIN is first identified on low power examination, which is the initial clue to diagnosis, given the contrast to the normal endocervical glands; it is not necessary to examine every endocervical gland under high power to look for CGIN. In high grade CGIN, the abnormal glands are confined to the pre-existing "normal" endocervical glandular field which, in itself, may be quite complicated. In some cases, there is accentuation of the normal lobular endocervical glandular architecture (Fig. 3.1). There is

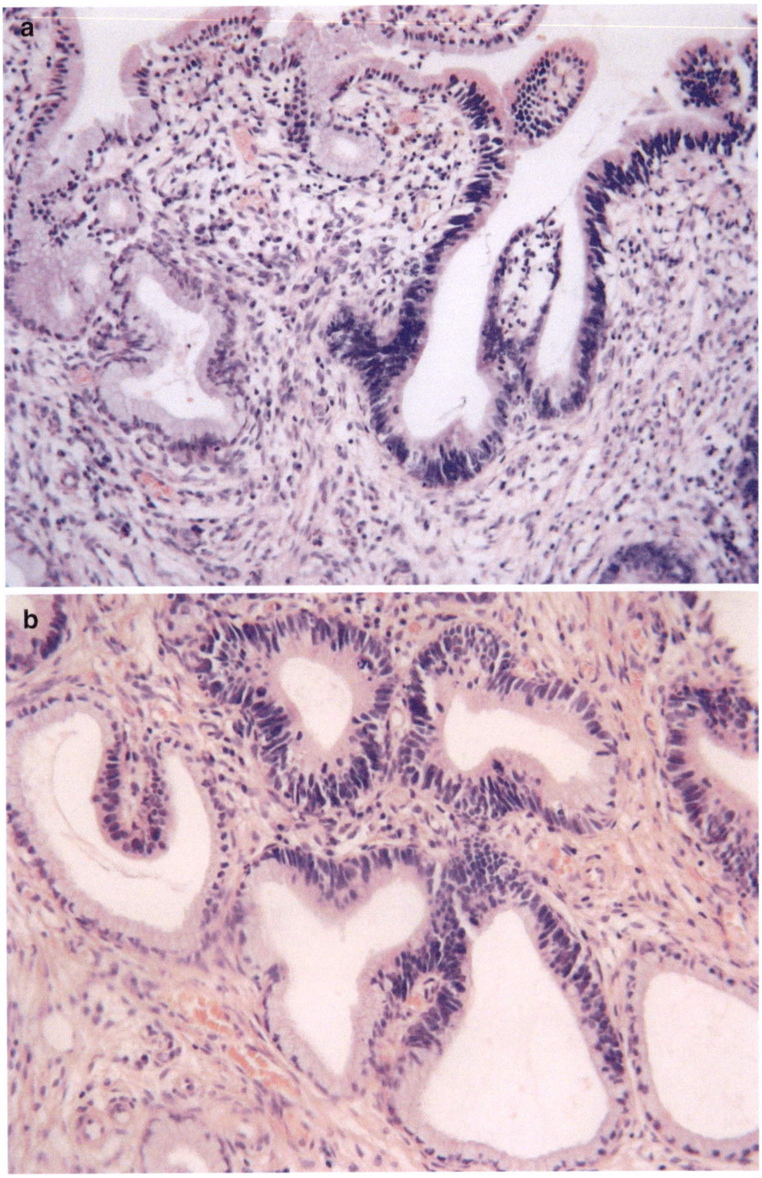

Fig. 3.2 Abrupt transition between normal endocervical glands and glands involved by high grade CGIN (**a**). Even within individual glands there may be a sharp demarcation between normal and high grade CGIN (**b**)

often an abrupt transition between normal and abnormal epithelium both within and between glands (Fig. 3.2). Usually both the surface and crypt epithelium is involved with mucin depletion, nuclear stratification (often with the long axis of the cells perpendicular to the base), atypia, hyperchromasia with coarse clumped chromatin and loss of polarity. There are usually easily identifiable mitotic figures, especially on the luminal aspect of the glands, sometimes with atypical mitoses; however, in some cases mitoses are relatively sparse. Apoptotic bodies are a characteristic and relatively constant feature and are usually seen in the non-luminal aspect of the glands (Fig. 3.3) [29–31]; sometimes they are numerous. In general, apoptotic bodies are more commonly seen and are more numerous in high grade CGIN than in invasive cervical adenocarcinomas. The combination of luminal mitoses and basal apoptotic bodies is a characteristic feature of high grade CGIN. Focal intraglandular papillae and a cribriform architecture may be seen in high grade CGIN (Fig. 3.4) but when these features are prominent and widespread, this should result in consideration of invasive adenocarcinoma; in those cases of CGIN with a

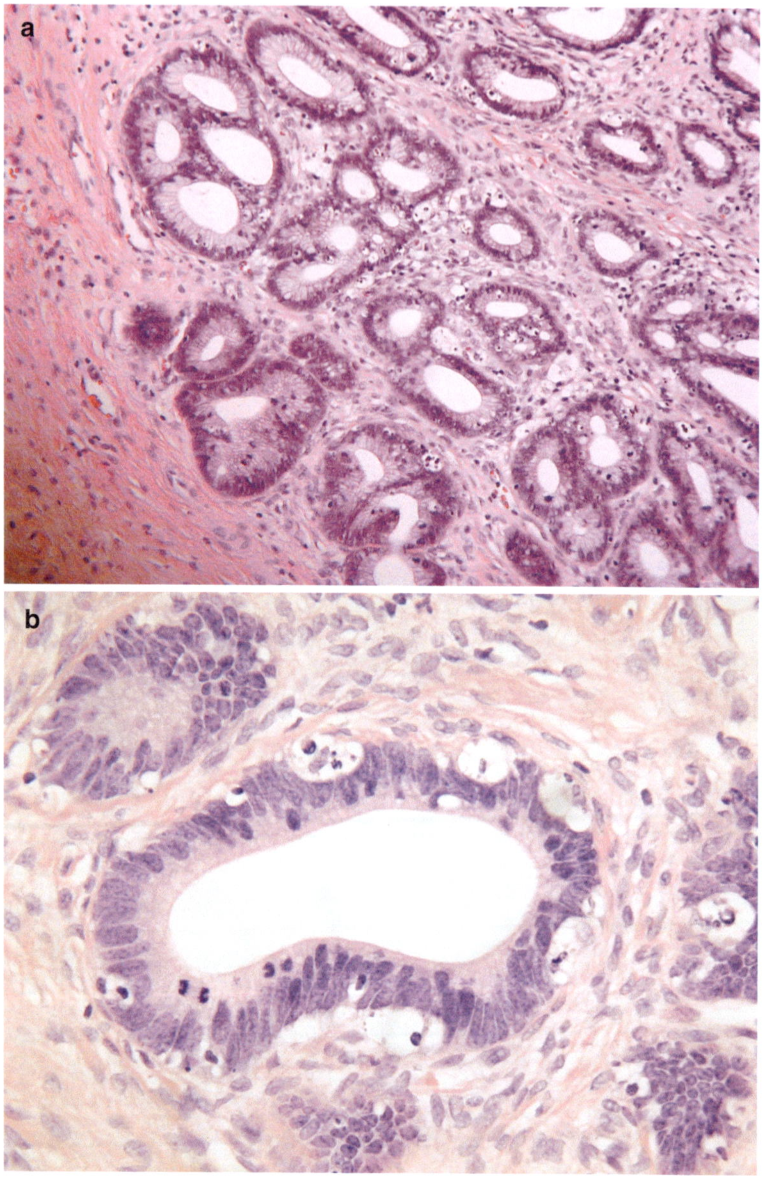

Fig. 3.3 Intermediate power (**a**) and high power (**b**) of high grade CGIN exhibiting nuclear hyperchromasia and atypia with luminal mitoses and basal apoptotic bodies

cribriform architecture, the glandular outlines should be round and not irregular. There may be inflammation of the stroma surrounding the glands in CGIN but there is no desmoplastic reaction. Since CGIN is confined to the pre-existing endocervical glandular field, it may also involve dilated crypts. Occasionally, CGIN involves a pre-existing benign endocervical glandular lesion such as papillary endocervicits, microglandular hyperplasia or tunnel clusters and this may result in diagnostic problems and consideration of adenocarcinoma for obvious reasons. The immunophenotype of high grade CGIN is discussed below (section on "Immunohistochemistry of premalignant endocervical glandular lesions").

As discussed, low grade CGIN is a much more uncommon and subtle lesion. The morphological features are similar to those of high grade CGIN but the cytological abnormalities are less marked.

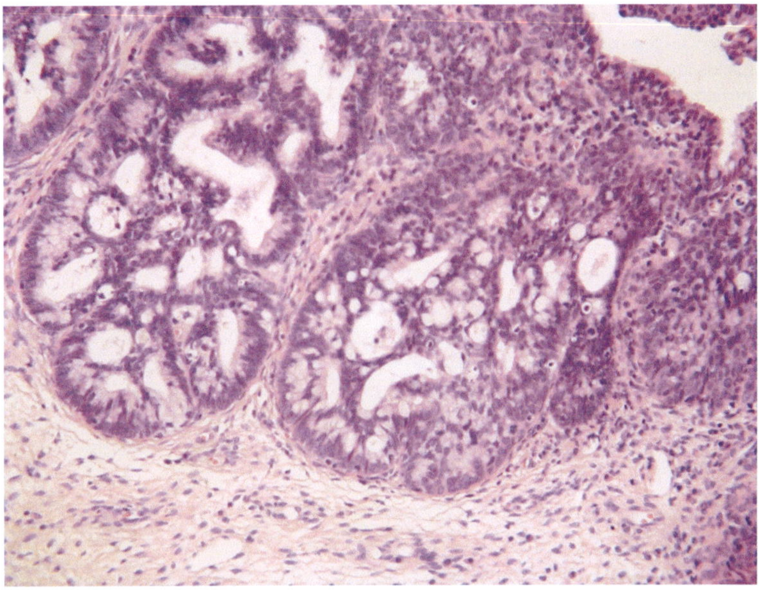

Fig. 3.4 High grade CGIN exhibiting focal cribriform architecture

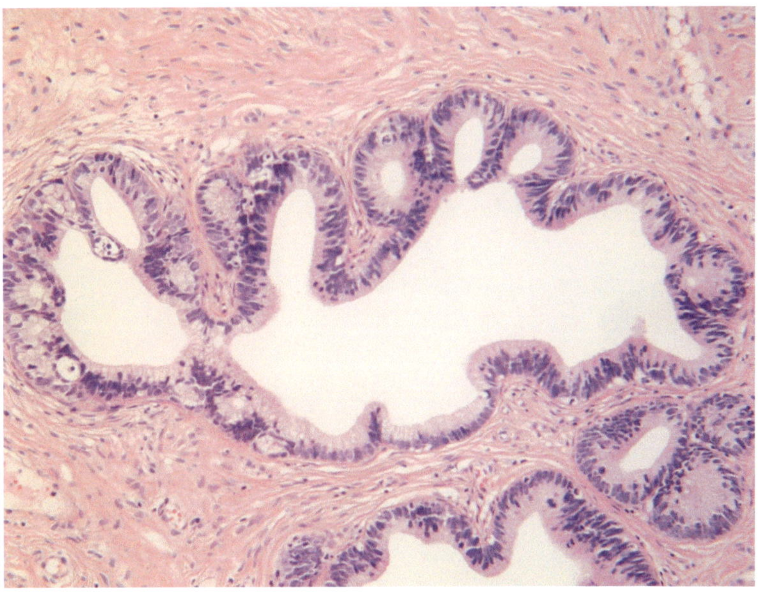

Fig. 3.5 Low grade CGIN with only mild nuclear atypia and occasional luminal mitoses and basal apoptotic bodies

There is usually nuclear hyperchromasia but there is only mild atypia, mucin depletion, nuclear stratification and loss of polarity (Fig. 3.5). Mitotic figures are usually present but not numerous. The presence of apoptotic bodies may be a useful diagnostic clue.

Superficial CGIN (superficial AIS) has been used as a term for CGIN which is confined to the surface mucosa and crypt openings (Fig. 3.6) [32]. It has been speculated that this represents an early form of CGIN occurring in a younger age group than more established CGIN. In contrast to the latter, in superficial CGIN there is usually only mild nuclear atypia with rare to absent apoptotic bodies. Given its superficial nature, the lesion may not be obvious at low power and may be overlooked, especially since the cytological abnormalities can be subtle; immunohistochemi-

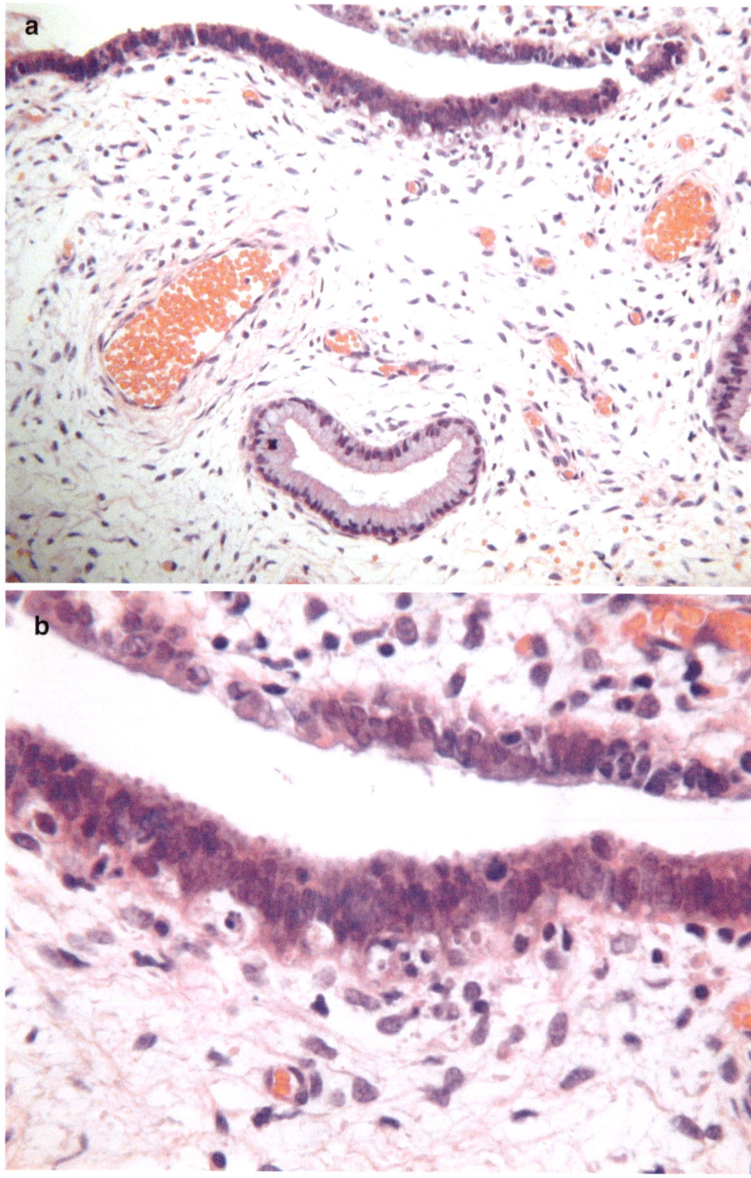

Fig. 3.6 Superficial high grade CGIN where abnormal glands are confined to the surface and superficial crypt openings (**a**). On high power, mitoses and apoptotic bodies are seen (**b**)

cal staining for p16 and MIB1 may assist in diagnosis (see below).

A scoring system for non-invasive endocervical glandular lesions to be used primarily in research practice has been proposed [33]. Using this system, a final numerical score is based on the summation of three individual scores given for nuclear atypia, stratification and the sum of mitoses and apoptoses [33]. While this scoring system may be useful in a research setting, it is of limited value in routine pathological practice.

Intestinal Type CGIN

After the usual type, the most common variant of CGIN is the intestinal type where goblet cells are present (Fig. 3.7). Paneth cells and/or neuroendocrine cells also occur more uncommonly [26, 34]. Intestinal type CGIN is usually associated with usual type; in one study, intestinal differentiation was present in 29 % of cases of CGIN, always in association with usual type [26]. When intestinal type epithelium with goblet

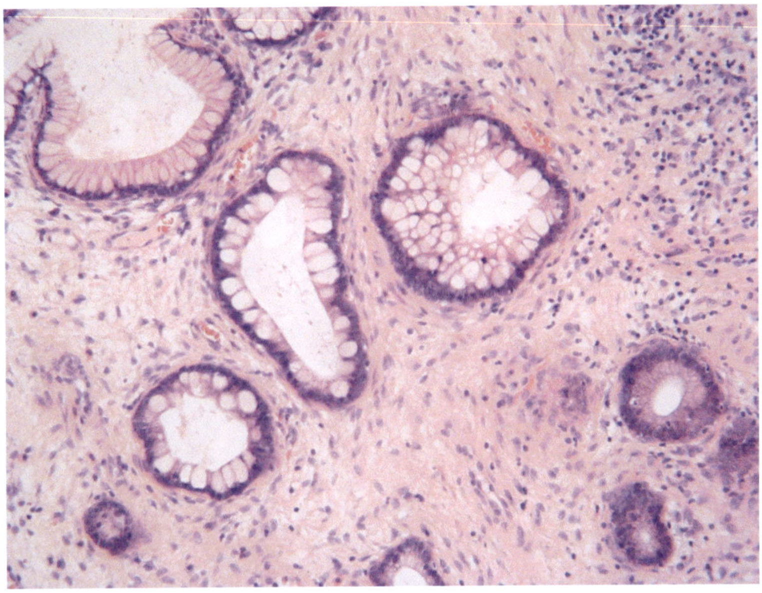

Fig. 3.7 Intestinal type CGIN characterised by the presence of goblet cells

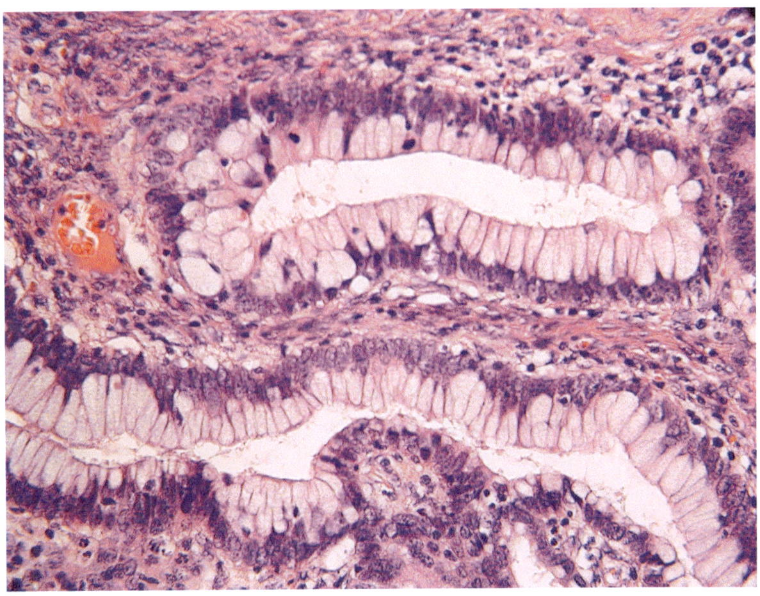

Fig. 3.8 Intestinal type CGIN where the nuclei are compressed by goblet cells

cells is present in the cervix, this almost always indicates a premalignant or malignant endocervical glandular lesion, although the nuclear features of malignancy may be subtle because of compression by intracytoplasmic mucin globules (Fig. 3.8). "Benign" intestinal metaplasia (unassociated with CGIN) rarely exists in the cervix, although it is occasionally seen in association with lobular endocervical glandular hyperplasia and other forms of gastric metaplasia (see Chap. 2, section on "Lobular endocervical glandular hyperplasia") [35, 36]. One study found that intestinal type CGIN is more likely than the usual type to be associated with early invasion [34].

Most cases of intestinal type CGIN are HPV-associated [37]. However, it has been suggested that a minority of examples of intestinal type CGIN are not HPV-associated [37]. In one study, cases of intestinal type CGIN which were not

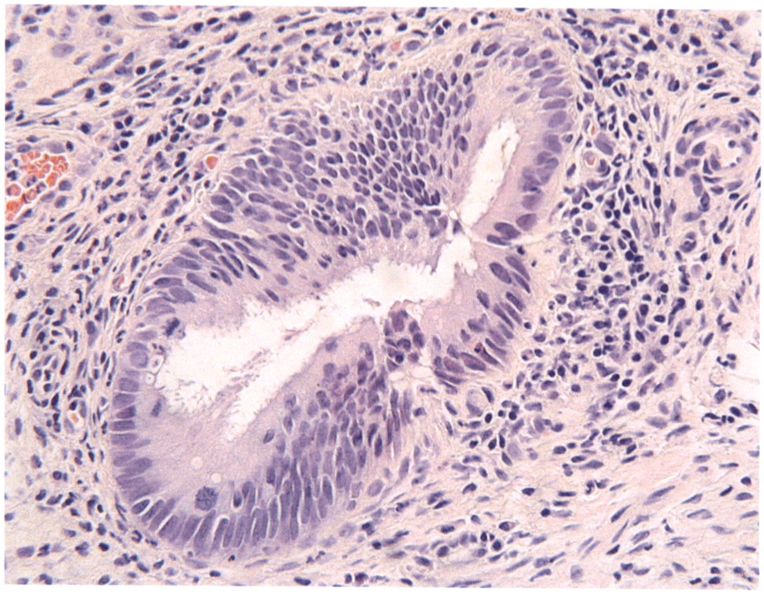

Fig. 3.9 Tubal type CGIN characterised by the presence of cilia

HPV-associated occurred in an older age group than HPV-associated CGIN, were less likely to express p16 diffusely and exhibited a lower MIB1 proliferation index [37].

Endometrioid Type CGIN

An endometrioid variant of CGIN (AIS) has been described. However, this is likely to merely represent usual type CGIN with marked depletion of intracytoplasmic mucin resulting in a pseudoendometrioid appearance. As such, it is doubtful whether a true endometrioid variant of CGIN exists or whether it could be distinguished from usual type.

Tubal (Ciliated) Type CGIN

Occasional examples of CGIN contain cilia and are referred to as being of tubal or ciliated type (Fig. 3.9) [38]. This uncommon variant of CGIN usually occurs in association with usual type. The main differential diagnosis is tuboendometrial metaplasia with a degree of nuclear atypia. Apoptotic bodies are a useful diagnostic clue in favour of CGIN but these should not be mistaken for the intraepithelial lymphocytes surrounded by a halo which are commonly seen in tuboendometrial metaplasia. It has been suggested that tubal type CGIN may arise from tuboendometrial metaplasia or atypical tuboendometrial metaplasia but there is no firm evidence for this. p16 may be useful in the distinction from tuboendometrial metaplasia in that CGIN is diffusely positive while tuboendometrial metaplasia is usually negative or exhibits patchy immunoreactivity. However, the immunophenotype of tubal type CGIN has not been studied given the rarity of the lesion. Given its rarity, caution should be exercised before making a diagnosis of tubal type CGIN. The nuclear features should unequivocally be those of a malignant lesion since tuboendometrial metaplasia may exhibit a significant degree of nuclear atypia.

Immunohistochemistry of Premalignant Endocervical Glandular Lesions

High grade CGIN is usually diffusely p16 positive (typically nuclear and cytoplasmic staining) secondary to the presence of high risk HPV (Fig. 3.10) [39–42]. The MIB1 proliferation index is typically in excess of 30 % (Fig. 3.11)

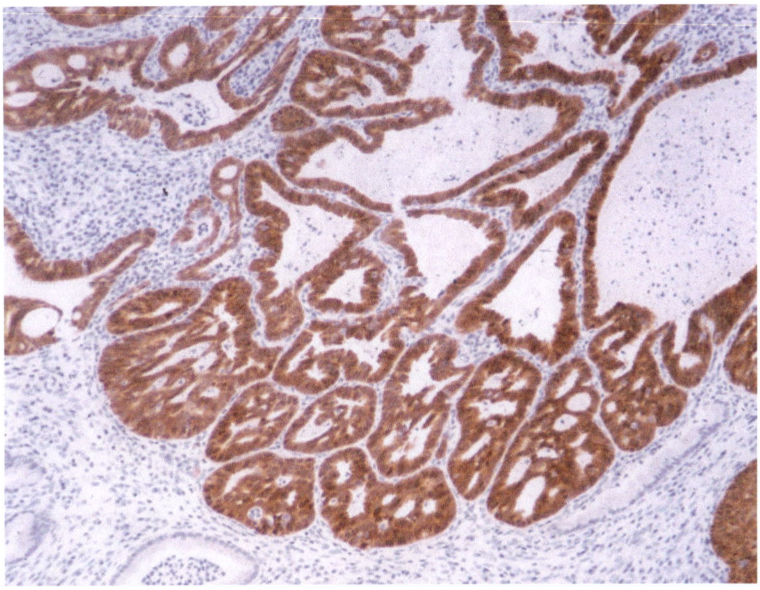

Fig. 3.10 High grade CGIN exhibiting diffuse nuclear and cytoplasmic staining with p16

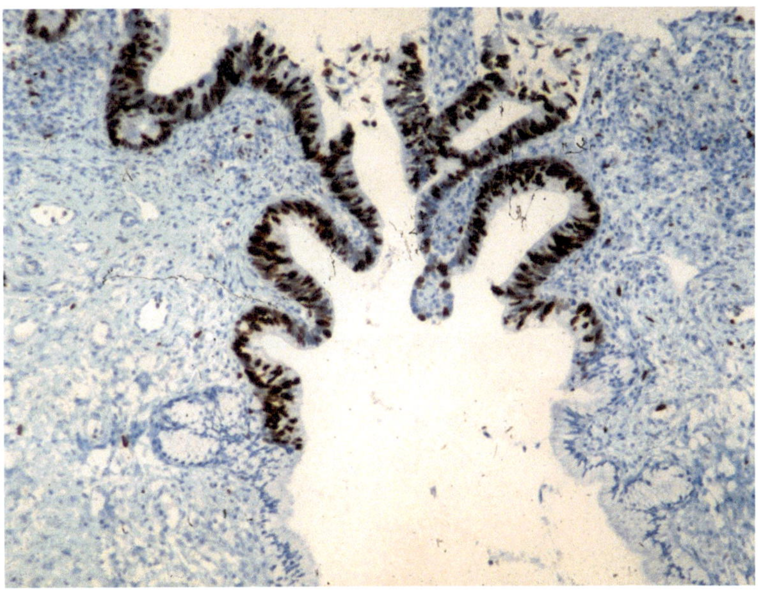

Fig. 3.11 High grade CGIN exhibiting a high MIB1 proliferation index

but is occasionally lower than this [39–41]. ProExC, a cocktail of antibodies against topoisomerase II alpha and minichromosome maintenance 2 proteins, is overexpressed [41, 43]. Bcl2 is negative or focally positive and this may be useful in the distinction from tuboendometrial metaplasia and superficial endometriosis which are usually diffusely positive [39, 40]. CEA is often, but not always, positive in high grade CGIN with cytoplasmic immunoreactivity, as opposed to luminal staining which may be seen in normal endocervical glands and benign glandular lesions (Fig. 3.12) [44]. Hormone receptors (ER and PR) and vimentin are usually negative or focally positive [44, 45]; this contrasts with tuboendometrial metaplasia and superficial endometriosis which are usually diffusely positive with hormone receptors and

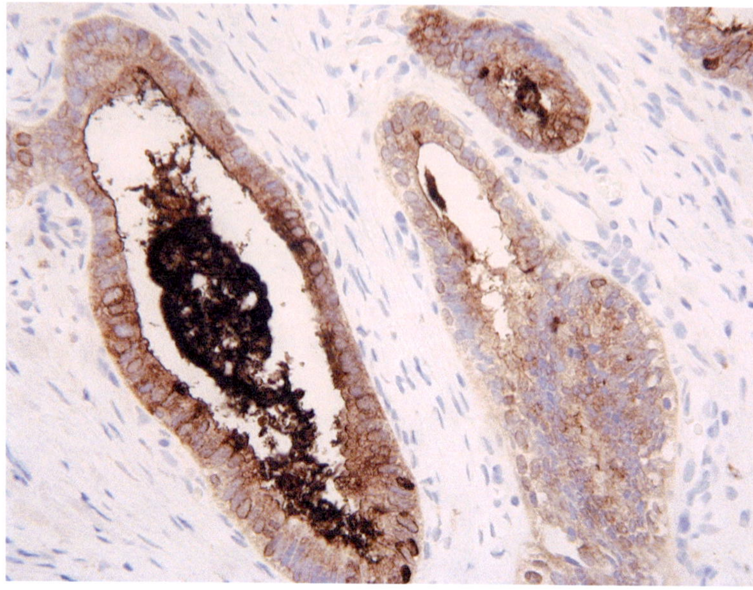

Fig. 3.12 High grade CGIN exhibiting diffuse staining with CEA

Table 3.2 Immunohistochemistry of high grade cervical glandular intraepithelial neoplasia and tuboendometrial metaplasia/superficial endometriosis

	High grade CGIN (adenocarcinoma in situ)	Tuboendometrial metaplasia/ superficial endometriosis
p16	Diffuse positive	Negative or focally positive
bcl2	Negative	Diffuse positive
MIB1	>30 %	<30 %
Vimentin	Negative	Diffuse positive
ER	Negative	Diffuse positive
CEA	Diffuse positive (cytoplasmic)	Negative or luminal staining
Cyclin D1	Negative	Positive
IMP3	Diffuse positive	Negative

This table lists the usual staining reactions but aberrant staining patterns may occur in individual cases

vimentin. Cyclin D1 is usually negative in CGIN but positive in normal endocervical glands and metaplastic endocervical glandular epithelium, including tuboendometrial metaplasia [46]. Insulin-like growth factor-II mRNA-binding protein 3 (IMP3) is often diffusely expressed in CGIN and negative in normal endocervical glands and tuboendometrial metaplasia [47]. Table 3.2 lists the staining patterns with various markers in high grade CGIN, in contrast to tuboendometrial metaplasia (and superficial endometriosis) which is often the main differential diagnosis.

Intestinal type CGIN is usually diffusely p16 positive, although some cases are only focally positive or even negative (discussed in section on "Intestinal type CGIN") [34, 37]. Analogous to other intestinal type lesions in the female genital tract, for example intestinal type ovarian mucinous neoplasms, intestinal type CGIN exhibits a partial enteric or hybrid immunophenotype in that, although it is usually diffusely CK7 positive, it is often also immunoreactive with the enteric marker CDX2 which is typically diffusely positive; CK20 is focally positive in some cases (Fig. 3.13) [34].

In contrast to high grade CGIN, the immunophenotype of low grade CGIN is not well studied, in part because of the problems in establishing this diagnosis. As stated, it is doubtful whether low grade CGIN should be diagnosed in the absence of diffuse staining with p16. The MIB1 proliferation index is variable and is usually only mildly elevated.

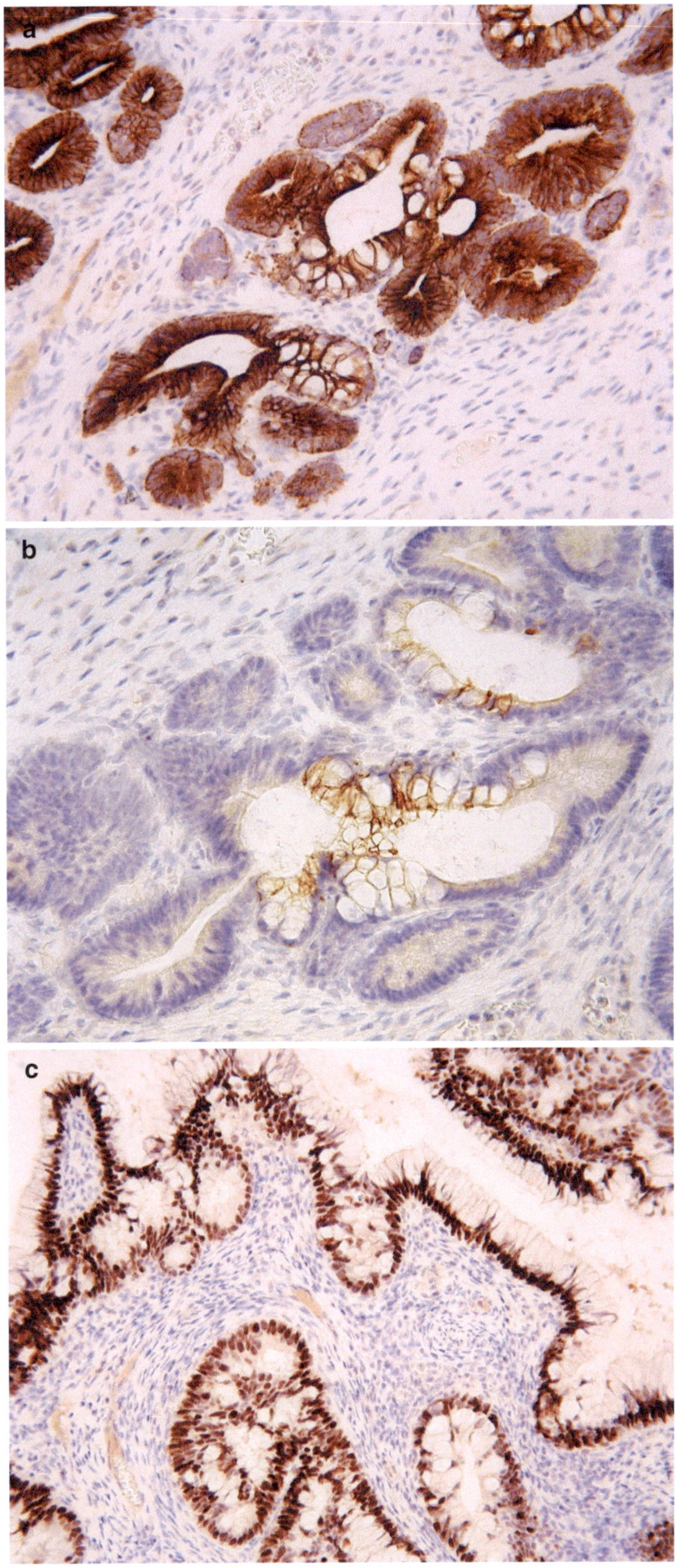

Fig. 3.13 Intestinal type CGIN which is diffusely positive with CK7 (**a**), focally positive with CK20 (**b**) and diffusely positive with CDX2 (**c**)

Differential Diagnosis of CGIN

The differential diagnosis of CGIN includes several of the benign endocervical glandular lesions discussed in the Chap. on 2. The most common of these lesions and the most likely to be confused with CGIN are tuboendometrial metaplasia and superficial endometriosis. The nuclei in CGIN are more hyperchromatic than in these two lesions and apoptotic bodies are a useful diagnostic feature of CGIN; these should not be confused with the intraepithelial lymphocytes surrounded by halos which are a characteristic feature of tuboendometrial metaplasia. In general, there are more mitoses in CGIN than in tuboendometrial metaplasia and superficial endometriosis, although this is not always the case since some cases of tuboendometrial metaplasia and superficial endometriosis exhibit easily identifiable mitotic activity. Cilia are present in tuboendometrial metaplasia which also characteristically contains a heterogenous population of cells, including ciliated and non-ciliated cells and lymphocytes. A combination of immunohistochemical markers including p16, bcl2 and MIB1 may also assist (Table 3.2) [39–42]. High grade CGIN is usually diffusely positive with p16, negative with bcl2 and exhibits a high MIB1 proliferation, usually in excess of 30 % and sometimes much higher. In contrast, tuboendometrial metaplasia and superficial endometriosis are usually negative or focally positive with p16 and exhibit diffuse cytoplasmic immunoreactivity with bcl2 [39–42]. The MIB1 proliferation is usually, but not always, less than 30 %; some cases of superficial endometriosis may exhibit a MIB1 proliferation index in excess of 30 %. Tuboendometrial metaplasia and endometriosis are usually vimentin positive and exhibit diffuse nuclear staining with ER and PR [44, 45]; in contrast, CGIN is usually vimentin negative and negative or focally positive with ER and PR. Most of the other benign endocervical glandular lesions are more likely to result in confusion with invasive adenocarcinoma than CGIN. On occasions, it may be difficult to distinguish high grade CGIN from invasive adenocarcinoma; this distinction is discussed in the Chap. on 4.

When endometrial adenocarcinoma involves the endocervical glands, the features may mimic CGIN. However, this is usually in the context of a patient with an endometrial adenocarcinoma in the same specimen and it is generally straightforward to ascertain that this represents cervical glandular involvement by endometrial adenocarcinoma and not an independent primary cervical glandular lesion. If there is doubt, immunohistochemistry may help in that CGIN is usually ER and vimentin negative or focally positive while CEA and p16 are usually diffusely positive; the converse immunophenotype is the rule with an endometrioid adenocarcinoma of the uterine corpus involving the cervix. Serous carcinomas of the uterine corpus exhibit aberrant p53 staining in that they are usually diffusely positive or more uncommonly completely negative ("all or nothing" staining) [48] while CGIN exhibits "wild-type" staining (focal, weak and heterogenous). Rarely, metastatic adenocarcinomas from other primary sites, most commonly serous carcinomas from the ovary or fallopian tube, are largely confined to the mucosal surface of the cervix and mimic CGIN; in such cases, the metastatic disease within the cervix is likely secondary to transtubal and transuterine spread [49]. Diffuse WT1 staining is useful in confirming a primary ovarian or tubal serous carcinoma [49].

Management of CGIN

Previously, because of the purported significant risk of skip lesions and extension high up the endocervical canal, most women diagnosed with CGIN underwent hysterectomy. However, hysterectomy is relatively infrequently undertaken nowadays in the management of CGIN and treatment is individualised. Many women with CGIN are young and wish to retain their fertility and in most cases, management is by local excision ensuring that the margins are clear. This may necessitate more than one local excision.

Cytological follow up is then undertaken. Some recommend cold knife cone biopsy rather than large loop excision of the transformation zone (LLETZ) for the local management of CGIN since a deeper loop can be excised and because of the potential interpretative problems associated with cautery artefact in LLETZ specimens, but many gynaecologists manage these patients with LLETZ. Hysterectomy may be undertaken in older women or in those with other pathology, such as uterine fibroids. If possible, local excision with clear margins should be undertaken prior to hysterectomy to ensure that invasion is not present. Hysterectomy may also be undertaken in younger women where fertility preservation is not an issue, especially when there is extensive CGIN. Some studies have found a poor correlation between the margin status in a local excision specimen and the risk of finding residual disease in the subsequent hysterectomy [50, 51]. In one study, 30 % of patients with a negative endocervical margin in the loop specimen had CGIN in the hysterectomy specimen while 56 % of patients with a positive endocervical margin had no CGIN in the hysterectomy [50]. However, local excision with clear margins and cytological follow up is routinely undertaken in the management of CGIN with good results. In a meta-analysis of 671 patients with CGIN (AIS) who were treated by local excision and followed up, only 2.6 % of patients with negative margins developed recurrent disease [51]. Invasive adenocarcinoma was more commonly associated with positive margins (5.2 %) compared with negative margins (0.1 %) [51]. There are occasional reports of invasive adenocarcinoma of cervical origin occurring in the vagina in patients who have undergone simple hysterectomy for CGIN [52, 53].

An important point is that CGIN is, in some cases, "colposcopically silent", especially since crypts may be involved rather than surface glands. In other words, the colposcopist may not see a lesion unless there is coexistent CIN. This raises management issues in that if a smear suggests a premalignant cervical glandular lesion, local excision may have to be performed in the absence of a colposcopically visible lesion.

Stratified Mucin Producing Intraepithelial Lesion (SMILE)

SMILE is a premalignant lesion which is not included in the 2003 WHO classification [6]. It is uncommon but not rare and is best discussed with and managed as for a premalignant cervical glandular lesion [54]. SMILE is usually, but not always, associated with CGIN and/or CIN and sometimes with an invasive squamous or glandular lesion and may be a marker of phenotypic instability. However, SMILE occasionally occurs in pure form unassociated with a premalignant or malignant squamous or glandular lesion. It has been variably suggested to be a form of adenosquamous carcinoma in situ or stratified CGIN [54] but is probably best regarded as a form of reserve cell dysplasia. If present in pure form, it should be managed as for CGIN and this should be stated on the pathology report; in other words, local excision should be undertaken and clear margins achieved.

Morphological and Immunohistochemical Features of SMILE

SMILE may involve both the surface and underlying crypt epithelium. There is morphological overlap with both CIN and CGIN. The epithelium is stratified similar to CIN but mucin, in the form of discrete vacuoles or cytoplasmic clearing, is present throughout the full epithelial thickness (Fig. 3.14) [54]. There is associated nuclear atypia and hyperchromasia. Mitotic figures are usually present but may not be conspicuous. Apototic bodies are seen in many cases and may be numerous. SMILE is p16 positive and exhibits a high MIB1 proliferation index; p63 is variable [54].

The main differential diagnosis is immature squamous metaplasia. In the latter, mucin is

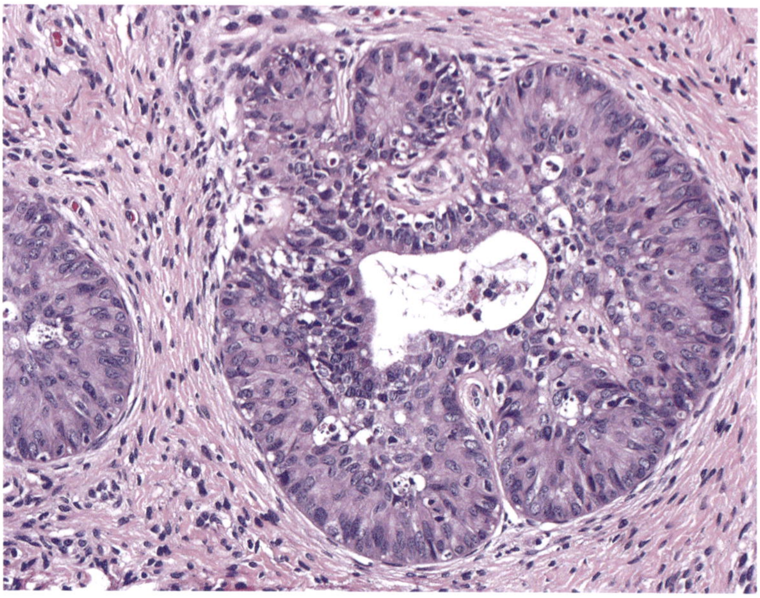

Fig. 3.14 SMILE involving an endocervical gland exhibits nuclear stratification with intracytoplasmic mucin globules

usually confined to the surface layer while in SMILE it is generally present throughout the full epithelial thickness. The nuclei are more atypical and hyperchromatic in SMILE than in immature squamous metaplasia. p16 may assist in that SMILE is positive while immature squamous metaplasia is generally negative. SMILE may also be confused with CIN involving immature metaplastic squamous epithelium and the distinction may be difficult, especially since both may be p16 positive; in CIN involving immature metaplastic squamous epithelium, the mucin is usually confined to the surface layers.

References

1. Friedell GA, McKay DG. Adenocarcinoma in situ of the endocervix. Cancer. 1953;6:887–97.
2. Sasieni P, Adams J. Changing rates of adenocarcinoma and adenosquamous carcinoma of the cervix in England. Lancet. 2001;357:1490–3.
3. Hemminki K, Li X, Vaittinen P. Time trends in the incidence of cervical and other genital squamous cell carcinomas and adenocarcinomas in Sweden, 1958–1996. Eur J Obstet Gynecol Reprod Biol. 2002;101:64–9.
4. Smith HO, Tiffany MF, Qualls CR, Key CR. The rising incidence of adenocarcinoma relative to squamous cell carcinoma of the uterine cervix in the United States- a 24 year population-based study. Gynecol Oncol. 2000;78:97–105.
5. Fox H, Buckley CH. Histopathology reporting in cervical screening. NHSCSP Publication, No 10; 1999.
6. Tavassoli FA, Devilee P, editors. World Health Organisation Classification of Tumours. Pathology and genetics. Tumours of the breast and female genital organs. Lyon: IARC Press; 2003.
7. Brown LJ, Wells M. Cervical glandular atypia associated with squamous intraepithelial neoplasia: a premalignant lesion. J Clin Pathol. 1986;39:22–8.
8. McCluggage WG. Endocervical glandular lesions: controversial aspects and ancillary techniques. J Clin Pathol. 2003;56:164–73.
9. Gloor E, Hurlmann J. Cervical intraepithelial glandular neoplasia (adenocarcinoma in situ and glandular dysplasia). Cancer. 1986;58:1272–80.
10. Houghton O, Jamison J, Wilson R, Carson J, McCluggage WG. p16 Immunoreactivity in unusual types of cervical adenocarcinoma does not reflect human papillomavirus infection. Histopathology. 2010;57:342–50.
11. Park KJ, Kiyokawa T, Soslow RA, et al. Unusual endocervical adenocarcinomas: an immunohistochemical analysis with molecular detection of human papillomavirus. Am J Surg Pathol. 2011;35:633–46.
12. Leary J, Jaworski R, Houghton R. In-situ hybridization using biotinylated DNA probes to human papillomavirus in adenocarcinoma-in-situ and endocervical glandular dysplasia of the uterine cervix. Pathology. 1991;23:85–9.
13. Tase T, Okagaki T, Clark BA, et al. Human papillomavirus DNA in adenocarcinoma in situ, microinvasive adenocarcinoma of the uterine cervix, and coexisting cervical squamous intraepithelial neoplasia. Int J Gynecol Pathol. 1989;8:8–17.
14. Thomas DB, Ray RM. Oral contraceptive and invasive adenocarcinomas and adenosquamous

carcinomas of the uterine cervix. The World Health Organization Collaborative Study of Neoplasia and Steroid Contraceptives. Am J Epidemiol. 1996;144: 281–9.

15. Jones MW, Silverberg SG. Cervical adenocarcinoma in young women: possible relationship to microglandular hyperplasia and use of oral contraceptives. Obstet Gynecol. 1989;73:984–9.
16. Kojima A, Mikami Y, Sudo T, et al. Gastric morphology and immunophenotype predict poor outcome in mucinous adenocarcinoma of the uterine cervix. Am J Surg Pathol. 2007;31:664–72.
17. Nara M, Hashi A, Murata S, et al. Lobular endocervical glandular hyperplasia as a presumed precursor of cervical adenocarcinoma independent of human papillomavirus infection. Gynecol Oncol. 2007;106: 289–98.
18. Kondo T, Hashi A, Murata S, et al. Endocervical adenocarcinomas associated with lobular endocervical glandular hyperplasia: a report of four cases with histochemical and immunohistochemical analyses. Mod Pathol. 2005;18:1199–210.
19. Goldstein NS, Ahmad E, Hussain M, Hankin RC, Perez-Reyes N. Endocervical glandular atypia: does a preneoplastic lesion of adenocarcinoma in situ exist? Am J Clin Pathol. 1998;110:200–9.
20. Ioffe OB, Sagae S, Moritani S, Dahmoush L, Chen TT, Silverberg SG. Symposium part 3: Should pathologists diagnose endocervical preneoplastic lesions "less than" adenocarcinoma in situ? Point Int J Gynecol Pathol. 2002;22:18–21.
21. Lee KR. Symposium part 3: Should pathologists diagnose endocervical preneoplastic lesions "less than" adenocarcinoma in situ? Counterpoint. Int J Gynecol Pathol. 2002;22:22–4.
22. Kurian K, Al-Nafussi A. Relation of cervical glandular intraepithelial neoplasia to microinvasive and invasive adenocarcinoma of the uterine cervix: a study of 121 cases. J Clin Pathol. 1999;52:112–7.
23. Lee KR, Sun D, Crum CP. Endocervical intraepithelial glandular atypia (dysplasia): A histopathologic, human papillomavirus, and MIB1 analysis of 25 cases. Hum Pathol. 2000;31:656–64.
24. Kurman RJ, Hedrick Ellenson L, Ronnett BM, editors. Chapter 5. Precursors of cervical adenocarcinoma. In: Blaustein's pathology of the female genital tract. 6th ed. Springer; New York: 2011, p. 225–8.
25. Ostor AG, Duncan A, Quinn M, Rome R. Adenocarcinoma in situ of the uterine cervix: an experience with 100 cases. Gynecol Oncol. 2000;79: 207–10.
26. Jaworski RC, Pacey NF, Greenberg ML, et al. The histologic diagnosis of adenocarcinoma in situ and related lesions of the cervix uteri. Cancer. 1988;61: 1171–81.
27. Chang MC, Nevadunsky NS, Viswanathan AN, Crum CP, Feltmate CM. Endocervical adenocarcinoma in situ with ovarian metastases: a unique variant with potential for long term survival. Int J Gynecol Pathol. 2010;29:88–92.
28. Yemelyanova A, Vang R, Seidman JD, Gravitt PE, Ronnett BM. Endocervical adenocarcinomas with prominent endometrial or endomyometrial involvement simulating primary endometrial carcinomas: utility of HPV DNA detection and immunohistochemical expression of p16 and hormone receptors to confirm the cervical origin of the corpus tumor. Am J Surg Pathol. 2009;33:914–24.
29. Al-Fehmi R, Qureshi F, Lawrence WG, Jacques SM. Apoptosis, proliferation, and expression of p53 and bcl-2 in endocervical glandular intraepithelial lesions and invasive endocervical adenocarcinoma. Int J Gynecol Pathol. 2004;23:1–6.
30. Moritani S, Ioffe OB, Sagae S, Dahmoush L, Silverberg SG, Hattori T. Mitotic activity and apotosis in endocervical glandular lesions. Int J Gynecol Pathol. 2002;21:125–33.
31. Biscotti CV, Hart WR. Apoptotic bodies. A consistent morphological feature of endocervical adenocarcinoma in situ. Am J Surg Pathol. 1998;22:434–9.
32. Witkiewicz A, Lee KR, Brodsky G, Cviko A, Brodsky J, Crum CP. Superficial (early) endocervical adenocarcinoma in situ: a study of twelve cases and comparison to conventional AIS. Am J Surg Pathol. 2005;29:1609–14.
33. Ioffe OB, Sagae S, Moritani S, Dahmoush L, Chen TT, Silverberg SG. Proposal of a new scoring scheme for the diagnosis of noninvasive endocervical glandular lesions. Am J Surg Pathol. 2003;27:452–60.
34. McCluggage WG, Shah R, Connolly LE, McBride HA. Intestinal-type cervical adenocarcinoma in situ and adenocarcinoma exhibit a partial immunophenotype with consistent expression of CDX2. Int J Gynecol Pathol. 2008;27:92–100.
35. Nicolae A, Goyenaga P, McCluggage WG, Preda O, Nogales FF. Endometrial intestinal metaplasia: a report of two cases, including one associated with cervical intestinal and pyloric metaplasia. Int J Gynecol Pathol. 2011;30:492–6.
36. Mikami Y, McCluggage WG. Endocervical glandular lesions exhibiting gastric differentiation: an emerging spectrum of benign, premalignant, and malignant lesions. Adv Anat Pathol. 2013;20:227–37.
37. Howitt BE, Herfs M, Brister K, Oliva E, Longtine J, Hecht JL, Nucci MR. Intestinal-type endocervical adenocarcinoma in situ. An immunophenotypically distinct subset of AIS affecting older women. Am J Surg Pathol. 2013;37:625–33.
38. Schlesinger C, Silverberg SG. Endocervical adenocarcinoma in situ of tubal type and its relation to atypical tubal metaplasia. Int J Gynecol Pathol. 1999;73:305–11.
39. McCluggage WG. Immunohistochemistry as a diagnostic aid in cervical pathology. Pathology. 2007;39: 97–111.
40. Cameron RI, Maxwell P, Jenkins D, McCluggage WG. Immunohistochemical staining with MIB1, bcl2 and p16 assists in the distinction of cervical glandular intraepithelial neoplasia from tubo-endometrial metaplasia, endometriosis and microglandular hyperplasia. Histopathology. 2002;41:313–21.

41. Negri G, Bellisano G, Carico E, et al. Usefulness of p16ink4a, ProEXC, and Ki-67 for the diagnosis of glandular dysplasia and adenocarcinoma of the cervix uteri. Int J Gynecol Pathol. 2011;30:407–13.
42. O'Neill CJ, McCluggage WG. p16 expression in the female genital tract and its value in diagnosis. Adv Anat Pathol. 2006;13:8–15.
43. Sanati S, Huettner P, Yiagan LR. Role of ProExC: a novel immunoperoxidase marker in the evaluation of dysplastic squamous and glandular lesions in cervical specimens. Int J Gynecol Pathol. 2010;29:79–87.
44. Marques T, Andrade LA, Vassallo J. Endocervical tubal metaplasia and adenocarcinoma in situ: role of immunohistochemistry for carcinoembryonic antigen and vimentin in differential diagnosis. Histopathology. 1996;28:549–50.
45. Stewart CJ, Little L. Diagnostic value and implications of vimentin expression in normal, reactive and neoplastic endocervical epithelium. Pathology. 2010; 42:217–33.
46. Little L, Stewart CJ. Cyclin D1 immunoreactivity in normal endocervix and diagnostic value in reactive and neoplastic endocervical lesions. Mod Pathol. 2010;23:611–8.
47. Li C, Rock KL, Woda BA, Jiang Z, Fraire AE, Dresser K. IMP3 is a novel biomarker for adenocarcinoma in situ of the uterine cervix: an immunohistochemical study in comparison with p16 (INK4a) expression. Mod Pathol. 2007;20:241–7.
48. McCluggage WG, Soslow RA, Gilks CB. Patterns of p53 immunoreactivity in endometrial carcinomas: 'all or nothing' staining is of importance. Histopathology. 2011;59:786–8.
49. McCluggage WG, Hurrell DP, Kennedy K. Metastatic carcinomas in the cervix mimicking primary cervical adenocarcinoma and adenocarcinoma in situ: report of a series of cases. Am J Surg Pathol. 2010;34: 735–41.
50. Goldstein NS, Mani A. The status and distance of cone biopsy margins as a predictor of excision adequacy for endocervical adenocarcinoma in situ. Am J Clin Pathol. 1998;109:727–32.
51. Salani R, Puri I, Bristow RE. Adenocarcinoma in situ of the uterine cervix: a metaanalysis of 1278 patients evaluating the predictive value of conisation margin status. Am J Obstet Gynecol. 2009;200:182e1–5.
52. Krivak TC, Retherford B, Voskuil S, Rose GS, Alagoz T. Recurrent invasive adenocarcinoma after hysterectomy for cervical adenocarcinoma in situ. Gynecol Oncol. 2000;77:334–5.
53. Hurrell DP, Jamison J, Dobbs SP, McCluggage WG. Cervical adenocarcinoma in situ recurring as vaginal adenocarcinoma 16 years after hysterectomy. Int J Gynecol Pathol. 2009;28:296–300.
54. Park JJ, Sun D, Quade BJ, et al. Stratified mucin producing intraepithelial lesions of the cervix: adenosquamous or columnar cell neoplasia? Am J Surg Pathol. 2000;24:1414–9.

Malignant Glandular Lesions of the Cervix

4

W. Glenn McCluggage

Abstract

Cervical adenocarcinomas are increasing in incidence and now account for approximately 25 % of cervical carcinomas in most developed countries. Most are associated with high risk human papillomavirus (HPV) infection and are of the usual endocervical type. However, a minor proportion of unusual morphological subtypes of cervical adenocarcinoma are not HPV associated. This chapter covers the clinicopathological features of the various subtypes of cervical adenocarcinoma.

Keywords

Cervix • Adenocarcinoma • Human papillomavirus

Introduction

As discussed in the Chap. 3, premalignant and malignant endocervical glandular lesions are increasing in incidence with adenocarcinomas now accounting for approximately 25 % of cervical carcinomas in most developed countries [1]. The mean age of patients with cervical adenocarcinoma in most series is between 44 and 54 years. Several morphological subtypes of cervical adenocarcinoma are recognized in the 2003 World Health Organization (WHO) classification [2] (modification in Table 4.1). Of these, by far the most common is the endocervical (or usual) type of mucinous adenocarcinoma which accounts for approximately 80 % of cervical adenocarcinomas. Some recently recognized subtypes of primary cervical adenocarcinoma, such as gastric type, are not currently recognized by the WHO but are discussed in this chapter. Although the association is less strong than with cervical squamous carcinoma, the majority of cervical adenocarcinomas are associated with high risk HPV, most commonly types 16 and 18; HPV 18 is proportionally more common than with invasive squamous carcinomas [3–9]. However, unusual morphological subtypes of cervical adenocarcinoma, such as adenoma malignum, gastric type, mesonephric and clear cell are mostly unrelated to HPV [3–6]. While diffuse p16 positivity has been regarded as a surrogate marker of the presence of high risk HPV, non-HPV related cervical adenocarcinomas may also be positive with this marker, although staining is usually focal rather than diffuse [3, 4].

W.G. McCluggage et al., *Cellular Pathology of Glandular Lesions and Uncommon Neoplasms of the Cervix*,
DOI 10.1007/978-1-4471-2210-4_4, © Springer-Verlag London 2014

Table 4.1 Modification of World Health Organization (WHO) classification of cervical adenocarcinomas [2]

Mucinous adenocarcinoma
Endocervical (usual) type
Intestinal
Signet-ring cell
Minimal deviation
Villoglandular
Gastric type (not included in WHO Classification)
Endometrioid adenocarcinoma
Clear cell adenocarcinoma
Serous adenocarcinoma
Mesonephric adenocarcinoma
Early invasive adenocarcinoma
Other epithelial tumours
Adenosquamous carcinoma
Mucoepidermoid carcinoma (not included in WHO classification)
Glassy cell carcinoma
Adenoid cystic carcinoma
Adenoid basal carcinoma
Carcinosarcoma
Mixed
Metastatic

Early Invasive Adenocarcinoma

Early invasive adenocarcinoma of the cervix is increasingly being diagnosed. While some of this increase may reflect the rising incidence of cervical adenocarcinoma in general or earlier detection due to improvements in cervical screening programmes, there is also probably better recognition by histopathologists of the features of early invasion in premalignant cervical glandular lesions; the features of early invasion may be subtle. It is recommended that the term microinvasive carcinoma is not used (for cervical squamous carcinomas, adenocarcinomas and other epithelial tumour types) but rather the tumour should be measured accurately and the appropriate FIGO stage provided. This is because the term microinvasive carcinoma does not appear in the FIGO staging system for cervical cancer [10]. Furthermore, the term microinvasive carcinoma has different in different places. In the United Kingdom, microinvasive carcinoma is considered to be synonymous with FIGO stage IA1 and IA2 disease in some institutions while in others the term is restricted to FIGO stage IA1 tumours. In the United States, the term is largely synonymous with stage IA1 disease. The Society of Gynecologic Oncology (SGO) has its own definition of microinvasive carcinoma which includes lesions up to a depth of 3 mm with no limit on the size of horizontal spread; neoplasms with lymphovascular invasion are excluded [11]. In order to avoid confusion, the British Association of Gynaecological Pathologists Working Group has recommended in the Royal College of Pathologists Dataset for Histological Reporting of Cervical Neoplasia a preference for avoiding the term microinvasive carcinoma and for using the specific FIGO stage as a descriptor [12, 13].

Morphological Features of Early Invasive Adenocarcinoma

Early invasion is, in general, more difficult to recognise in cervical glandular than squamous lesions and it is likely that there is significant interobserver variability in the diagnosis of early invasive adenocarcinoma. This is because there is often an admixture of cervical glandular intraepithelial neoplasia (CGIN) and adenocarcinoma and sometimes it is not straightforward to ascertain whether invasion is present and where CGIN ends and early invasion starts. This also makes accurate measurement of early invasive adenocarcinoma problematic (discussed below). However, there are a number of morphological features which help to distinguish CGIN from invasive adenocarcinoma [14, 15]. Simplistically, the distinction between CGIN and adenocarcinoma is based on the glandular architecture being too complex in the latter to conform to the normal endocervical glandular field; however, this in itself can be problematic in that the "normal" endocervical glandular architecture may be complex. It should also be recognised that, although rare, CGIN may involve a pre-existing

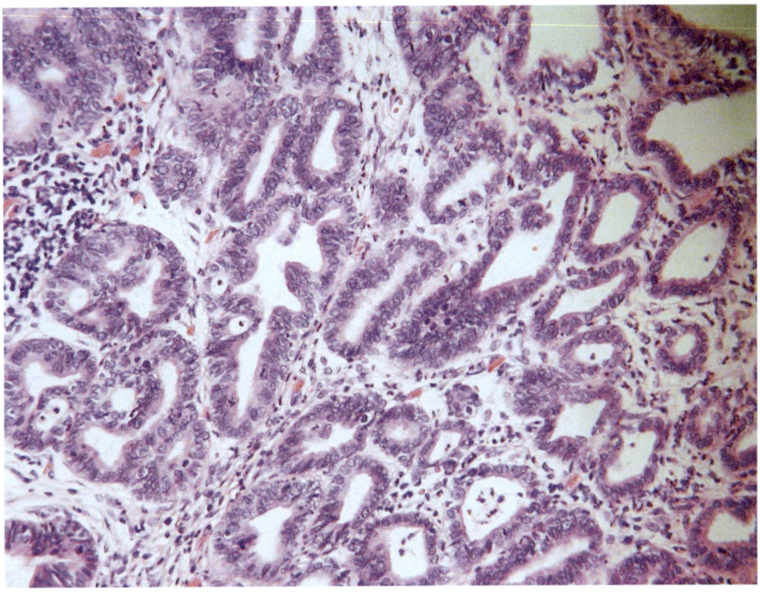

Fig. 4.1 Small adenocarcinoma with an obvious infiltrative growth pattern

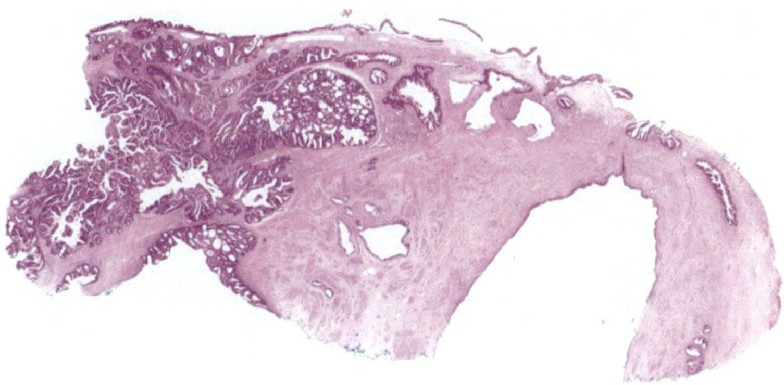

Fig. 4.2 Cervical adenocarcinoma where there is no obvious infiltrative growth pattern but the overall architecture is too complicated to conform to the normal endocervical glandular field

benign endocervical glandular lesion, for example microglandular hyperplasia, where the architecture may be complex and this can result in obvious diagnostic difficulties.

In some cases, although the adenocarcinoma is small there is an obvious infiltrative growth pattern which is often best appreciated on low power with irregular angulated or "crab-like" glands infiltrating the stroma with or without an associated desmoplastic, oedematous or inflammatory reaction (Fig. 4.1). This infiltrative pattern contrasts with CGIN where there is preservation of the normal lobular architecture, although the lobular architecture may be "accentuated". There are other cases where, although there is no obvious infiltrative growth pattern or stromal reaction, a diagnosis of invasion is made on the sheer glandular architectural complexity which is beyond that compatible with the normal endocervical glandular field (Fig. 4.2). In such cases, there are often papillary, cribriform, labyrinthine and solid growth patterns [14, 15]. Although minor papillary and/or cribriform areas may be present in CGIN, any appreciable amount of papillary or cribriform architecture should suggest adenocarcinoma. Another morphological pattern of early invasion is the presence of small buds, glands or solid nests of cells with abundant

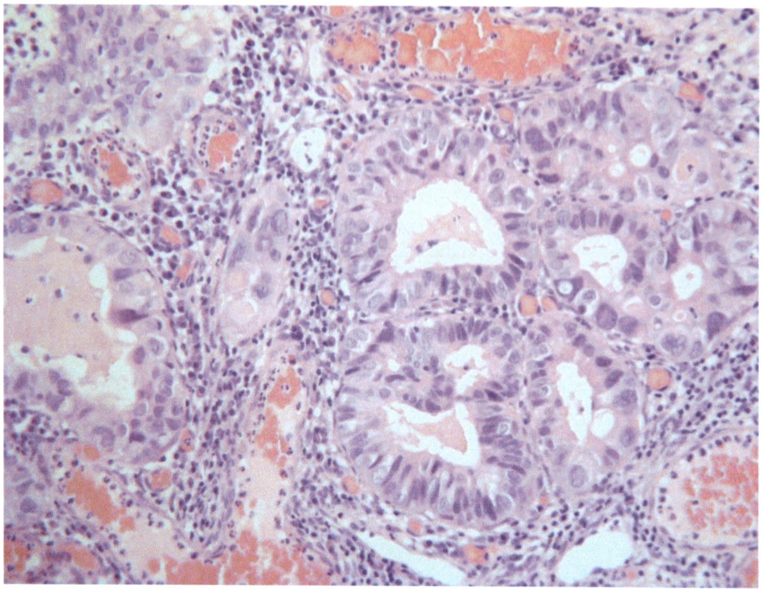

Fig. 4.3 Early invasive adenocarcinoma where small buds of cells with a squamoid appearance emanate from glands involved by CGIN

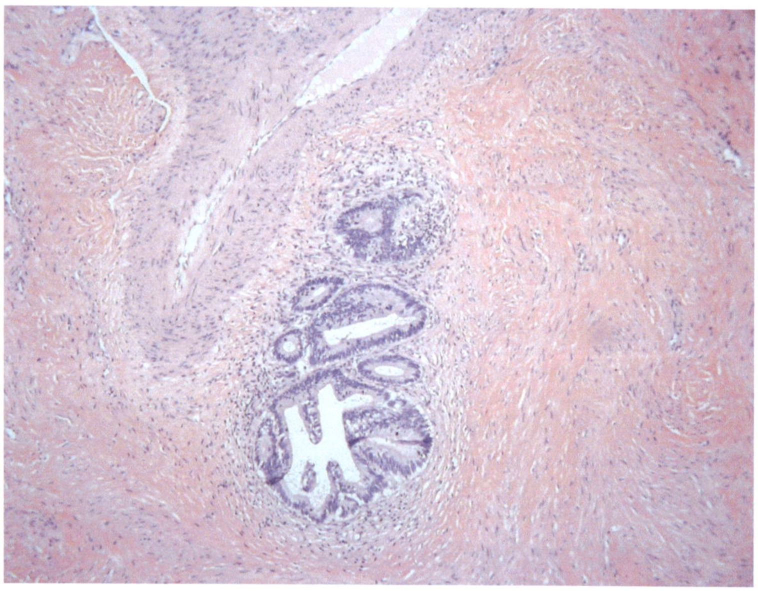

Fig. 4.4 Close proximity of glands to thick walled stromal blood vessels may be helpful in confirming an invasive adenocarcinoma

eosinophilic cytoplasm (squamoid appearance) that emanate from glands involved by obvious CGIN (Fig. 4.3) [16]. This "squamoid" change is analogous to that often seen with early invasive squamous carcinoma. The cells with a squamoid appearance often have enlarged nuclei with prominent nucleoli and may be surrounded by an inflammatory reaction. Close proximity of abnormal glands to thick-walled stromal blood vessels may also be useful in helping to confirm an invasive lesion (Fig. 4.4), especially in cases where there is little in the way of a stromal response [17]. A stromal inflammatory, oedematous or desmoplastic response is not always apparent in early invasive adenocarcinomas, or indeed in some overt adenocarcinomas, but may be useful when present. However, it should be noted that the glands of CGIN may be surrounded by an inflammatory or oedematous stroma; as such, a true desmoplastic stromal reaction is more useful in diagnosing invasion than inflammation or oedema. Lymphovascular space invasion may be seen but is relatively uncommon in early invasive adenocarcinomas [18].

In general, immunohistochemistry is of little value in the diagnosis of early invasion in cervical glandular lesions. The value of basement membrane markers, such as laminin and type IV collagen, has been investigated but, although the results of various studies are somewhat contradictory [19, 20], these markers are of limited use in individual cases. Although the basement membrane is generally uniform and intact in CGIN (diffuse expression of these markers) and focally deficient in early invasive adenocarcinoma (focal loss of these markers), there are exceptions in that these proteins may be focally lost in some cases of CGIN and conversely invasive adenocarcinomas, even in lymph node metastases, may produce them. One study found that α smooth muscle actin was of some value in the distinction between CGIN and invasive adenocarcinoma in that there is an increase in staining surrounding invasive glands, probably secondary to stromal desmoplasia [21]; however, this marker is unlikely to be of value in individual problematic cases.

Measurement of Early Invasive Adenocarcinoma

The measurement of small invasive adenocarcinomas may be extremely difficult because of the problems in recognising early invasion and in ascertaining which foci constitute CGIN and which represent invasion. It cases where there is doubt, it is best to err on the side of caution and measure the whole of the lesion which is considered to possibly represent invasion. The depth of invasion of a cervical carcinoma is generally measured from the deepest point of invasion to the basement membrane of the surface or crypt epithelium from which the tumour arises. However, this may be extremely difficult with glandular lesions and, especially in cases where a diagnosis of invasion is made on the presence of extreme architectural complexity, measurement should be from the surface to the deepest aspect of the lesion; as such, tumour thickness rather than depth of invasion is measured in these cases and it is recognised that this may overestimate the depth of invasion [22]. The lesion should also be measured from one lateral extent to the other on the slide on which the extent is greatest and, as with other carcinomas, the third dimension is calculated by multiplying the number of blocks involved by the thickness of the blocks (calculated from the macroscopic description of the specimen). As with squamous lesions, there may be difficulties in measuring cases with multifocal or possible multifocal invasion, although multifocal invasion appears more uncommon in cervical adenocarcinomas than squamous carcinomas. If the multiple foci of invasion are clearly separate, these can be regarded as multifocal early invasive adenocarcinomas. In such cases, each individual focus of invasion is measured rather than the width of the whole lesion. However, as stated, this is relatively uncommon in adenocarcinomas and, if the foci are not clearly separate, the width of the whole lesion should be taken as the horizontal measurement [12].

FIGO stage 1A adenocarcinoma cannot be diagnosed in an incompletely excised lesion with CGIN or adenocarcinoma at a margin. With a small adenocarcinoma which is completely excised by LLETZ or cone, the closest margin should be stated and the distance of the adenocarcinoma and CGIN from the margin provided on the pathology report. The presence or absence of lymphovascular invasion should also be documented.

Management of Early Invasive Adenocarcinoma

Management of early invasive adenocarcinoma is individualised and depends on multiple factors such as the age of the patient, the tumour stage and precise measurements, parity, fertility issues and the patient's wishes. There is good evidence that FIGO stage 1A1 adenocarcinomas can be treated by local excision (more than one local excision may be necessary to ensure the margins are clear of premalignant and malignant disease) with clear margins and follow up [18, 23–27]. Radical hysterectomy with pelvic lymph node dissection is usually undertaken for FIGO 1A2 and small 1B1 adenocarcinomas, although trachelectomy is an option for such neoplasms when fertility preservation is an issue. If simple hysterectomy is being undertaken for a FIGO stage 1A1 adenocarcinoma, local excision with clear margins should be achieved before hysterectomy in order to ensure that a larger focus of invasion is not present. Studies have shown an extremely low risk of lymph node and parametrial involvement and of tumour recurrence or metastasis in cervical adenocarcinomas 2 cm or less in maximum dimension raising the possibility that such tumours could be safely treated by local excision [18, 23–27]; however, such management is not in widespread use and carefully designed studies are necessary to determine the efficacy and safety of such methods of treatment. In a literature review of 1,170 stage 1A cervical adenocarcinomas, there was no difference in survival between stage 1A1 and 1A2 neoplasms [26].

Cervical Adenocarcinoma

Gross Features of Primary Cervical Adenocarcinomas

There are no specific gross features of any of the morphological subtypes of primary cervical adenocarcinoma. A mass is usually present which may be polypoid, ulcerated or result in a "barrel-shaped" cervix. In some cases, there is little or no mucosal abnormality but diffuse thickening of the cervical wall. Cystic areas may be present, especially in adenoma malignum. Mesonephric adenocarcinomas usually arise deep within the lateral wall of the cervix from mesonephric remnants. However, at diagnosis, a location deep within the cervical wall is generally no longer apparent. Small adenocarcinomas may not be visible grossly. In larger neoplasms, there may be obvious gross invasion of the uterine corpus and/or extension outside the uterus.

Usual Type Cervical Adenocarcinoma (Mucinous Adenocarcinoma of Endocervical Type)

As discussed, this is the most common subtype of cervical adenocarcinoma. These neoplasms are referred to as mucinous adenocarcinoma of endocervical type by the WHO [2] but these are not overtly mucinous and others refer to these as usual type cervical adenocarcinoma which is the preferred designation [14, 15]. They are often associated with and arise from CGIN. CIN may also be present. Most of these neoplasms are HPV- associated. An association with hormonal use has also been suggested but this is not generally accepted [28]. As stated, most examples of this tumour type are not overtly mucinous and contain relatively inconspicuous intracytoplasmic mucin, although special stains may reveal sparse apical and intracytoplasmic accumulation [14, 15]. Architecturally, these neoplasms are often relatively well differentiated with glandular formation throughout much of the tumour (Fig. 4.5). Solid areas may occur but are relatively uncommon. The nuclei are hyperchromatic, sometimes with nucleoli, and there is often prominent mitotic and apoptotic activity, even when the neoplasms are architecturally well differentiated. The mitoses typically have a predominant luminal location and the apoptotic bodies are situated at the base of the cells (Fig. 4.6). The cytoplasm is usually lightly eosinophilic and ranges from scant to abundant. The glandular profiles are complex and at low power there is usually an obviously infiltrative growth pattern with angulated, branched, budded or cribriform glands, sometimes with "crab-like" profiles (Fig. 4.7). Some cases have a papillary architecture, especially towards the surface (Fig. 4.8),

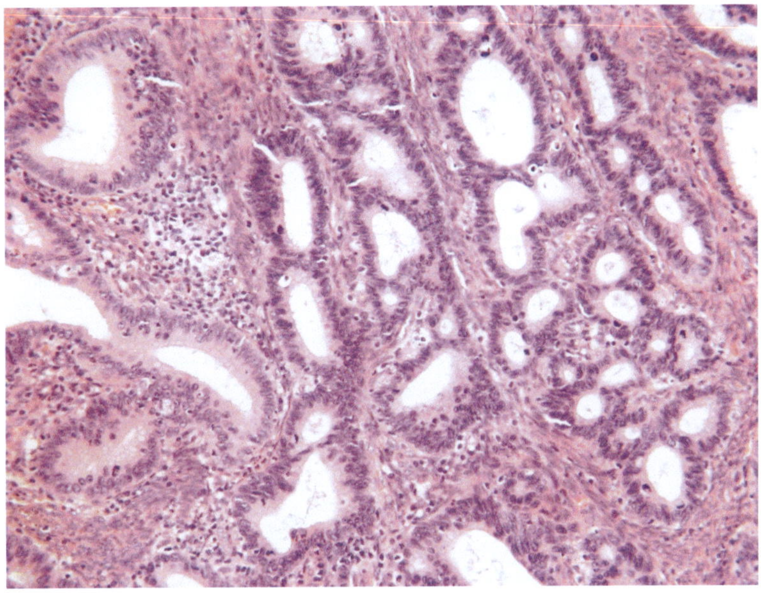

Fig. 4.5 Well differentiated cervical adenocarcinoma with good glandular differentiation

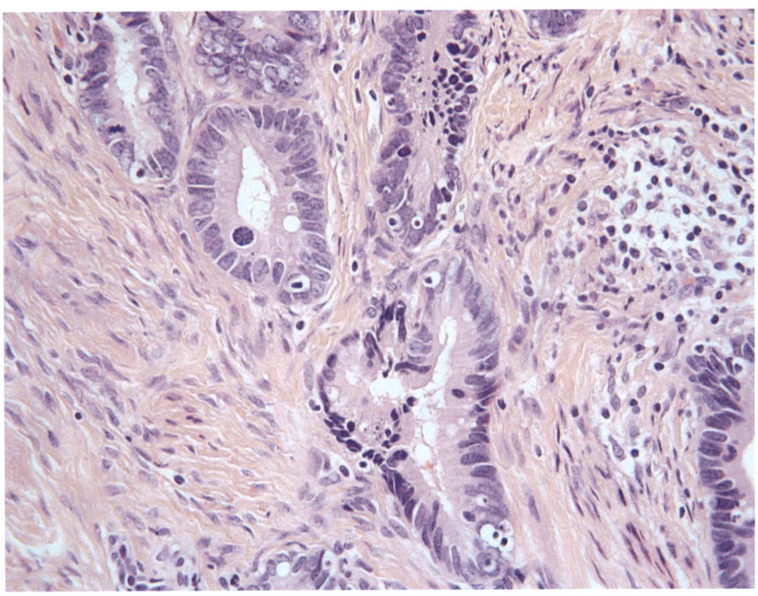

Fig. 4.6 Cervical adenocarcinoma containing luminal mitoses and basal apoptotic bodies

and should not be mistaken for other types of cervical adenocarcinoma which characteristically form papillae such as serous and villoglandular (see below). Intraluminal papillae occur in some cases. In some papillary variants of usual endocervical type adenocarcinoma, the tumour is predominantly located on the mucosal surface with an exophytic growth pattern and little in the way of stromal invasion. Such cases should not be diagnosed as CGIN but as exophytic adenocarcinomas since the architecture is too complex to conform to the normal endocervical glandular field. Even though there is no underlying stromal invasion, the tumour thickness and horizontal extent should be measured and the FIGO stage determined from these measurements. A stromal

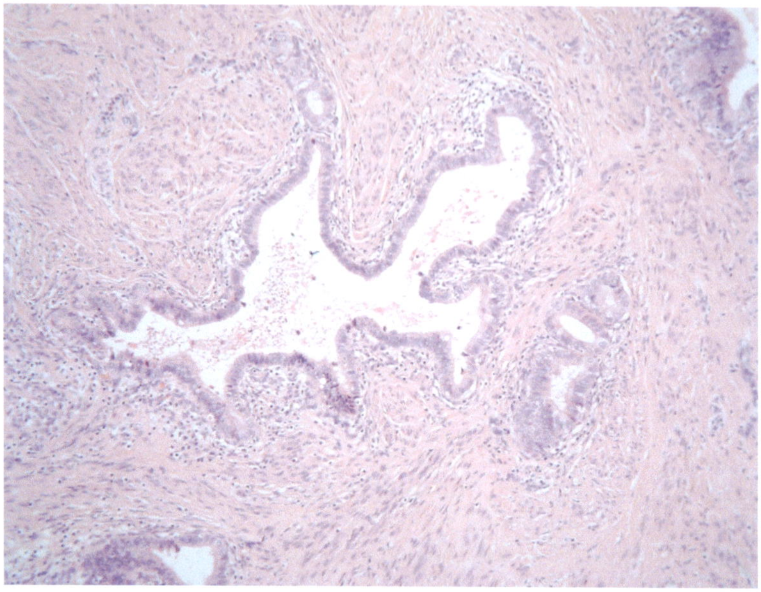

Fig. 4.7 Cervical adenocarcinoma with angulated and crab-like glands

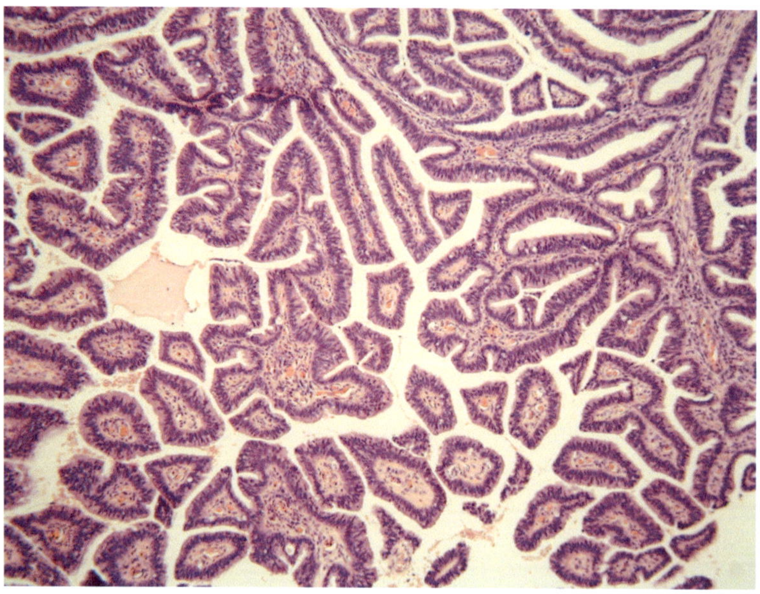

Fig. 4.8 Cervical adenocarcinoma with prominent papillary architecture

desmoplastic, inflammatory or oedematous reaction is usually present at least focally but some usual endocervical type adenocarcinomas are characterized by a so-called "naked" pattern of invasion and melt through the stroma without eliciting a reaction (Fig. 4.9). Lymphovascular and perineural invasion are often seen.

A rare microcystic variant of usual type adenocarcinoma has been described which at low power resembles dilated benign glands or tunnel clusters (Fig. 4.10) [29]. This variant of adenocarcinoma is distinguished from benign lesions by the presence, at least focally, of some combination of nuclear atypia, a stromal response, significant mitotic and apoptotic activity and cribriform foci [29]. Areas of typical adenocarcinoma may also be present. Occasional examples of usual type adenocarcinoma have a prominent microglandular architecture, sometimes with conspicuous acute inflammatory cells, and may mimic microglandular hyperplasia [30]. This phenomenon, which is more

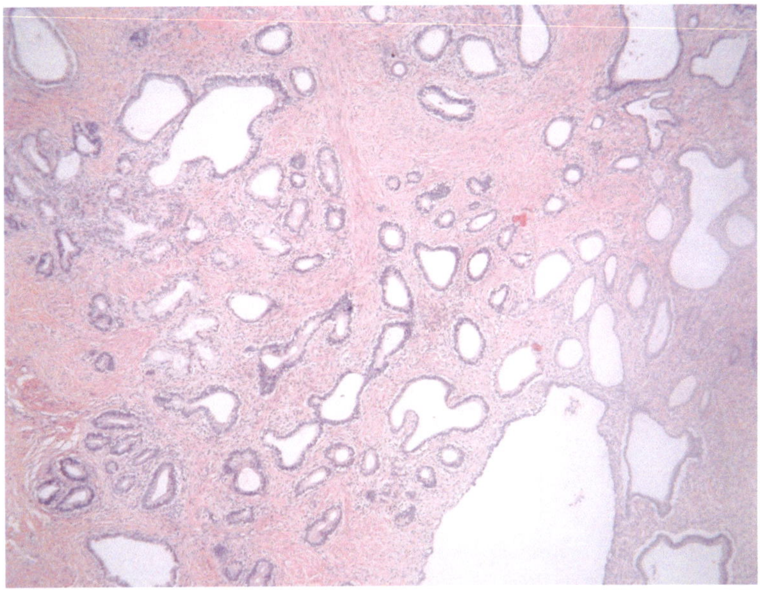

Fig. 4.9 Cervical adenocarcinoma exhibiting "naked" pattern of invasion with no stromal response

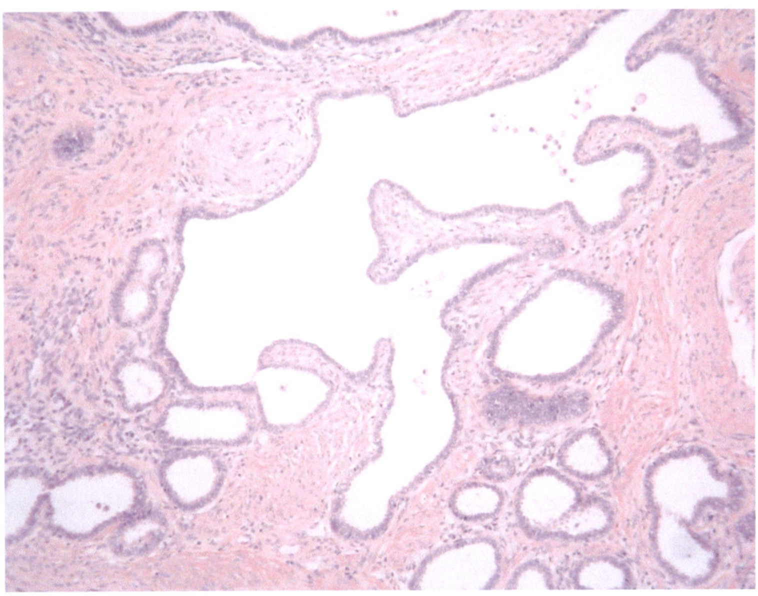

Fig. 4.10 Micocystic variant of cervical adenocarcinoma

commonly seen in adenocarcinomas of the uterine corpus, is rare and is usually a focal finding. A rare variant has been described containing areas resembling breast lobular carcinoma with Indian-file, nested and targetoid growth patterns and intracytoplasmic lumina (Fig. 4.11); these neoplasms exhibit loss of E-cadherin staining which may account for the morphological appearances [31]. Choriocarcinomatous and hepatoid differentiation have rarely been reported [32, 33]. Occasional cervical neoplasms consist of an admixture of adenocarcinoma and a neuroendocrine carcinoma, either of small cell or large cell type.

There is no universal grading system for cervical adenocarcinomas but it has been recommended that these neoplasms are graded using the FIGO system for endometrial adenocarcinomas [12]. Others use nuclear grading systems. A poorly differentiated cervical carcinoma with no evidence of squamous differentiation (intercellular bridges or keratinisation) but

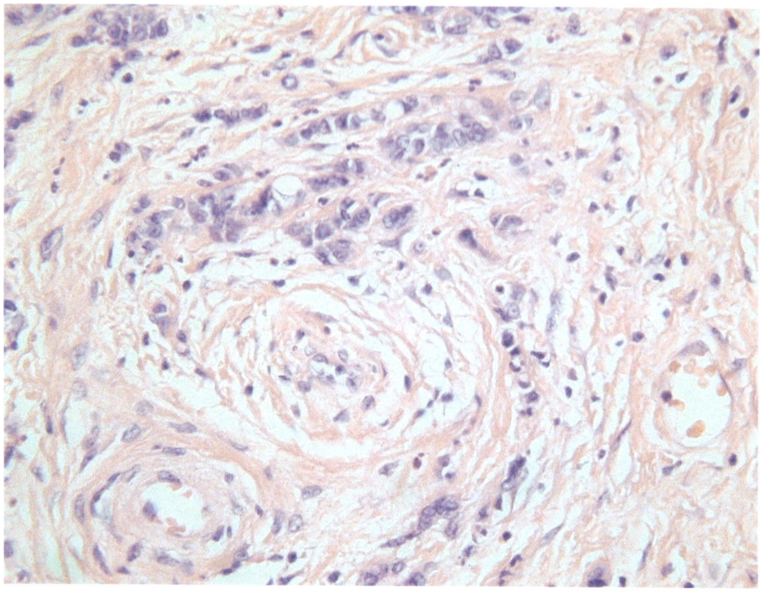

Fig. 4.11 Cervical adenocarcinoma resembling breast lobular carcinoma

with conspicuous intracytoplasmic mucin, as demonstrated by mucin stains, should be categorized as a poorly differentiated adenocarcinoma [2] (Fig. 4.12a, b).

Most usual endocervical type adenocarcinomas are diffusely positive with CK7, CEA (cytoplasmic staining) and p16 (Fig. 4.13a, b). ER, PR and vimentin are usually negative or focally positive but occasional cases exhibit diffuse immunoreactivity, especially with ER; those cases which are diffusely immunoreactive with ER tend to be well differentiated but this is not invariable [34–38]. A panel of markers comprising CEA, p16, ER and vimentin, along with molecular tests for HPV, may be useful in the distinction between a usual endocervical type adenocarcinoma and a low grade endometrioid adenocarcinoma of the uterine corpus [34–38] (see section on "Distinction between endometrial and cervical adenocarcinoma"). Scattered chromogranin positive neuroendocrine cells are found in some usual endocervical type adenocarcinomas [39].

Occasional usual endocervical-type adenocarcinomas, some with limited tumour within the cervix, result in prominent endometrial or endo/myometrial involvement and may simulate a primary endometrial adenocarcinoma, even to the extent that there are foci which resemble atypical endometrial hyperplasia [40]. Such cases may be misdiagnosed as a primary endometrial adenocarcinoma with cervical extension or independent synchronous neoplasms. In such cases, molecular studies to look for HPV and immunohistochemistry may be useful in proving that this represents a primary cervical adenocarcinoma with extension to the uterine corpus (see section on "Distinction between endometrial and cervical adenocarcinoma").

Another peculiar scenario which may result in diagnostic confusion is the ability of metastatic cervical adenocarcinomas in the ovary to mimic primary ovarian neoplasms of endometrioid or mucinous type. Some of these cases, similar to metastatic adenocarcinomas from other organs, exhibit a pronounced maturation phenomenon and contain areas mimicking borderline or even benign ovarian neoplasia (Fig. 4.14) [41, 42]. On occasions, the primary adenocarcinoma in the cervix is very small or even not recognisably invasive and the ovarian neoplasm may be discovered before there is known to be a lesion in the cervix [41, 42]. In such cases, the ovarian involvement may be secondary to transuterine and transtubal spread and the prognosis is relatively favourable compared to other stage IV cervical adenocarcinomas [41, 42]. Clues that one is dealing with a metastasis (these may not all be present) include the fact that the ovarian neoplasms are often bilateral and exhibit prominent surface involvement. There is often a "hybrid" of endometrioid and mucinous features. Extensive sampling often

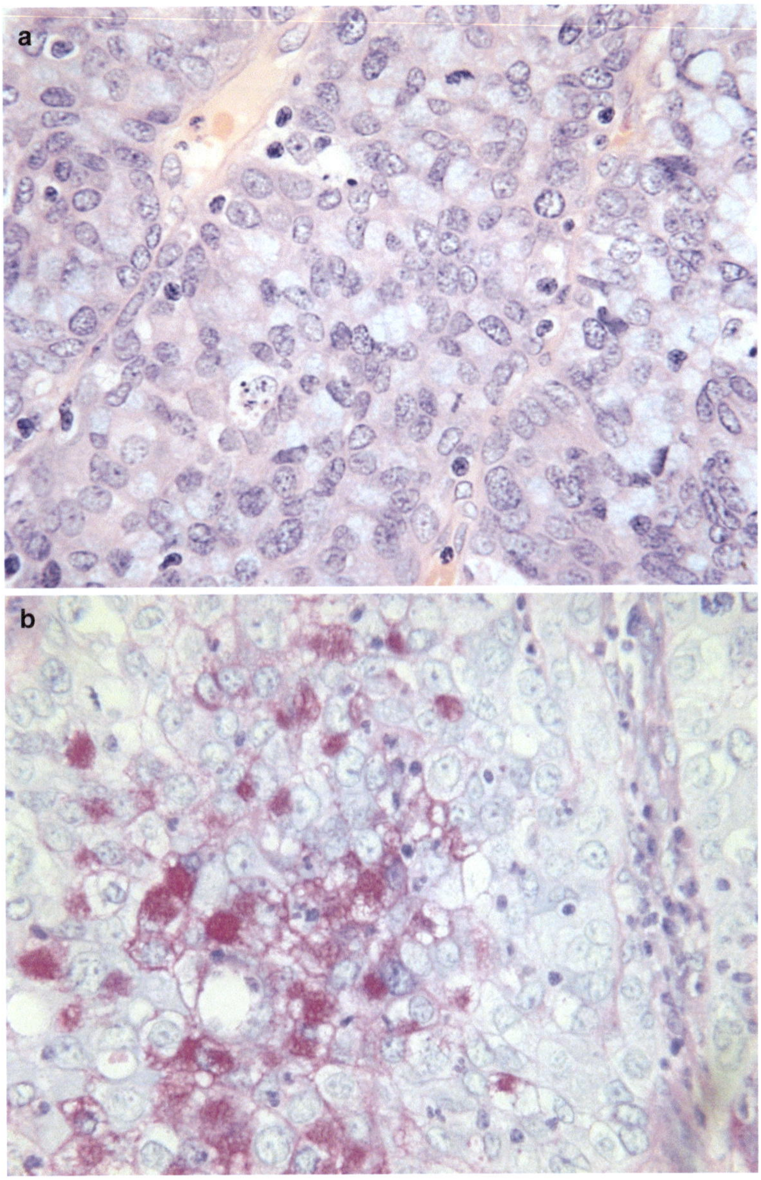

Fig. 4.12 Poorly differentiated cervical adenocarcinoma with intracytoplasmic mucin (**a**). Mucin stain in poorly differentiated cervical adenocarcinoma (**b**)

reveals foci more suggestive of a secondary such as destructive stromal invasion or extensive lymphovascular involvement. There may also be endometrial or endo/myometrial involvement. Molecular studies to demonstrate HPV and diffuse p16 staining may be of value in helping to confirm a cervical primary. ER staining may also assist when the differential includes a primary ovarian endometrioid neoplasm since the latter are usually diffusely positive while primary cervical adenocarcinomas are usually negative or exhibit focal immunoreactivity.

Management and Prognosis of Cervical Adenocarcinomas

The management of cervical adenocarcinomas is similar to corresponding stage cervical squamous carcinomas and the morphological subtype of adenocarcinoma does not play any significant role in affecting the management. Stage 1A1 adenocarcinomas can be managed by local excision (see section on "Management of early invasive adenocarcinoma") while radical hysterectomy and pelvic lymph node dissection is usually undertaken for stage 1A2 and 1B1 and

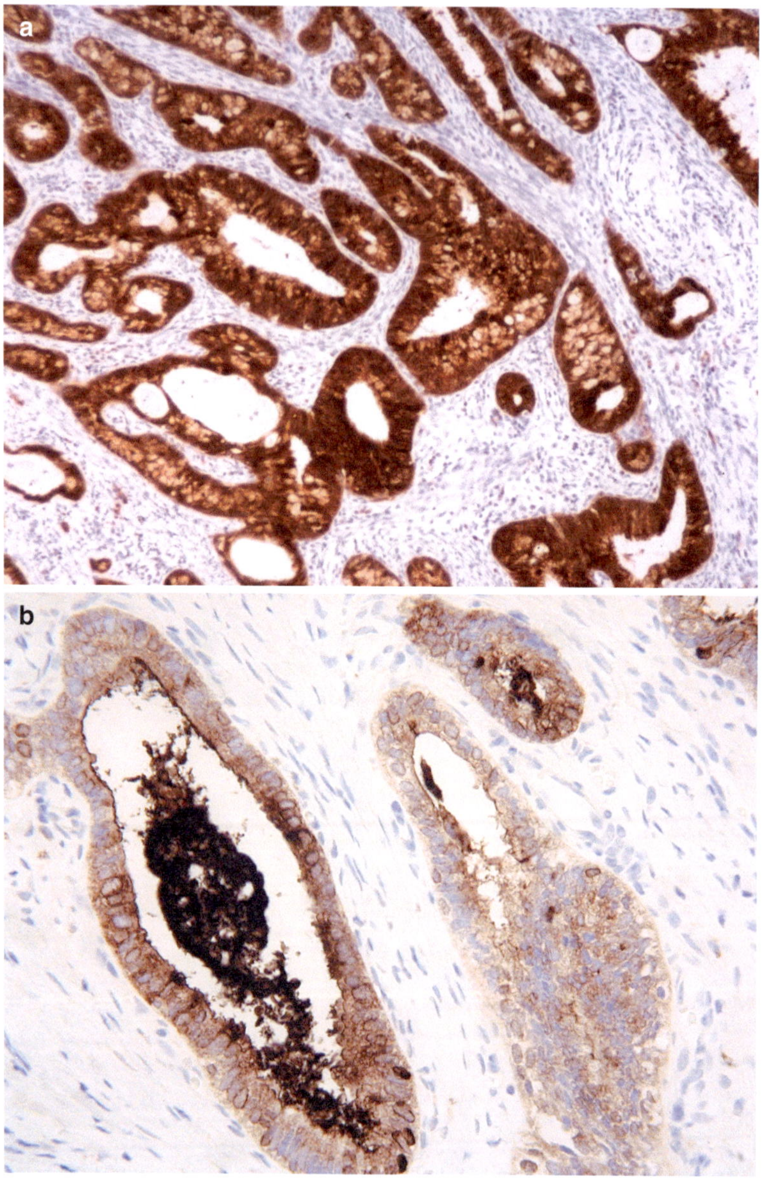

Fig. 4.13 Cervical adenocarcinoma which is diffusely positive with p16 (**a**) and CEA (**b**)

sometimes stage 2A. Primary chemoradiation is usually administered for stage 1B2, 2B and above. It is controversial whether cervical adenocarcinomas have a worse prognosis stage for stage compared to squamous carcinomas and this is not proven. In a large study published in abstract form of 230 cases of cervical adenocarcinoma of all morphological subtypes, Eftekhar et al. found a 5 year survival of 76.6 % for all stages. The 5 year survival was 100, 89, 83, 49, 34 and 3.3 % for stage 1A, 1B1, 1B2, 2, 3 and 4 respectively [43]. The survival rate was 92, 73 and 66 % respectively for well, moderate and poorly differentiated adenocarcinomas. Patients with negative lymph nodes had a 5 year survival of 92 % compared to 65 % for those with positive nodes. In another study [44], the 5 year survival rates were 80.1, 59.7, 6.3 and 0.0 % respectively for patients with stage 1, 2, 3 and 4 cervical adenocarcinoma; the overall 5 year survival rate was 59.0 %. Univariate analysis indicated a poor prognosis for non-exophytic tumours, tumour diameter >4 cm, advanced clinical stage, mucinous adenocarcinoma and clear cell carcinoma and

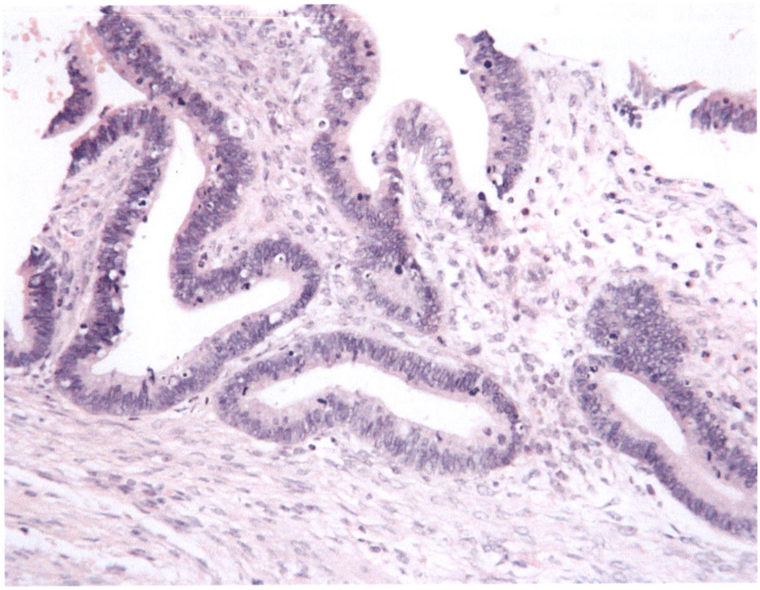

Fig. 4.14 Metastatic cervical adenocarcinoma in ovary exhibiting maturation phenomenon with areas resembling a benign or borderline mucinous neoplasm of the ovary

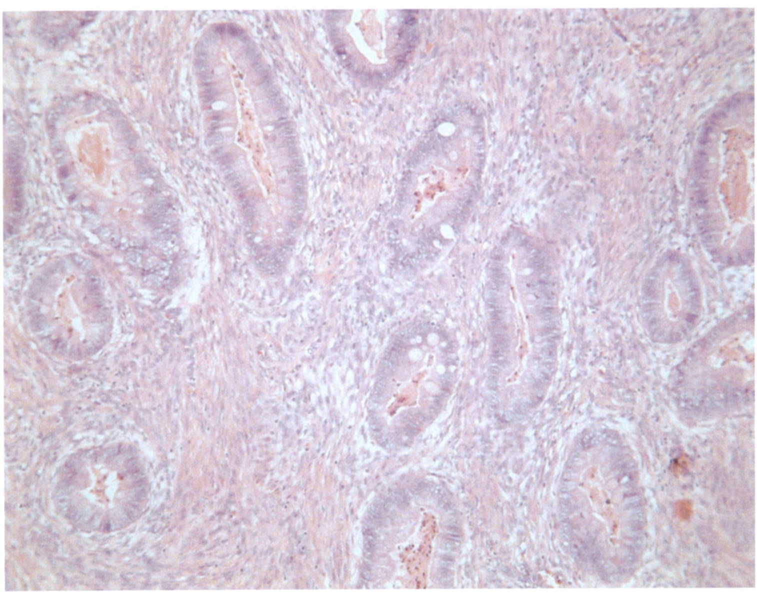

Fig. 4.15 Intestinal type cervical adenocarcinoma with goblet cells

poorly differentiated tumour. The prognosis was also related to lymph node metastasis and deep myometrial invasion. Multivariate analysis indicated that in addition to clinical stage, myometrial invasion, lymph node metastasis and tumour shape were also independent prognostic factors [44]. The prognosis of the more unusual morphological subtypes of cervical adenocarcinoma, some of which probably have a worse outcome than usual endocervical type adenocarcinomas, is discussed in the appropriate sections.

Intestinal Type Mucinous Adenocarcinoma

This is an uncommon variant of primary cervical adenocarcinoma which is not well described in the literature and which morphologically resembles a colorectal adenocarcinoma. Some, but probably not all, arise from a villous adenoma. Morphologically, these neoplasms are characterized by goblet cells and "dirty" necrosis (Fig. 4.15) [45–49]. Paneth and neuroendocrine

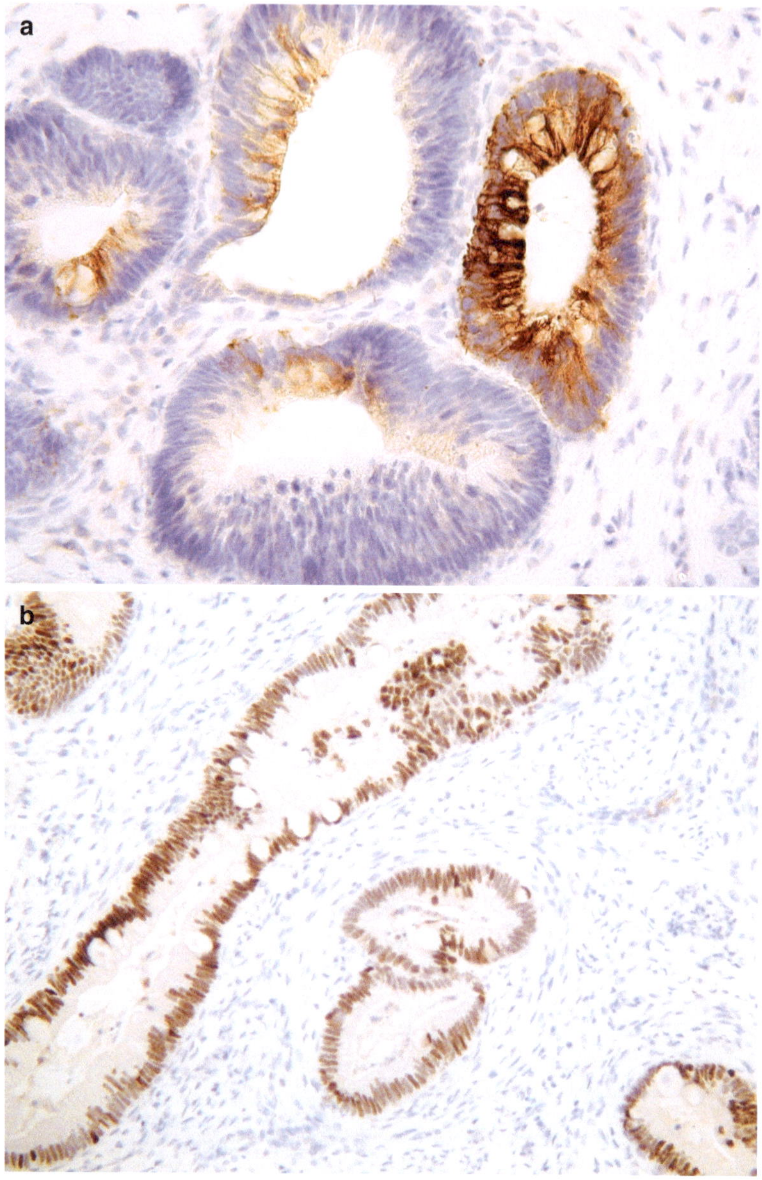

Fig. 4.16 Intestinal type cervical adenocarcinoma exhibiting focal staining with CK20 (**a**) and diffuse staining with CDX2 (**b**)

cells may be present. There is no adjacent CGIN. These neoplasms differ from those usual endocervical-type adenocarcinomas which arise from intestinal type CGIN. Only a small number of intestinal-type cervical adenocarcinomas have been studied by immunohistochemistry and most have been diffusely positive with CK7 and focally or diffusely positive with CK20 and CDX2 (Fig. 4.16a, b) [46, 48]. p16 staining has been variable [46, 48]. These tumours are probably not associated with HPV.

Intestinal type cervical adenocarcinoma is distinguished from metastasis or direct spread from a colorectal primary by a combination of clinical and pathological parameters, including history, radiological appearances and pattern of cervical involvement. Colorectal adenocarcinomas involving the cervix are often predominantly located within the deep cervical stroma underlying normal endocervical glands. Immunohistochemistry may assist in that primary cervical intestinal-type adenocarcinoma is

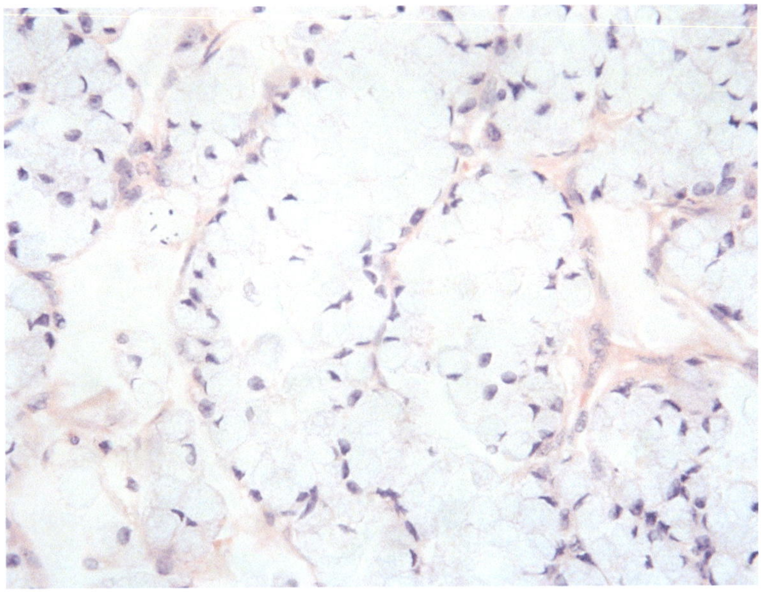

Fig. 4.17 Primary cervical adenocarcinoma with signet ring cells

usually diffusely CK7 positive and only focally positive with CK20 while colorectal metastasis is usually diffusely positive with CK20 and CK7 negative, although rectal primaries may be CK7 positive [50]. Enteric type mucins (o-acetylated sialomucins) have been demonstrated in some primary cervical adenocarcinomas, including those not exhibiting any morphological evidence of intestinal differentiation [51].

Signet-Ring Cell Mucinous Adenocarcinoma

Primary cervical adenocarcinomas with a component of signet ring cells are very rare [52, 53]. The signet ring cells may be present throughout the tumour but are more commonly a focal phenomenon, usually in association with a usual endocervical-type adenocarcinoma (Fig. 4.17). If the entire neoplasm is composed of signet ring cells, a metastasis from the breast, stomach or elsewhere should be excluded. CK7, CEA and p16 are usually positive. Rare cervical squamous carcinomas may contain signet ring cells [54], as can clear cell carcinoma. Diathermy can result in signet ring-stromal cells but the nuclei are not atypical and epithelial markers are negative [55].

Mucinous Variant of Minimal Deviation Adenocarcinoma (Adenoma Malignum)

The mucinous variant of minimal deviation adenocarcinoma (MDA) (adenoma malignum) is a rare, but well known, type of cervical adenocarcinoma accounting for approximately 1–2 % of all primary cervical adenocarcinomas and occurring over a wide age range [56]. The term MDA was proposed by Silverberg and Hurt in 1975 [57]. There is a well known association with Peutz-Jeghers syndrome, although a minority of tumours occurs in patients with this syndrome. This is an autosomal dominant syndrome characterised by intestinal hamartomatous polyps in association with mucocutaneous melanocytic macules and caused by germ-line mutation of the LKB1 (STK11) gene [58]. Abnormalities of LKB1 have been identified in some sporadic cases of cervical MDA unassociated with Peutz-Jeghers syndrome. For example, in one study somatic mutations involving this gene were demonstrated in 6 of 11 (55 %) cases of MDA [59]. MDAs with the mutation had a significantly poorer prognosis that those without. In another study, loss of heterozygosity of LKB1 was demonstrated in cases of MDA [60]. Cervical MDA is not related to HPV [3–5, 61, 62] and it has been

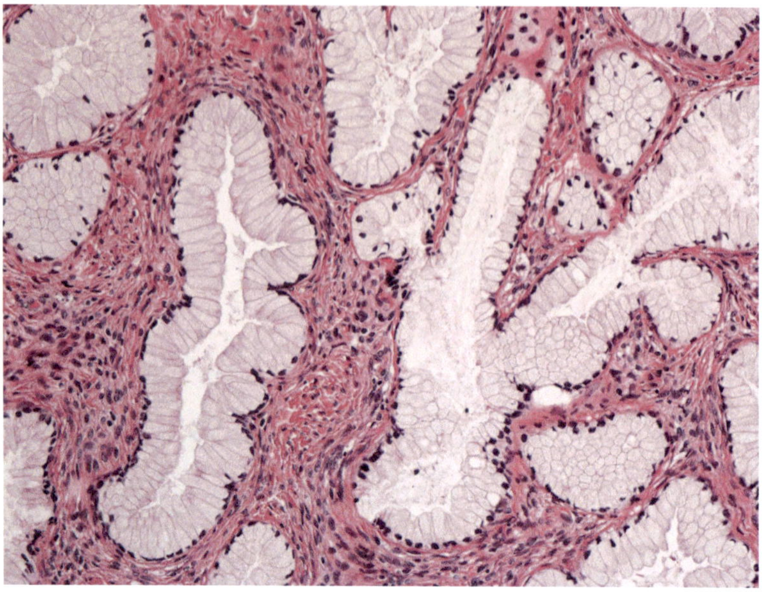

Fig. 4.18 Minimal deviation adenocarcinoma of mucinous type (adenoma malignum) composed of glands lined by bland mucinous epithelium

suggested that these neoplasms arise in some cases from the benign endocervical glandular lesion, lobular endocervical glandular hyperplasia [62–64].

In most cases, presentation is with symptoms similar to other cervical tumours, such as abnormal vaginal bleeding, but some patients present with profuse mucoid vaginal discharge. Clinically and grossly the cervix may be normal (making diagnosis difficult) or firm, enlarged and indurated. Cystic areas are present in some neoplasms. Radiological examination may reveal diffuse enlargement of the cervix with cystic areas [65].

Histologically, MDA is characterized by an extremely well differentiated appearance and a haphazard arrangement of glands with irregular profiles which usually deeply infiltrate the cervical stroma (Fig. 4.18). There is an absence of the normal lobular endocervical glandular architecture, irregular spacing and claw or crab-shaped profiles. The glands are usually highly variable in size and shape; some may be cystic or exhibit papillary infolding. Most of the tumour cells contain abundant intracytoplasmic mucin with basal nuclei and exhibit minimal cytological atypia, mitotic and apoptotic activity. Stromal desmoplasia is usually present at least focally and is useful in confirming a malignant process (Fig. 4.19). Proximity of glands to thick walled stromal blood vessels may also be a useful diagnostic clue in helping to confirm a malignant process. Extensive sampling often reveals focal areas of overt nuclear atypia (Fig. 4.20). Perineural and lymphovascular space invasion also facilitate the diagnosis and help to exclude a benign lesion. In some cases, focal areas in keeping with lobular endocervical glandular hyperplasia or atypical lobular endocervical glandular hyperplasia are present (see Chap. 2, section on "Lobular endocervical glandular hyperplasia") and it has been suggested that this represents a precursor lesion to some cases of MDA [62, 63].

Because of the bland morphological features, there is a risk of underdiagnosis and mistaking MDA for normal endocervical glands or a benign endocervical glandular lesion, especially on a small biopsy specimen. However, there is also a risk of overdiagnosis of MDA since various benign endocervical glandular lesions, including lobular and diffuse endocervical glandular hyperplasia and others, may somewhat resemble MDA. It is helpful that most of the benign endocervical glandular lesions do not form a mass, although occasionally lobular

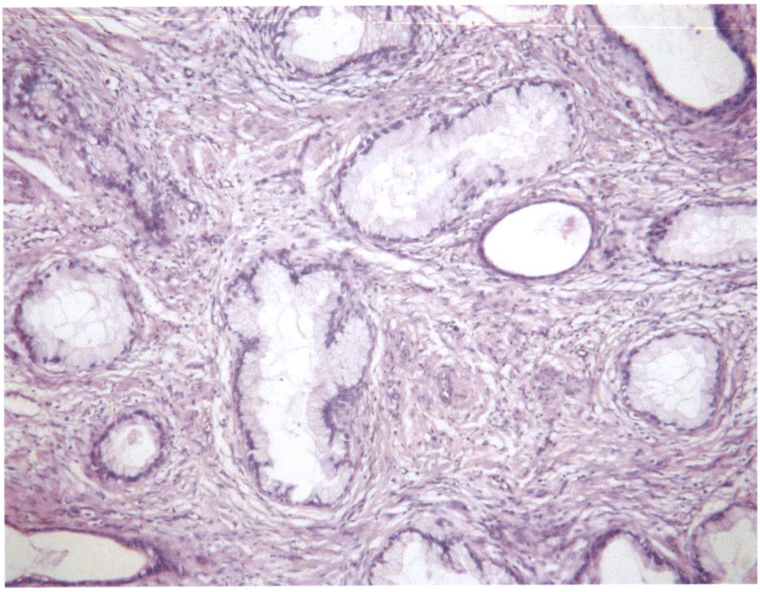

Fig. 4.19 Minimal deviation adenocarcinoma of mucinous type (adenoma malignum) consisting of bland glands with abundant intracytoplasmic mucin and surrounded by a desmoplastic stromal response

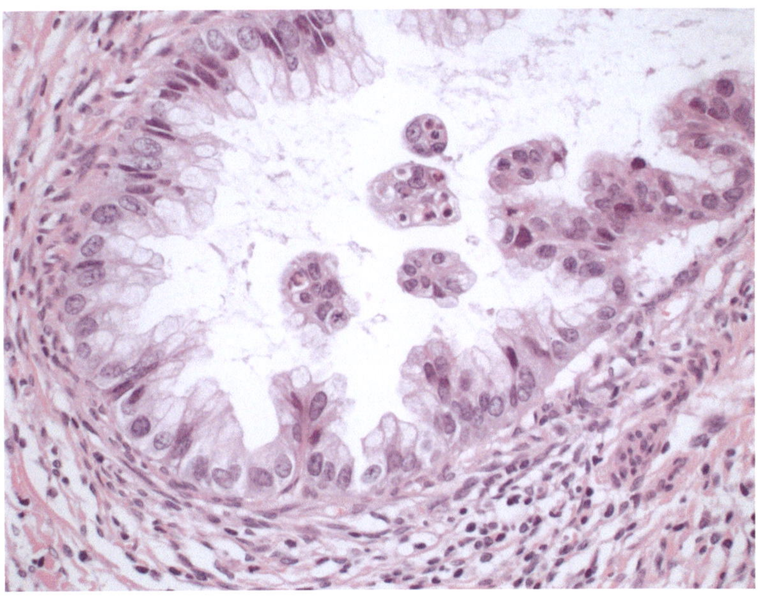

Fig. 4.20 Minimal deviation adenocarcinoma of mucinous type (adenoma malignum) with focal areas exhibiting nuclear atypia

endocervical glandular hyperplasia forms a grossly visible lesion [64].

Some usual endocervical-type adenocarcinomas are well differentiated without marked nuclear atypia. These should not be misdiagnosed as MDA which is a highly differentiated adenocarcinoma characterized by the presence of cells with abundant intracytoplasmic mucin and little mitotic or apoptotic activity. It has been shown that there is significant interobserver variability amongst pathologists in the diagnosis of MDA [66].

MDA is considered to belong to a spectrum of benign, premalignant and malignant endocervical glandular lesions which exhibit gastric (pyloric) differentiation (see Table 2.1- Chap. 2) [65]. Other lesions considered to be part of this spectrum include type A tunnel clusters,

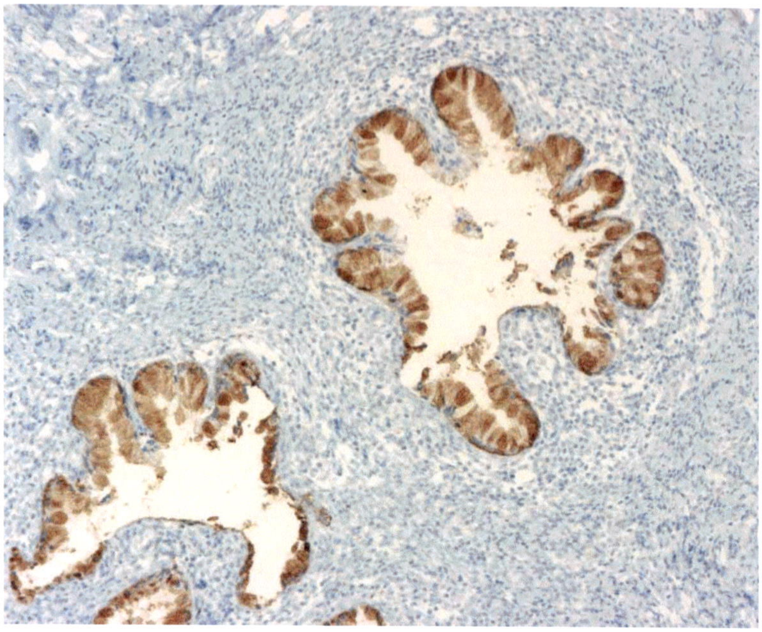

Fig. 4.21 Minimal deviation adenocarcinoma of mucinous type (adenoma malignum) which is positive with HIK1083

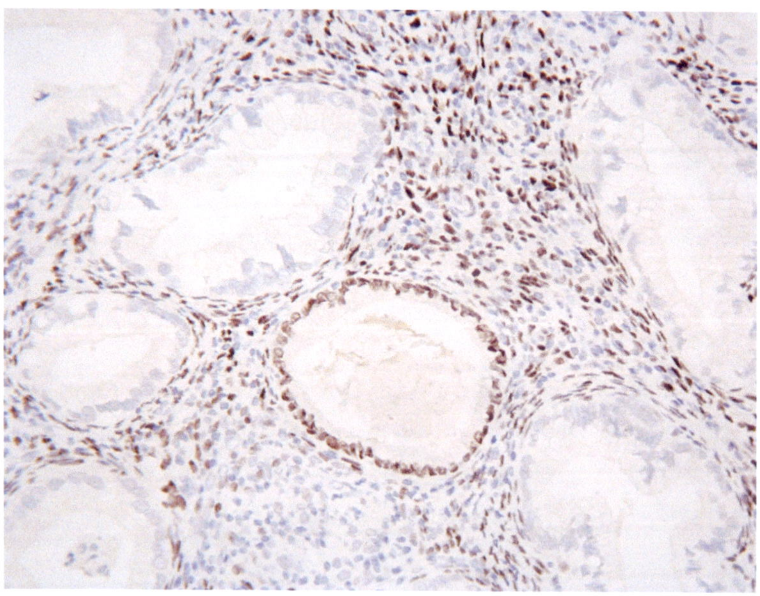

Fig. 4.22 Minimal deviation adenocarcinoma of mucinous type (adenoma malignum) which is ER negative. A benign endocervical gland is positive

simple gastric metaplasia, lobular endocervical glandular hyperplasia (complex gastric metaplasia) and gastric type adenocarcinoma [65, 67]. Immunohistochemically, MDA is often positive with HIK1083 and MUC6 (Fig. 4.21) [68–70], markers of pyloric gland mucins, although these markers are not, at present, in widespread use and are not totally specific for gastric type lesions. CEA is usually positive with cytoplasmic immunoreactivity, although this is not always the case and staining with this marker may be focal [34, 71]; only diffuse cytoplasmic staining is diagnostically useful in the distinction from benign endocervical glands since the latter may exhibit luminal immunoreactivity. p16 is usually negative or focally positive [3–5, 34]. ER and PR are usually negative (Fig. 4.22) and CA125 is negative or focally

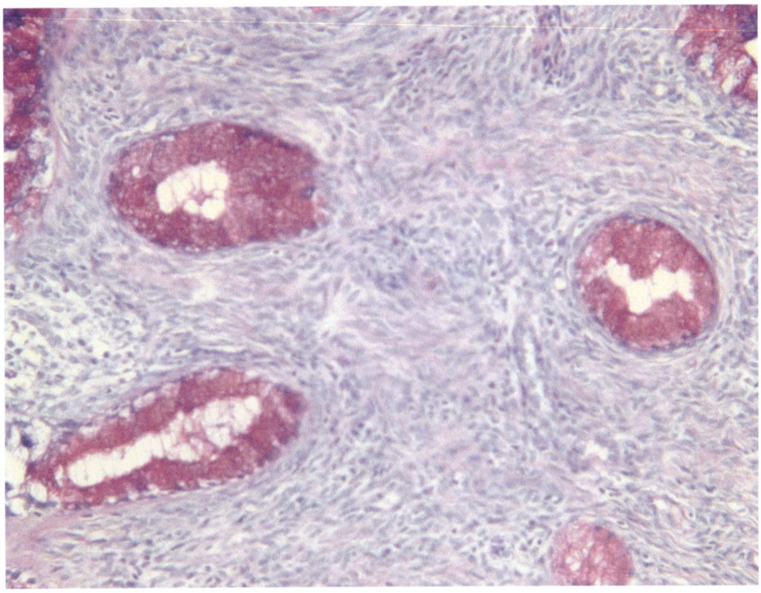

Fig. 4.23 Minimal deviation adenocarcinoma of mucinous type (adenoma malignum) stains red with combined alcian blue/PAS

positive [69]. In contrast to the situation with benign endocervical glandular lesions, the desmoplastic stroma surrounding the glands of MDA is predominantly smooth muscle actin positive and ER negative [72]. A component of neuroendocrine cells is often seen in MDA when neuroendocrine markers are performed [56]. The tumour cells contain neutral mucins and stain red with combined Alcian-blue/PAS while normal endocervical glands stain a purple-violet colour due to their admixture of acid and neutral mucins (Fig. 4.23) [73]; however, in practice there is some overlap in the staining patterns.

In cases of MDA with or without Peutz-Jeghers syndrome, mucinous lesions are occasionally present elsewhere in the genital tract, such as the ovary and fallopian tube; in such cases, it may be difficult to ascertain whether these represent independent synchronous lesions or bland metastasis from the cervical tumour [74, 75].

Overall, MDA has a poor prognosis, although it is not clear whether the prognosis is worse stage for stage compared to usual endocervical type adenocarcinomas. It is possible that the poor prognosis is due to a delay in diagnosis in some cases. In a literature review performed some years ago, it was found that only 30 % of patients (all stages) and 50 % of patients with stage 1 tumours were alive and disease free after 5 years [56].

Gastric Type Cervical Adenocarcinoma

This variant of cervical adenocarcinoma has been described by Japanese investigators and is not included in the 2003 WHO classification of cervical neoplasms [76]. It is an uncommon, but not rare, type of primary cervical adenocarcinoma and, like MDA, is not HPV related and is considered to exhibit gastric differentiation [3–5, 77]. It may be more common in Japanese than Western populations. Other features in common with MDA include the fact that some cases are associated with and possibly arise from lobular endocervical glandular hyperplasia and occasional occurrence in patients with Peutz-Jeghers syndrome. However, in contrast to MDA, primary gastric type adenocarcinoma is characterized by obvious malignant cytological features.

Histologically, gastric type adenocarcinoma is characterised by tumour cells with atypical nuclei and abundant clear or eosinophilic cytoplasm, typically with distinct cell borders (Fig. 4.24) [76]. There is sometimes a marked associated

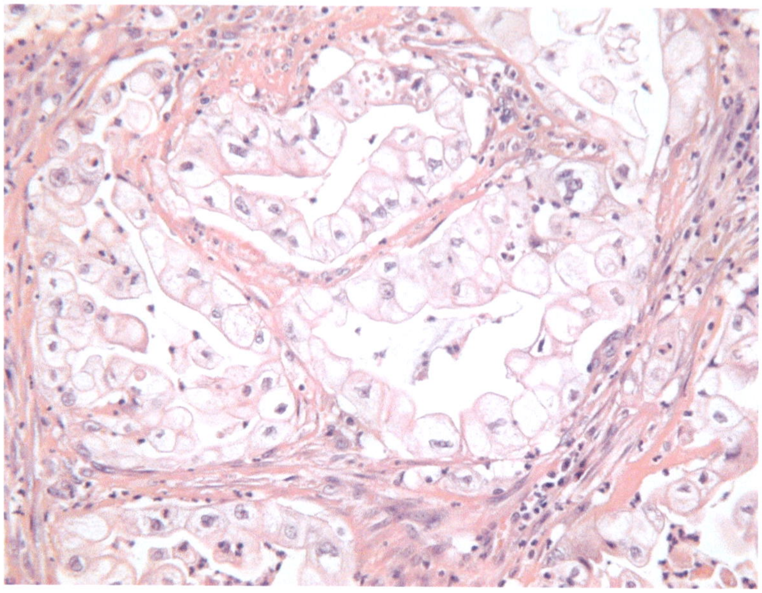

Fig. 4.24 Gastric type cervical adenocarcinoma with abundant clear cytoplasm and prominent cells membranes

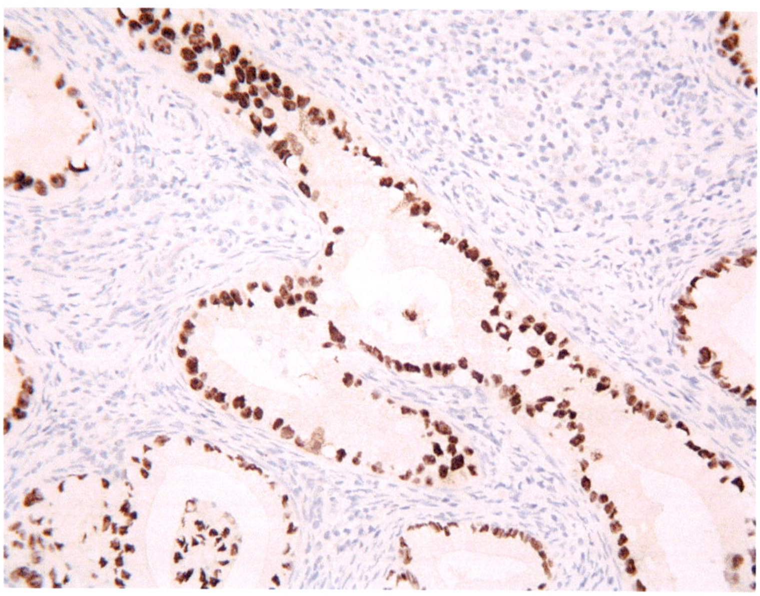

Fig. 4.25 Gastric type cervical adenocarcinoma exhibiting diffuse nuclear staining with p53

inflammatory infiltrate, including lymphocytes, neutrophils and eosinophils. The tumour cells are often positive with HIK1083 and MUC6, markers of pyloric gland mucins [76]. They may be diffusely p53 (Fig. 4.25) and CEA positive and p16 is usually negative or focally positive [3–5, 76]. ER and PR are negative.

Occasional neoplasms with an admixture of MDA and gastric type adenocarcinoma have been reported and it is likely that these constitute a spectrum of malignancies exhibiting gastric differentiation [78].

Although the clinical features have not been extensively studied, it is thought that gastric type adenocarcinoma is associated with aggressive behaviour and a poor prognosis, including a possible propensity for peritoneal and adnexal dissemination [76]. Kojima et al. found that gastric

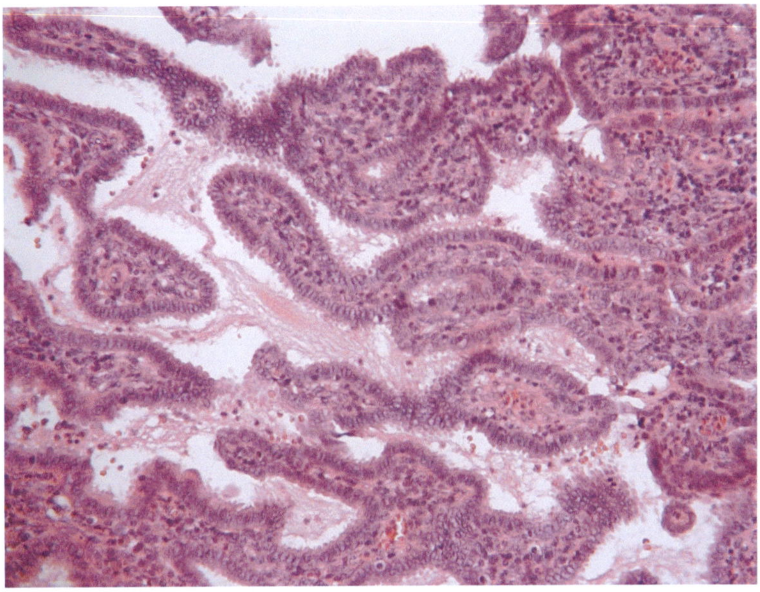

Fig. 4.26 Villoglandular cervical adenocarcinoma with pronounced papillary architecture and little in the way of nuclear atypia

type adenocarcinomas had a 5 year disease free survival of 30 % compared to 74 % for usual endocervical-type adenocarcinomas [76].

Villoglandular Adenocarcinoma

Villoglandular adenocarcinoma is a very uncommon and probably overdiagnosed variant of primary cervical adenocarcinoma which most commonly occurs in relatively young patients (average age 35) [79, 80]. It is likely that there is significant interobserver variability amongst pathologists in the diagnosis of villoglandular adenocarcinoma [81] and this diagnosis should not be made with any cervical adenocarcinoma with a papillary architecture since usual endocervical type adenocarcinomas, serous adenocarcinomas and other variants may have a focal or diffuse papillary architecture, especially towards the surface. Villoglandular adenocarcinomas are HPV related neoplasms [82] and it has been suggested that there is an association with hormonal preparations (67 % of patients in one series-79).

Grossly, villoglandular adenocarcinomas are exophytic polypoid lesions. Morphologically they are characterized by thick or thin papillae covered by columnar epithelium which generally contains little intracellular mucin (Fig. 4.26). Atypia is mild or at the most moderate. Mitoses are usually present but are not prominent. The cores of the papillae typically contain conspicuous numbers of inflammatory cells. There may be associated CGIN. Some cases are almost entirely exophytic with little or no invasion of the underlying tissues, although this is not always the case. Examples in which there is no invasion of the underlying cervical stroma may be misdiagnosed as CGIN but the overall architecture is too complex to conform to the normal endocervical glandular field. In those cases which exhibit invasion of the stroma, the "invasive" component may have a papillary architecture, comprising elongated branching glands, or resemble a usual endocervical-type adenocarcinoma. Measurement of those lesions which do not exhibit significant invasion of the stroma may be difficult but the tumour thickness should be measured as well as the lateral extent. A definitive diagnosis of villoglandular adenocarcinoma should only be made in an excision specimen since foci resembling villoglandular adenocarcinoma can be seen in other papillary adenocarcinomas.

In most cases, the tumour is confined to the cervix at diagnosis and villoglandular adenocarcinomas are widely assumed to have a good prognosis, although there are few large studies with long term follow up [79, 80, 83]. It has been

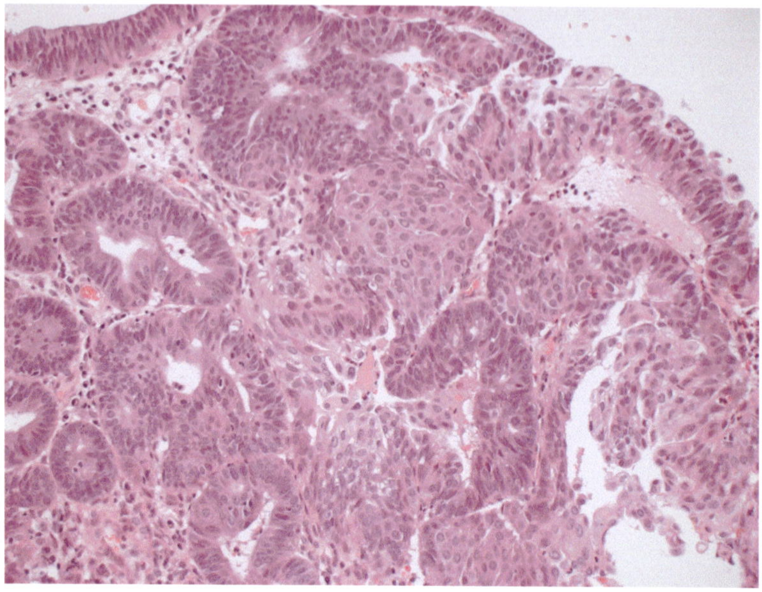

Fig. 4.27 Endometrioid adenocarcinoma of the cervix with bland squamous elements in the form of morules

suggested that conservative management, in the form of local excision, suffices in some patients. However, management should be individualized and those tumours which exhibit significant stromal invasion should be managed as for usual endocervical-type adenocarcinomas, especially since there are few reported case series with significant follow up. Conservative management should probably be reserved for those neoplasms which are purely villoglandular in type, confined to the surface or exhibit only superficial invasion of the stroma and in which there is no lymphovascular invasion.

Endometrioid Adenocarcinoma

Some authorities previously considered that endometrioid adenocarcinomas of the cervix are common and account for up to 30 % of primary cervical adenocarcinomas [84, 85]. However, most cases diagnosed as primary cervical endometrioid adenocarcinomas probably represent usual endocervical type adenocarcinomas with minimal intracytoplasmic mucin, resulting in a pseudoendometrioid appearance, and true primary endometrioid adenocarcinomas of the cervix are rare. The diagnosis should probably be reserved for neoplasms which contain morphologically bland squamous elements (Fig. 4.27) [86], these being common in primary endometrioid adenocarcinomas of the uterine corpus and ovary. Primary endometrioid adenocarcinomas of the cervix are characterized by simple to complex glands lined by endometrioid type epithelium with stratified nuclei and minimal intracytoplasmic mucin and squamous elements in the form of morules or keratinizing squamous epithelium. When classical endometrioid features are present, spread from a primary neoplasm in the uterine corpus should be excluded.

A very rare endometrioid subtype of minimal deviation adenocarcinoma has been described characterized by the presence of morphologically bland endometrioid-type glands, some of which may be cystically dilated, infiltrating the stroma with little in the way of a stromal response (Fig. 4.28) [87, 88]. Some of the glands may be ciliated or exhibit apical snouts. This should be distinguished from endometriosis, tuboendometrial metaplasia and cervical involvement by endometrial adenocarcinoma.

Due to the paucity of reported cases of well characterized true endometrioid adenocarcinomas of the cervix, the immunophenotype of these neoplasms is not well described. However, one study found that, similar to their counterparts in

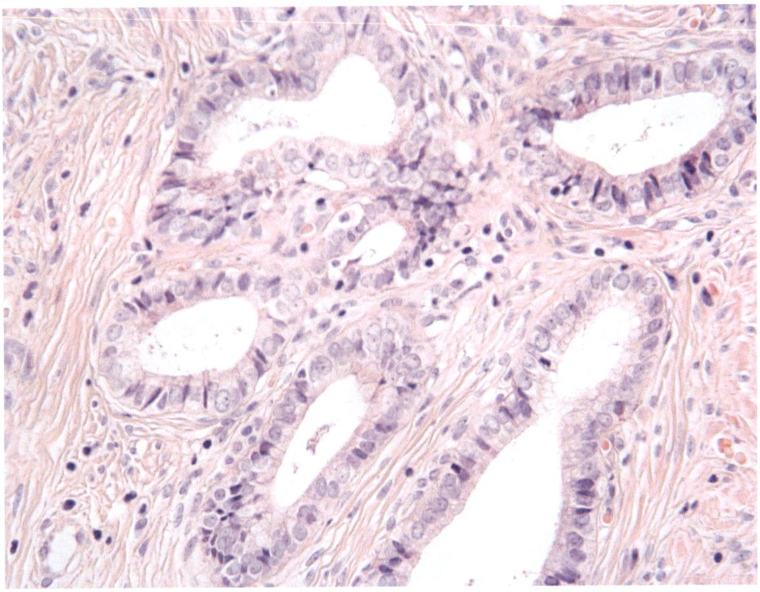

Fig. 4.28 Minimal deviation variant of endometrioid adenocarcinoma lined by bland endometrioid type glands

the uterine corpus, primary endometrioid adenocarcinomas of the cervix were usually vimentin positive [89]. The behaviour of these neoplasms does not differ from usual endocervical type adenocarcinomas.

Clear Cell Adenocarcinoma (Clear Cell Carcinoma)

Clear cell carcinomas are uncommon primary cervical neoplasms, accounting for 2–4 % of cervical adenocarcinomas. There is a bimodal age distribution with peaks at 26 and 71 years [90]. As with the corresponding vaginal neoplasms, there is an association with intrauterine exposure to diethylstilbestrol (DES) [91]. This association was generally in cases diagnosed prior to 1990 and nowadays most women with a primary cervical clear cell carcinoma have not had intrauterine exposure to DES [90, 92]. Those neoplasms associated with DES exposure typically occur in young females (peak age 19) and there may be coexistent vaginal adenosis and congenital malformations of the genital tract. Cervical clear cell carcinomas are usually not HPV associated.

Morphologically, these neoplasms are identical to their vaginal, endometrial and ovarian counterparts [93]. Solid, tubulocystic and papillary growth patterns are characteristic and a proportion of the tumour cells have abundant clear, glycogen rich cytoplasm with prominent cell membranes (Fig. 4.29). Hobnail cells, eosinophilic hyalinised stromal cores, eosinophilic hyaline globules and intraluminal mucin are present in some cases. Signet ring cells may be present.

Before diagnosing a primary cervical clear cell carcinoma, spread from a neoplasm in the uterine corpus should be excluded, especially in older women. There are no immunohistochemical markers which facilitate the distinction between a primary clear cell carcinoma of the uterine corpus, cervix or elsewhere in the female genital tract. The differential diagnosis of clear cell carcinoma of the cervix may include benign lesions such as mesonephric hyperplasia, microglandular hyperplasia and Arias Stella reaction and malignant neoplasms such as mesonephric adenocarcinoma, gastric type adenocarcinoma, squamous carcinoma or adenosquamous carcinoma with a clear cell squamous component, yolk sac tumour and alveolar soft part sarcoma. The usual presence of a tumour mass helps to exclude the various benign lesions. Immunohistochemically, clear cell carcinoma is usually p16, ER, PR and CEA negative. CA125 and hepatocyte nuclear factor 1-beta are typically positive.

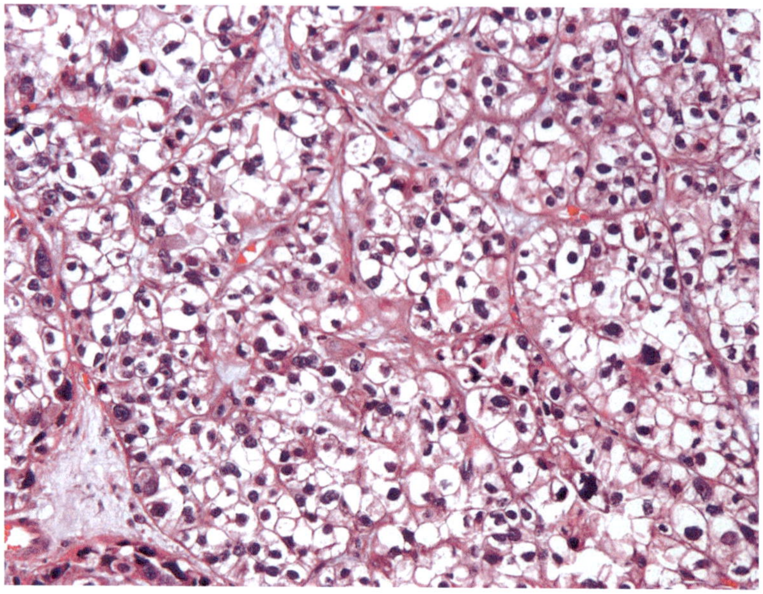

Fig. 4.29 Clear cell carcinoma of cervix with solid growth pattern

The prognosis is considered to be relatively poor and possibly worse than usual endocervical type adenocarcinomas, although due to a paucity of studies with long term follow up, this is not proven.

Serous Adenocarcinoma

Serous adenocarcinomas of the cervix are extremely rare. They have been considered to account for approximately 3 % of primary cervical adenocarcinomas but are probably even rarer than this and caution should be exercised before making this diagnosis given its rarity as a primary cervical neoplasm [94]. Overall, they occur in a younger age group than uterine corpus serous carcinoma and a bimodal age distribution was found in one study with one peak <40 years and the other >65 years [94]. These neoplasms are usually associated with high risk HPV [3–5]. Before making a diagnosis of pure primary serous adenocarcinoma of the cervix, spread from a neoplasm within the uterine corpus or elsewhere in the female genital tract should be excluded.

The morphological features are similar to primary endometrial, ovarian, tubal and peritoneal serous adenocarcinomas. These neoplasms are characterised by a focal, predominant or exclusive papillary architecture with marked nuclear atypia and abundant mitotic activity (Fig. 4.30). Detached epithelial buds and psammoma bodies may be present. There may also be glandular formations and slit-like spaces and occasional neoplasms are predominantly or purely glandular in type. Sometimes there is a component of usual endocervical-type adenocarcinoma and CGIN may be present. Serous adenocarcinomas of the cervix are usually diffusely positive with p16 while p53 is variable [94, 95]. WT1 is usually negative. A diagnosis of primary cervical serous adenocarcinoma should only be made when the classical morphological features of a serous malignancy are present and not with any adenocarcinoma with a predominantly papillary architecture and significant nuclear atypia. Indeed, it is probable that some or even most cases reported as primary serous adenocarcinoma of the cervix represent usual cervical type adenocarcinomas with a papillary or slit-like architecture and marked nuclear atypia. The differential diagnosis of primary cervical serous adenocarcinoma may include villoglandular adenocarcinoma, papillary variants of usual endocervical type adenocarcinoma, mesonephric adenocarcinoma and metastatic serous adenocarcinoma from elsewhere within the female genital tract,

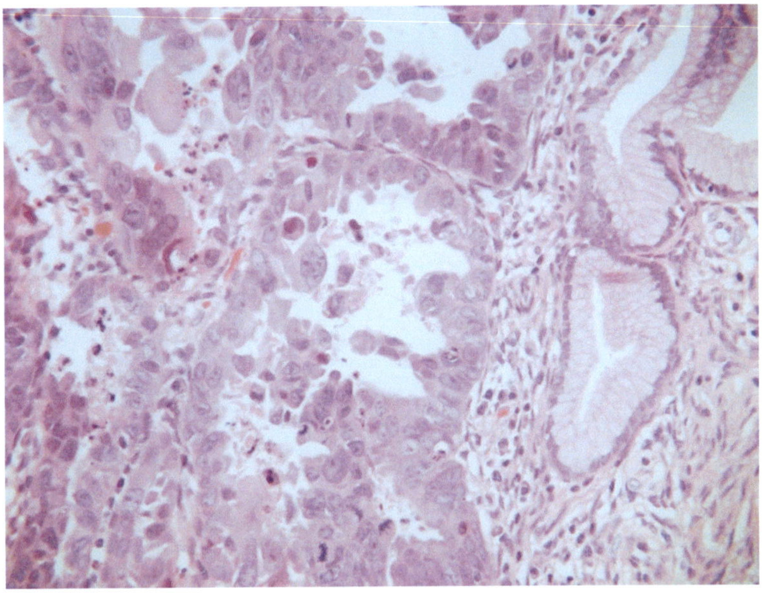

Fig. 4.30 Serous adenocarcinoma of the cervix with papillary architecture and marked nuclear atypia

especially the uterine corpus but also the ovary or fallopian tube.

Due to the limited number of reported well characterized cases with long term follow-up, the behaviour is not well established. It is controversial whether primary cervical serous adenocarcinomas, similar to their uterine corpus counterparts, are associated with a poor prognosis, although some behave aggressively.

Mesonephric Adenocarcinoma

Mesonephric adenocarcinomas of the cervix are rare and are thought to arise from mesonephric remnants in the lateral wall of the cervix [96–99]. However, when mesonephric adenocarcinomas become clinically apparent, they may involve any quadrant of the cervix and a location in the lateral wall is usually no longer apparent. Sometimes, they have a completely intramural location, expanding the cervical wall, while in other cases they present as polypoid or ulcerated neoplasms. They are not associated with HPV [3–5].

Morphologically, mesonephric adenocarcinomas are characterized by a varied and heterogenous appearance, often with multiple different architectural arrangements (Fig. 4.31). This admixture of patterns, while a somewhat characteristic feature of mesonephric adenocarcinoma, may also result in diagnostic confusion since a variety of other types of adenocarcinoma can be mimicked. The most common architectural pattern is closely packed small tubules, some of which may be dilated, lined by cuboidal or columnar mucin-free cells. Occasionally a proportion of the tubules are markedly dilated resulting in a resemblance to thyroid tissue. Other patterns include ductal, papillary, retiform, solid, sex cord-like and sarcomatoid [96–99]. Sometimes, at least focally, the nuclear features are relatively bland but in most cases significant nuclear atypia and mitotic activity can be found in some areas. Eosinophilic luminal material, referred to as colloid-like, is characteristically present, especially in the small tubular areas, although this is not specific for mesonephric adenocarcinomas. Focally, there may be clearing of the cytoplasm. A spindle cell sarcomatous component may be present, usually resembling endometrial stromal sarcoma or non-specific sarcoma; heterologous elements, including rhabdomyoblasts and cartilage, have been present in occasional cases [96, 97]. In some, but not all, cases benign mesonephric remnants are identified, although it may be difficult to distinguish between foci of well differentiated tumour and benign mesonephric remnants. There is no associated CIN or CGIN.

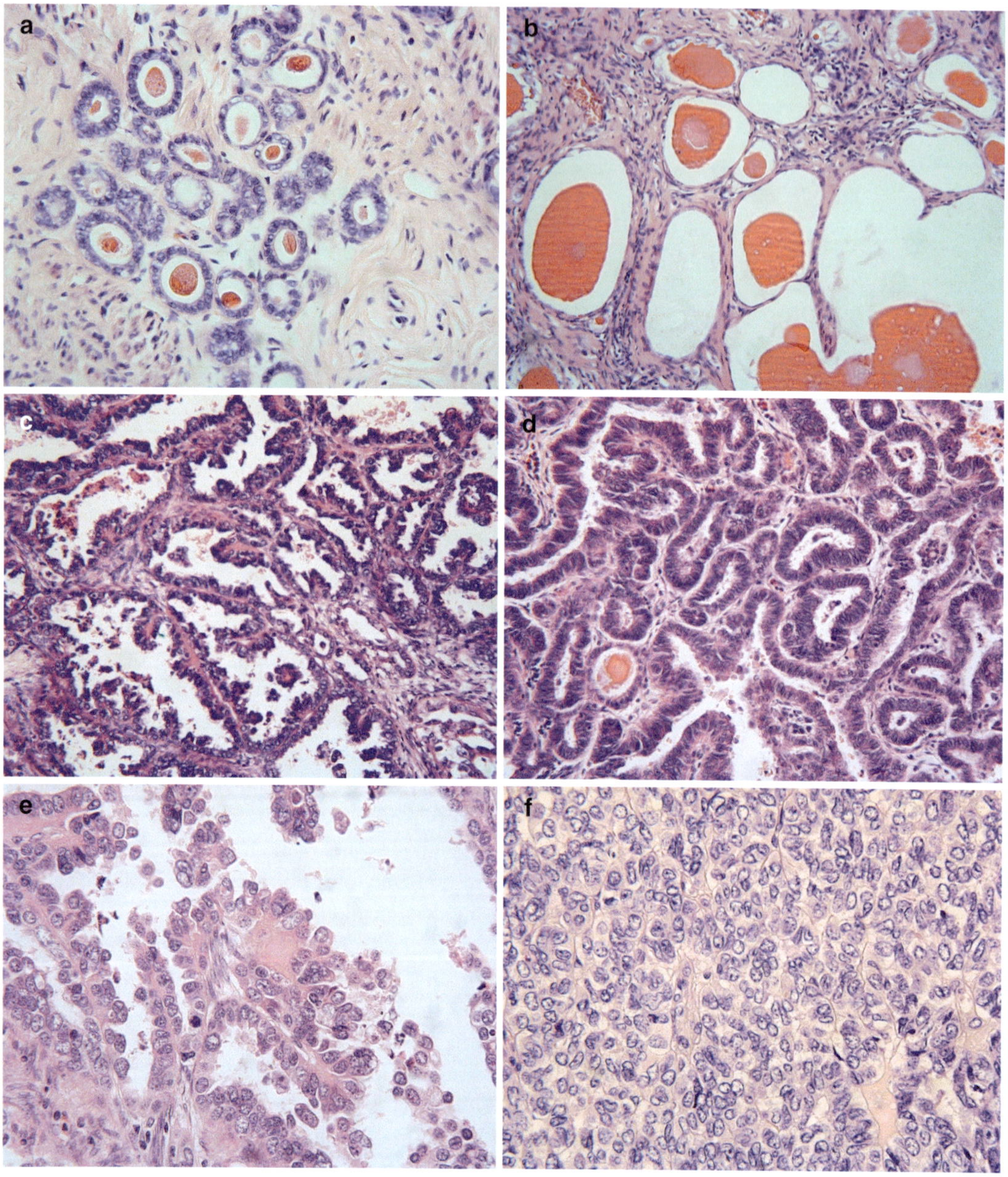

Fig. 4.31 Various architectural patterns in mesonephric adenocarcinomas. Small tubular areas (**a**), dilated tubules (**b**), slit-like spaces mimicking serous adenocarcinoma (**c**), duct-like structures mimicking endometrioid adenocarcinoma (**d**), areas mimicking clear cell carcinoma (**e**) and solid areas (**f**)

Immunohistochemically, AE1/3, CK7, EMA, CD10 (luminal pattern of immunoreactivity) and vimentin are typically positive (Fig. 4.32) but the immunophenotype is variable and there is no specific marker of mesonephric adenocarcinoma, the diagnosis largely being based on the morphological appearances [99–101]. Inhibin and calretinin may be focally positive [96–98]. ER, PR and CEA are usually negative [99–101]. Other markers which may be positive in mesonephric adenocarcinoma include PAX8, CA125, HMGA2, TTF1 and hepatocyte nuclear factor 1-beta [99].

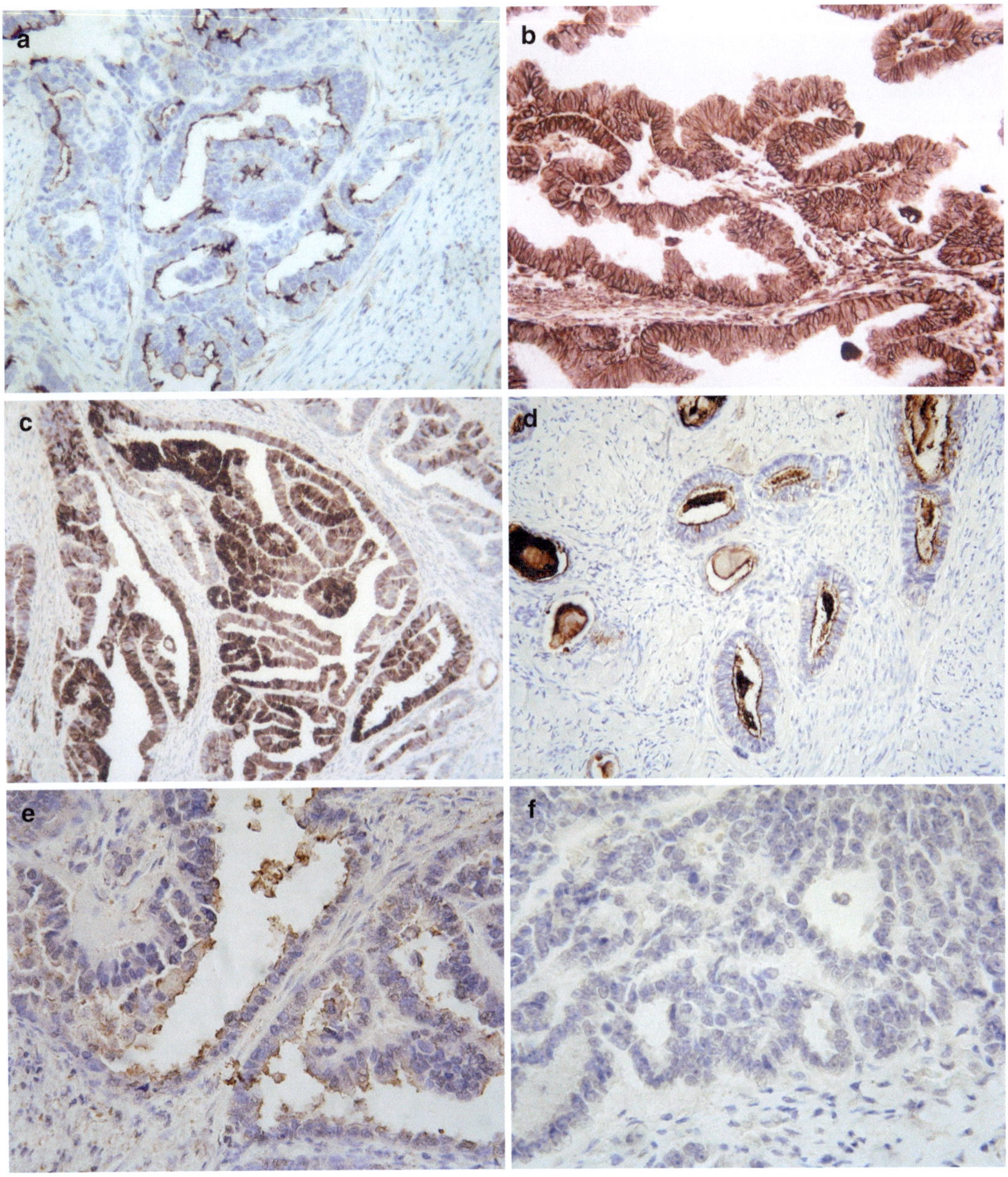

Fig. 4.32 Mesonephric adenocarcinomas exhibiting luminal positivity with CD10 (**a**), cytoplasmic staining with vimentin (**b**), cytoplasmic staining with calretinin (**c**), luminal staining with CA125 (**d**), cytoplasmic staining with inhibin (**e**) and totally negative staining with ER (**f**)

The differential diagnosis may include mesonephric hyperplasia. This distinction may be particularly problematic since mesonephric hyperplasia can be extremely florid and involve much of the cervix. Furthermore, some mesonephric adenocarcinomas are morphologically relatively bland, at least focally. Of diagnostic value is the fact that mesonephric hyperplasia does not usually result in a mass lesion [102]; indeed, one should be wary of diagnosing mesonephric adenocarcinoma in the absence of a tumorous mass. Extension beyond the cervix,

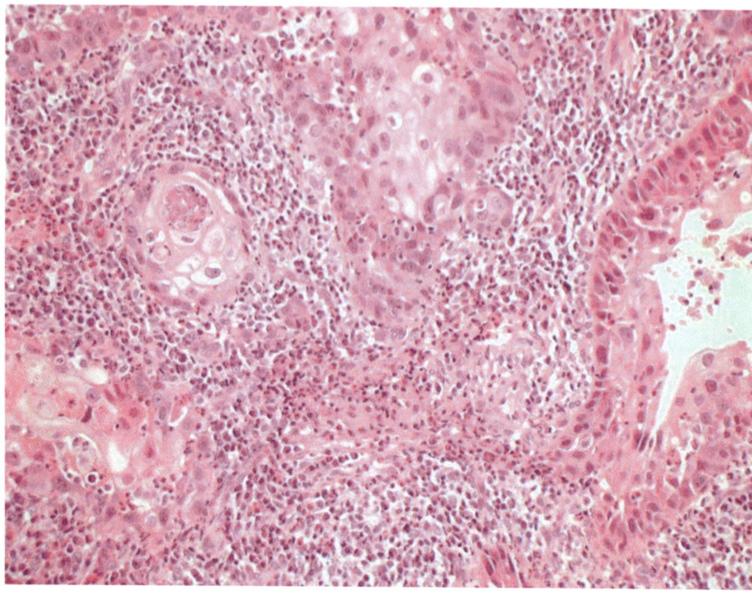

Fig. 4.33 Adenosquamous carcinoma of cervix containing malignant squamous and glandular elements

significant nuclear atypia or mitotic activity and vascular or perineural infiltration are suggestive of adenocarcinoma. The different architectural patterns may suggest a clear cell carcinoma; however, in most cases, the overall morphological appearances are significantly different between the two neoplasms and any appreciable component of clear cells, hobnail cells or eosinophilic stromal hyalinization is in favour of a clear cell carcinoma. Foci within some mesonephric adenocarcinomas may resemble an endometrioid or serous adenocarcinoma but again the overall morphological appearances are significantly different between these neoplasms. Those cases with a spindle cell component may be misdiagnosed as a Mullerian carcinosarcoma but recognition of the mesonephric features of the epithelial element helps to establish the diagnosis and the spindle cell component is usually more bland than in Mullerian carcinosarcomas. Misdiagnosis as a usual endocervical type adenocarcinoma may also occur.

Due to their uncommon nature, it is not clear whether cervical mesonephric adenocarcinomas have a different behaviour from usual endocervical-type adenocarcinomas, although it has been suggested that may have a propensity for late recurrence and metastasis [96].

Adenosquamous Carcinoma

Adenosquamous carcinoma of the cervix is uncommon, but not rare, accounting for approximately 4 % of cervical carcinomas [103, 104]. In order to establish this diagnosis, the tumour should be composed of an admixture of malignant glandular and squamous elements both morphologically recognisable on examination of routine haematoxylin and eosin stained sections (Fig. 4.33) [2]. Usually the glandular element is of the usual endocervical type. Scattered mucin containing cells may be present in an otherwise typical squamous carcinoma and this should not be termed adenosquamous carcinoma [2]. Poorly differentiated carcinomas resembling poorly differentiated squamous carcinoma but with many mucin containing cells and lacking intercellular bridges or keratinisation should be diagnosed as poorly differentiated adenocarcinoma [2]. Adenosquamous carcinoma should be distinguished from endometrioid adenocarcinoma with benign squamous elements, although these are extremely rare within the cervix. Occasionally spatially separate adenocarcinoma and squamous carcinoma coexist within the cervix and this should not be diagnosed as adenosquamous carcinoma. Occasional cases of adenosquamous carcinoma are characterized by abundant clear cytoplasm within the squamous component, potentially mimicking a clear cell carcinoma [105]. Adenosquamous carcinomas are graded as well, moderately or poorly differentiated according to the degree of differentiation of the squamous and glandular components. It has been suggested that adenosquamous carcinomas have a worse prognosis than similar stage and grade squamous and adenocarcinomas but this is controversial and not proven [103, 104, 106–108].

Mucoepidermoid Carcinoma

Mucoepidermoid carcinoma of the cervix is a controversial entity [109] and is not included in the 2003 WHO classification of cervical neoplasms [2]. By strict morphological criteria, the tumour is identical histologically to salivary gland mucoepidermoid carcinoma and is characterized by nests containing an admixture of three cell types (epidermoid/squamoid, intermediate and mucin containing) in the absence of overt glandular differentiation. Mucoepidermoid carcinoma of the major and minor salivary glands harbours a characteristic t(11;19)(q21;p13) chromosomal translocation, a rearrangement that results in fusion of the cyclic adenosine 3′,5′ monophosphate coactivator CRTC1 to the Notch coactivator MAML2 [109]. Similar molecular abnormalities have been demonstrated in a small number of cervical tumours morphologically in keeping with mucoepidermoid carcinoma [109]. These molecular abnormalities were not found in cervical adenosquamous carcinomas. This demonstrates that cervical neoplasms defined as mucoepidermoid carcinoma by strict morphologic criteria harbour genetic aberrations involving the genes characteristically rearranged in mucoepidermoid carcinoma of the salivary glands and suggests that cervical mucoepidermoid carcinoma is an entity distinct from conventional adenosquamous carcinoma. Since drug therapy is being developed to target the genes rearranged in salivary gland mucoepidermoid carcinoma, this underscores the importance of correct classification.

Glassy Cell Carcinoma

Glassy cell carcinoma is an extremely rare and somewhat controversial cervical neoplasm [110–112]. It is considered a variant of adenosquamous carcinoma and is HPV related (usually HPV 18). It may occur in pure form or be admixed with a usual endocervical type adenocarcinoma, squamous carcinoma or adenosquamous carcinoma. There is likely to be significant interobserver variability in the diagnosis of this tumour type. Morphologically, glassy cell carcinoma is characterized by large cells with abundant eosinophilic ground-glass cytoplasm, distinct cell borders, large nuclei, macronucleoli and a high mitotic rate. There may be single cell keratinisation and there is often intense stromal inflammation typically including abundant eosinophils. Glassy cell carcinoma is generally thought to have a poor prognosis but this has been disputed and, given the rarity of this tumour type and the problems in diagnosis, the behaviour has not been proven to be significantly different to squamous carcinoma, adenocarcinoma or adenosquamous carcinoma [110–112].

Adenoid Cystic Carcinoma

Adenoid cystic carcinoma of the cervix is rare, accounting for less than 1 % of cervical adenocarcinomas, and mainly occurs in postmenopausal women [113–115]. It has been speculated that these neoplasms are more common in black than Caucasian women. Most examples are HPV-related, usually type 16 [116, 117]. The morphological features are similar to those of the corresponding salivary gland tumour (Fig. 4.34). The neoplasm is composed of rounded cuboidal cells with hyperchromatic nuclei and a high nuclear to cytoplasmic ratio. Necrosis and high mitotic activity are usual. Various architectural patterns are present, including cribriform, acinar, nested, trabecular and corded arrangements. Peripheral palisading is usually present as well as PAS positive extracellular hyaline basement membrane material. Foci of squamous differentiation with keratinisation may be seen focally.

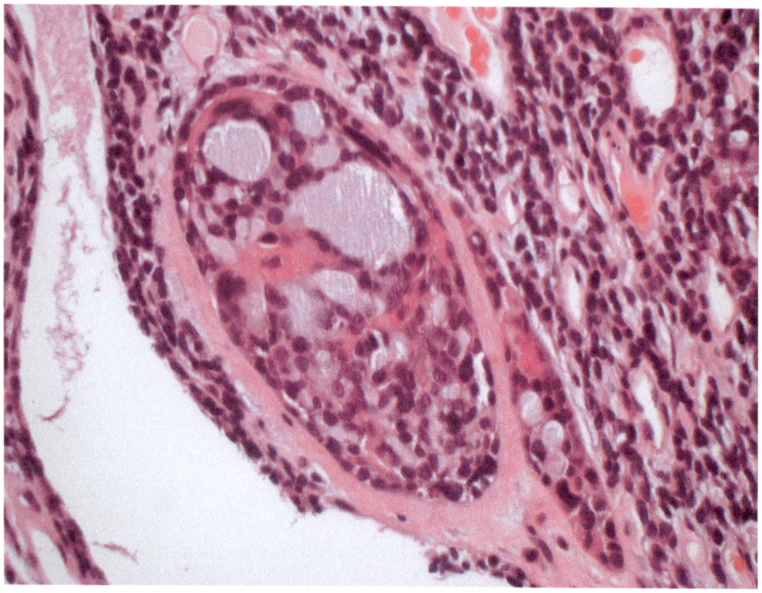

Fig. 4.34 Adenoid cystic carcinoma with cribriform architecture

Similar to the salivary gland, a solid variant has been described and the presence of basement membrane material between tumour cells is a useful clue to the diagnosis [118]. Lymphovascular invasion is common and there is usually a fibroblastic or somewhat myxoid stromal component. In some cases, there are microscopic foci resembling adenoid basal carcinoma (see below) and occasional neoplasms contain typical areas of both adenoid cystic and adenoid basal carcinoma [114, 119, 120]. In some cervical carcinosarcomas, the epithelial element is adenoid cystic in type. In one reported case of cervical adenoid cystic carcinoma, there was ultrastructural evidence of neuroendocrine differentiation [115]. These neoplasms have a poor prognosis with a propensity for haematogenous spread. The differential diagnosis may include adenoid basal carcinoma, small cell and large cell neuroendocrine carcinoma and non keratinizing variants of squamous carcinoma.

It is controversial whether so-called adenoid cystic carcinomas of the cervix are morphologically identical to salivary gland adenoid cystic carcinomas or are merely "adenoid cystic-like". In one study, it was considered that the cervical neoplasms exhibited more necrosis, mitotic activity and nuclear atypia than the corresponding salivary neoplasms and S100 positive myoepithelial cells were not found, suggesting that that these may be "adenoid cystic-like" rather than true adenoid cystic carcinomas [113]. However, in another study, most of the neoplasms were S100 positive, suggesting myoepithelial differentiation [114]. p16 is usually diffusely positive [117] while CD117 (c-kit) immunoreactivity has been demonstrated in a small number of cervical adenoid cystic carcinomas, similar to the salivary gland counterpart; in that study, adenoid basal carcinomas were CD117 negative [121].

Adenoid Basal Carcinoma

Adenoid basal carcinoma is uncommon and mainly occurs in postmenopausal women [113, 114, 117, 119]. Like adenoid cystic carcinoma, it has been suggested that this neoplasm has a propensity to arise in black women. In contrast to other primary cervical carcinomas, there is typically no cervical enlargement and adenoid basal carcinoma is usually an incidental microscopic finding unless associated with another type of cervical carcinoma. Most cases are HPV related, usually type 16, and in mixed neoplasms the same HPV type has been demonstrated in the adenoid basal carcinoma component and the other neoplastic element [117].

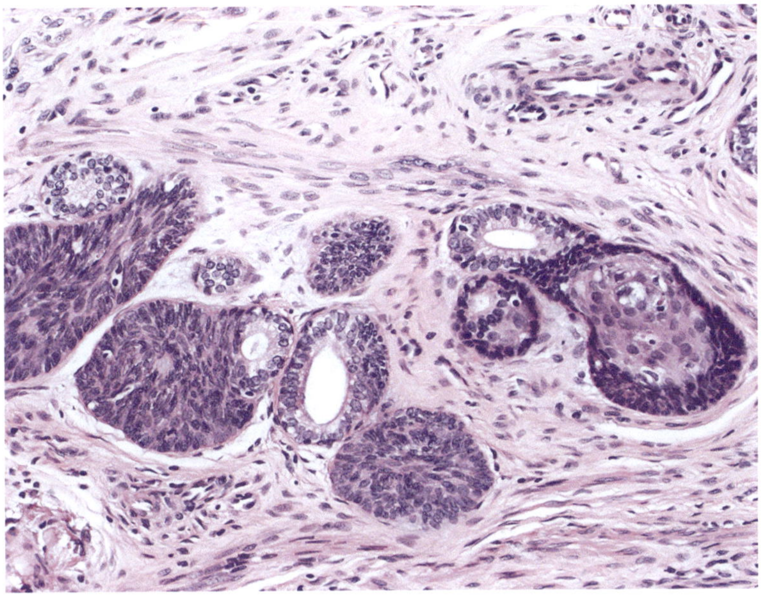

Fig. 4.35 Adenoid basal carcinoma with small nests of basaloid cells with central lumina

Morphologically, adenoid basal carcinoma is characterized by small round or oval nests of bland, mitotically inactive cells, sometimes with peripheral palisading (Fig. 4.35). The cytoplasm is scant resulting in a basaloid appearance. Foci of squamous differentiation may be present within the nests and some of the nests can have a transitional appearance. Glandular structures may also be present lined by mucinous epithelium, basaloid or flattened cells. There is usually no stromal reaction and the depth of stromal invasion is generally <10 mm. There is commonly associated CIN and/or another type of carcinoma. This is most commonly squamous carcinoma but adenocarcinoma, adenosquamous carcinoma or adenoid cystic carcinoma may also occur [117]. In such cases, the proportions of the two components should be documented in the pathology report.

The prognosis is excellent when adenoid basal carcinoma occurs in pure form and because of this it has been suggested that this tumour type be renamed adenoid basal epithelioma, although this term is not recommended [117, 120]. Adenoid basal carcinoma can be treated conservatively with local excision as long as a more aggressive tumour type is not present. The prognosis is worse if associated with another neoplastic type and, in such cases, the prognosis is related to the other tumour type.

It is important to distinguish adenoid basal carcinoma from adenoid cystic carcinoma.

In contrast to adenoid basal carcinoma, adenoid cystic carcinoma is associated with a tumour mass and is characterised by the presence of basement membrane material, necrosis, significant mitotic activity and often lymphovascular space involvement. Adenoid basal carcinomas are CD117 (c-kit) negative, in contrast to adenoid cystic carcinomas which may be positive [121]. As stated earlier, foci resembling adenoid basal carcinoma may be present in some adenoid cystic carcinomas. Adenoid basal carcinoma should also be distinguished from adenoid basal hyperplasia. The latter is also usually an incidental microscopic finding, most commonly in postmenopausal women, consisting of microscopic bud-like proliferations of basal cells with bland nuclear features emanating from the surface squamous or glandular epithelium [120]. Squamous differentiation and gland-like spaces may be present in some of the buds. There is no stromal reaction and the overlying epithelium is normal. It has been suggested that some of these proliferations represent early adenoid basal carcinomas, although this is not proven [120]. So-called ectopic prostatic tissue may also enter into the differential diagnosis of adenoid basal carcinoma but the former is usually located more deeply within the stroma and is usually positive with prostatic markers.

Mixed Adenocarcinomas

Mixed adenocarcinomas are defined as neoplasms containing more than one morphological subtype of adenocarcinoma. They are extremely rare within the cervix. According to the WHO, a mixed tumour is only diagnosed when the minor component accounts for at least 10 % of the neoplasm [2]. However, in practice, even if the non-dominant component accounts for less than 10 %, a mixed adenocarcinoma is diagnosed. With a mixed adenocarcinoma, the proportion of each component should be documented in the pathology report.

Metastatic Adenocarcinoma

Metastatic adenocarcinomas involving the cervix are uncommon [122]. The most common extra-cervical tumour to involve the cervix is endometrial carcinoma which involves the cervix by direct spread. Endometrial carcinomas may involve the glandular surface, crypt epithelium, stroma, vascular spaces or a combination. The diagnosis is usually straightforward if there is a known endometrial carcinoma (usually in the same specimen) and if there is deep stromal involvement and/or lymphovascular permeation. However, there are multiple problems in the evaluation of cervical involvement in endometrial carcinoma and one study showed significant interobserver variability in the assessment of this, even amongst specialist gynecological pathologists [123]. One basic problem is that the junction between the lower uterine segment/isthmus and the endocervix is not clearly defined. There are no histological landmarks which clearly delineate the junction and here there is an admixture of ciliated lower uterine segment endometrial glands and mucinous endocervical glands. It has been suggested that the uppermost mucinous gland be taken as the junction between the cervix and the lower uterine segment [123] while in another study it was suggested that the lowest ciliated gland be taken as that junction [124].

Endocervical glandular involvement by endometrial carcinoma may be subtle and difficult to recognise, especially if it involves the surface and forms a monolayer and is not continuous with the neoplasm in the uterine corpus. Because of this, there is a risk of the pathologist missing subtle endocervical glandular involvement. Problems may also arise in the distinction between endocervical surface involvement and so-called "floaters" or artefactual tumour incorporation [125]. With "floaters" within the endocervical canal, it is usually relatively straightforward to ascertain that this does not represent true cervical involvement. However, problems arise when tumour is closely applied to the endocervical surface or embedded in granulation tissue secondary to implantation. Although cervical glandular involvement by endometrial carcinoma does not now denote stage II disease, this being defined by cervical stromal involvement in the 2009 FIGO staging system [10], many oncologists still administer vault brachytherapy when there is endocervical glandular involvement by endometrial carcinoma and so its recognition by pathologists is important.

There can also be significant problems in deciding whether tumour is confined to the cervical glandular epithelium or also involves the stroma. This is in part because normal endocervical epithelium as well as lining the surface invaginates to form crypts which lie within the superficial cervical stroma. Thus, tumour may be present within the cervical stroma but still be confined to the glandular epithelium; it can be difficult in such cases to decide whether the neoplasm within the stroma is confined to pre-existing glandular elements, especially since endometrial adenocarcinomas invading the cervical stroma may infiltrate as widely spaced glands which do not elicit a stromal reaction.

As discussed, there is a risk of missing focal microscopic endocervical surface involvement by endometrial carcinoma. The opposite scenario is that there may be reactive changes involving the endocervical epithelium secondary to recent endometrial biopsy or curettage [126]. This is not

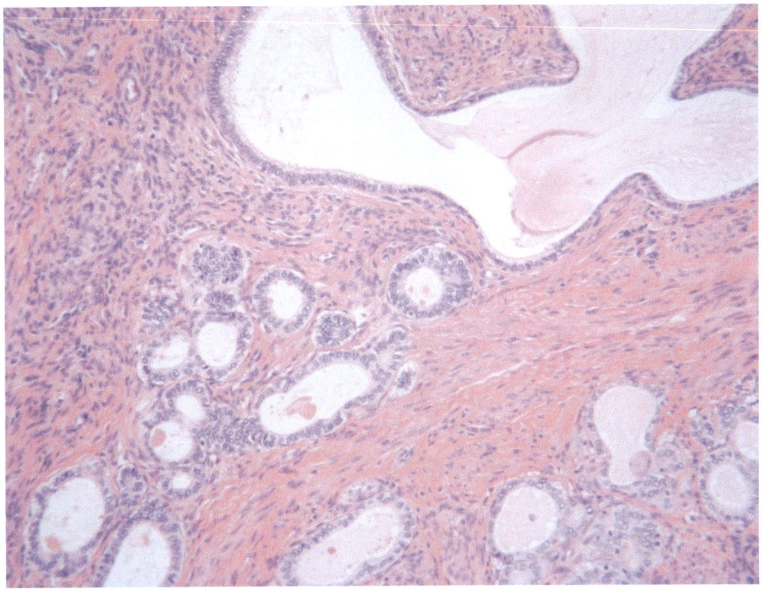

Fig. 4.36 Subtle "burrowing" pattern of cervical stromal invasion by endometrioid adenocarcinoma of the uterine corpus

uncommon and has been termed atypical reactive proliferation of the endocervix [126]. When the changes are florid, this has the potential to be misdiagnosed as endocervical surface involvement by tumour [126]. The histological features, not all of which are present in every case, include nuclear stratification and multilayering with short micropapillary processes, squamoid change, hobnail cells and mild cytological atypia. Other features which may be present are surface erosion, clearing of the cytoplasm, fibrin deposition, an inflammatory infiltrate, fibrosis of the subepithelial tissue and extreme vascularity with a granulation tissue-like appearance [126]; when benign glandular elements become entrapped within the fibrous stroma, the features may even mimic cervical stromal invasion by tumour. Tubal or tuboendometrial metaplasia of the endocervical glands or superficial endometriosis in a patient with an endometrial carcinoma may also be mistaken for tumour involvement.

In most cases, cervical stromal involvement by endometrial carcinoma is easily recognised microscopically. However, a subtle "burrowing" pattern of cervical stromal involvement occasionally occurs which can result in misdiagnosis [127, 128]. With this burrowing pattern, the tumour infiltrates as "naked" widely spaced, often cytologically bland, glands which lie beneath normal endocervical glands and do not elicit a stromal reaction (Fig. 4.36). At low power, the infiltrating glands, given their location and morphological features, can be misdiagnosed as mesonephric remnants, especially since they may have a somewhat linear arrangement and contain luminal eosinophilic "colloid-like" material, both features of cervical mesonephric remnants [127, 128]. As well as mesonephric remnants, this pattern of infiltration may be misdiagnosed as a primary endocervical adenocarcinoma, CGIN, tuboendometrial metaplasia or tunnel clusters since some of the glands may be dilated. Occasional serous carcinomas of the uterine corpus also infiltrate the cervical stroma as widely spaced glands without eliciting a stromal reaction; in such cases, the nuclear features are usually high grade.

Neoplasms from other sites in the female genital tract, such as the ovary or fallopian tube, may also involve the cervix [122]. In most of these cases, there is a known primary neoplasm elsewhere and there is predominant involvement of the outer aspects of the cervix, often with obvious lymphovascular permeation. However, a small series of metastatic adenocarcinomas involving the cervix with predominant or exclusive mucosal involvement which mimicked a small primary cervical adenocarcinoma or high grade CGIN has

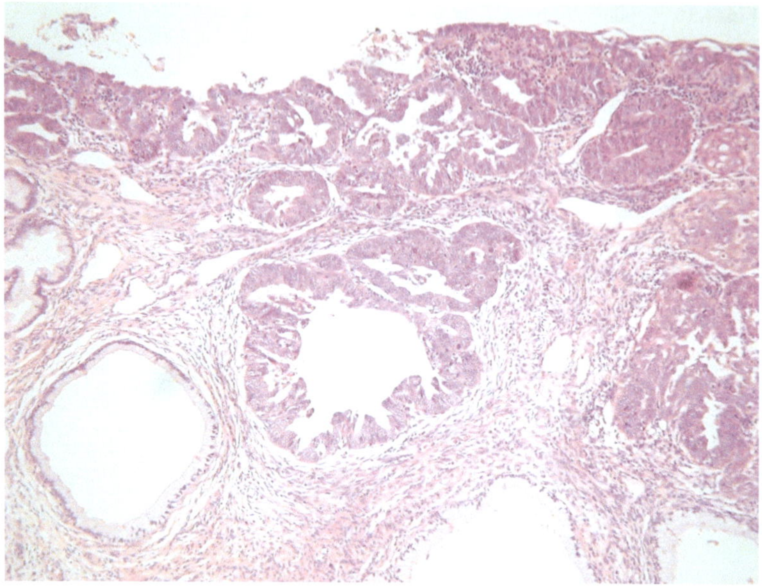

Fig. 4.37 Metastatic ovarian high grade serous adenocarcinoma involving mucosa of cervix and mimicking CGIN

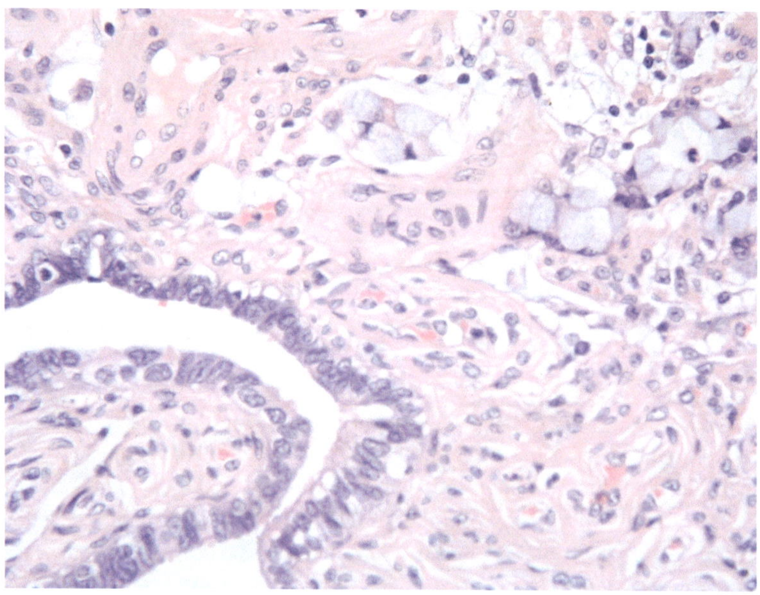

Fig. 4.38 Metastatic gastric signet ring adenocarcinoma infiltrating around pre-existing benign endocervical glands

been reported (Fig. 4.37) [129]; most of these represented primary ovarian or tubal high grade serous adenocarcinomas but one was from a pancreatic primary. A case of a low grade ovarian serous adenocarcinoma presenting in the cervix and misdiagnosed as a primary cervical adenocarcinoma has been reported [130].

Other metastatic adenocarcinomas which uncommonly involve the cervix include colorectum (often by direct extension), breast, stomach, pancreas and urinary bladder (Fig. 4.38) [122]. In such cases, predominant involvement of the deep cervical stroma, often with prominent lymphovascular permeation, and a relative absence of mucosal involvement is often a clue to the diagnosis, as is infiltration around pre-existing benign glandular elements and an absence of CGIN. Some characteristic morphological features also raise the possibility of metastasis from a specific site. For example, extensive "dirty" necrosis raises the possibility of a colorectal primary, an Indian file arrangement of a breast lobular carcinoma and signet ring cells a gastric or breast primary. However, all these features are occasionally seen in primary cervical adenocarcinomas. The radiological appearances, a known history of a primary neoplasm elsewhere and immunohistochemistry may also help in determining the primary site.

Distinction Between Endometrial and Cervical Adenocarcinoma

There are a number of scenarios where an issue may arise as to whether an adenocarcinoma is primary in the uterine corpus or cervix, for example when adenocarcinoma is present in both endometrial and cervical biopsies. This is of importance in that a simple hysterectomy is usually performed for an endometrial cancer (although modified radical hysterectomy is often undertaken when it is known preoperatively that an endometrial carcinoma involves the cervix) whereas radical hysterectomy or primary chemoradiation is generally undertaken for a cervical carcinoma. Preoperative imaging may or may not assist in determining the tumour origin. Problems may also occur in a hysterectomy specimen where tumour involves both the uterine corpus and the cervix and the choice of adjuvant therapy may depend on the site of origin. Sometimes the cervix is biopsied for a suspected cervical neoplasm and this contains an unsuspected endometrial adenocarcinoma. Another scenario is that occasional cervical adenocarcinomas may result in prominent endometrial or endomyometrial involvement and simulate primary endometrial adenocarcinoma or even atypical hyperplasia [40]. Typically the morphology is somewhat different between a usual endocervical-type adenocarcinoma and an endometrial adenocarcinoma of endometrioid type. Foam cells and squamous elements are more common in the latter neoplasms while cervical adenocarcinomas are often more mitotically and apoptotically active. Identification of a precursor lesion such as atypical endometrial hyperplasia or CGIN may

Table 4.2 Immunohistochemical markers and other ancillary tests useful in distinction between low grade endometrioid adenocarcinoma of uterine corpus and usual endocervical type adenocarcinoma

	Endometrioid adenocarcinoma of uterine corpus	Usual endocervical type adenocarcinoma
Estrogen receptor (ER)	Diffusely positive	Negative or focally positive
Vimentin	Diffusely positive	Negative or focally positive
p16	Negative or focally positive ("mosaic" pattern)	Diffusely positive
Monoclonal carcinoembryonic antigen (CEA)	Negative or focally positive	Diffusely positive
Human papillomavirus (HPV) studies	Negative	Positive

These are the most common staining patterns but in individual cases, aberrant or unexpected staining reactions may occur

also help, but there may be considerable histological overlap.

A panel of markers comprising ER, vimentin, p16 and monoclonal CEA may be of value [35–38] (Table 4.2). Endometrial adenocarcinomas of endometrioid type, especially when low grade, typically exhibit diffuse nuclear ER and cytoplasmic vimentin positivity. CEA is usually negative or focally positive, although the squamous elements which are common in these neoplasms, may be immunoreactive. In contrast, cervical adenocarcinomas are usually, but not always, CEA positive. Vimentin is usually negative and ER is typically negative or there is focal weak positivity; however, occasional well differentiated cervical adenocarcinomas exhibit diffuse staining with ER. Cervical adenocarcinomas typically exhibit diffuse p16 positivity (usually a combination of nuclear and cytoplasmic staining) due to the presence of high risk HPV while endometrial adenocarcinomas of endometrioid type are typically negative or more commonly focally positive. Some examples of the latter neoplasm exhibit quite diffuse p16 immunoreactivity but even then staining is usually patchy with positive foci admixed with areas of negative staining, a so-called mosaic staining pattern. The squamous elements of endometrioid adenocarcinomas may be p16 positive. Molecular studies for HPV may also be of value since usual endocervical-type adenocarcinomas are typically positive whereas endometrial adenocarcinomas are almost always negative. The panel of markers discussed (Table 4.2) also assists in cases of subtle cervical stromal invasion by endometrioid adenocarcinoma of the uterine corpus [127, 128]. Rarely, an endometrioid adenocarcinoma of the uterine corpus and a premalignant or malignant endocervical glandular lesion coexist and the aforementioned panel of markers helps to clarify the relationship between the two neoplasms.

Uterine serous carcinoma (similar to ovarian high grade serous carcinoma) is often diffusely positive with p16, due to non-HPV related mechanisms [131, 132], and it is stressed that the panel of markers discussed is only of value in distinguishing a usual endocervical type adenocarcinoma from an endometrial adenocarcinoma of endometrioid type. When uterine serous carcinoma is present in a cervical biopsy and the panel of markers discussed is performed in an attempt to distinguish between an endometrial and a cervical origin, the pattern of diffuse p16 staining and negative or focal immunoreactivity with ER typical of many uterine serous carcinomas may result in misdiagnosis as a cervical primary with resultant inappropriate management. In this scenario, p53 staining and HPV studies may be of value in that most uterine serous carcinomas exhibit aberrant p53 staining (diffusely positive or more uncommonly totally negative- [133, 134]) and are HPV negative whereas most cervical adenocarcinomas exhibit wild-type p53 staining (focal, weak and heterogenous pattern) and are HPV positive.

The question also arises as to the immunophenotype of a mucinous adenocarcinoma of the endometrium and an endometrioid adenocarcinoma of the cervix; in other words, is the immunophenotype more dependent on the site of origin or the pattern of differentiation? One study which addressed this issue found that if a tumour exhibited diffuse positivity with ER and vimentin then it was almost certainly of endometrial origin [89]. Some mucinous adenocarcinomas or endometrioid adenocarcinomas with mucinous differentiation arising in the endometrium may be vimentin negative and CEA positive, this immunophenotype overlapping with that of a cervical adenocarcinoma. However, these endometrial neoplasms are typically ER positive and p16 negative or focally positive. It is emphasised that in an individual tumour, unexpected staining reactions may occur with one or more of the markers discussed. This can result in potential diagnostic problems and illustrates that the immunohistochemistry is always to be interpreted in light of the clinical, radiological, gross pathological and microscopic findings.

References

1. Sasieni P, Adams J. Changing rates of adenocarcinoma and adenosquamous carcinoma of the cervix in England. Lancet. 2001;357:1490–3.
2. Tavassoli FA, Devilee P, World Health Organisation Classification of Tumours. Pathology and genetics. Tumours of the breast and female genital organs. Lyon: IARC Press; 2003.
3. Houghton O, Jamison J, Wilson R, Carson J, McCluggage WG. p16 Immunoreactivity in unusual types of cervical adenocarcinoma does not reflect human papillomavirus infection. Histopathology. 2010;57:342–50.
4. Park KJ, Kiyokawa T, Soslow RA, et al. Unusual endocervical adenocarcinomas: an immunohistochemical analysis with molecular detection of human papillomavirus. Am J Surg Pathol. 2011;35:633–46.
5. Pirog EC, Kleter B, Olgac S, et al. Prevalence of human papillomavirus DNA in different histological subtypes of cervical adenocarcinoma. Am J Pathol. 2000;157:1055–62.
6. Hee JA, Kim KR, Kim IS. Prevalence of human papillomavirus DNA in various histological subtypes of cervical adenocarcinoma: a population-based study. Mod Pathol. 2005;18:528–34.
7. Duggan MA, McGregor SE, Benoit JL, et al. The human papillomavirus status of invasive cervical adenocarcinoma: a clinicopathological and outcome analysis. Hum Pathol. 1995;26:319–25.
8. Tenti P, Romagnoli S, Silini E, et al. Human papillomavirus types 16 and 18 infection in infiltrating adenocarcinoma of the cervix: PCR analysis of 138 cases and correlation with histologic type and grade. Am J Clin Pathol. 1996;106:52–6.
9. Skylderg BM, Murray E, Lambkin H, et al. Adenocarcinoma of the uterine cervix in Ireland and

Sweden: human papillomavirus infection and biologic alterations. Mod Pathol. 1999;12:675–82.
10. Pecorelli S. Revised FIGO staging for carcinoma of the vulva, cervix, and endometrium. Int J Gynaecol Obstet. 2009;105:103–4.
11. Creasman WT. New gynecologic cancer staging. Gynecol Oncol. 1995;58:198–202.
12. Hirschowitz L, Ganesan R, Singh N, McCluggage WG. Dataset for the histological reporting of cervical neoplasia. London: Royal College of Pathologists; 2011.
13. McCluggage WG. Ten problematic issues identified by pathology review for multidisciplinary gynaecological oncology meetings. J Clin Pathol. 2012;65: 293–301.
14. McCluggage WG. Endocervical glandular lesions: controversial aspects and ancillary techniques. J Clin Pathol. 2003;56:164–73.
15. Young RH, Clement PB. Endocervical adenocarcinoma and its variants: their morphology and differential diagnosis. Histopathology. 2002;41:185–207.
16. Rollason TP, Cullimore J, Bradgate MG. A suggested columnar cell morphological equivalent of squamous carcinoma in situ with early stromal invasion. Int J Gynecol Pathol. 1989;8:230–6.
17. Wheeler DT, Kurman RJ. The relationship of glands to thick-wall blood vessels as a marker of invasion in endocervical adenocarcinoma. Int J Gynecol Pathol. 2005;24:125–30.
18. Al-Kalbani M, McVeigh G, Nagar H, McCluggage WG. Do FIGO stage 1A and small (≤2 cm) 1B1 adenocarcinomas have a good prognosis and warrant less radical surgery? Int J Gynecol Cancer. 2012;26: 291–8.
19. Negri G, Romano F, Vittadello F, et al. Laminin-5 gamma 2 chain immunohistochemistry facilitates the assessment of invasiveness and improves the diagnostic reproducibility of glandular lesions of the cérvix uteri. Hum Pathol. 2006;37:704–10.
20. Yavner DL, Dwyer IM, Hancock WW, Ehrmann RC. Basement membrane of cervical adenocarcinoma: an immunoperoxidase study of laminin and type IV collagen. Obstet Gynecol. 1990;76:1014–9.
21. Jordan SM, Watanabe T, Osann K, Monk BJ, Lin F, Rutgers JK. Desmoplastic stromal response as defined by positive α-smooth muscle actin staining is predictive of invasion in adenocarcinoma of the uterine cervix. Int J Gynecol Pathol. 2012;31:369–76.
22. Ostor AG. Early invasive adenocarcinoma of the uterine cervix. Int J Gynecol Pathol. 2000;19:29–38.
23. Ceballos KM, Shaw D, Daya D. Microinvasive cervical adenocarcinoma (FIGO stage 1A tumors): results of surgical staging and outcome analysis. Am J Surg Pathol. 2006;30:370–4.
24. Reynolds EA, Tierney K, Keeney G, et al. Analysis of outcomes of microinvasive adenocarcinoma of the uterine cervix by treatment type. Obstet Gynecol. 2010;116:1150–7.
25. Balega J, Michael H, Hurteau J, et al. The risk of nodal metastasis in early adenocarcinoma of the uterine cervix. Int J Gynecol Cancer. 2004;14:104–9.
26. Smith HO, Qualls CR, Romero AA, et al. Is there a difference in survival for 1A1 and 1A2 adenocarcinoma of the uterine cervix? Gynecol Oncol. 2002;85:229–41.
27. Yahata T, Nishino K, Kashima K, et al. Conservative treatment of stage 1A1 adenocarcinoma of the uterine cervix with a long-term follow-up. Int J Gynecol Cancer. 2010;20:1063–6.
28. Smith JS, Green J, de Gonzalez Berrington A, et al. Cervical cancer and use of hormonal contraceptives: a systematic review. Lancet. 2003;361:1159–67.
29. Tambouret R, Bell DA, Young RH. Microcystic endocervical adenocarcinomas: a report of eight cases. Am J Surg Pathol. 2000;24:369–74.
30. Young RH, Scully RE. Uterine carcinomas simulating microglandular hyperplasia: a report of six cases. Am J Surg Pathol. 1992;16:1092–7.
31. Mansor S, McCluggage WG. Cervical adenocarcinoma resembling breast lobular carcinoma: a hitherto undescribed variant of primary cervical adenocarcinoma. Int J Gynecol Pathol. 2010;29:594–9.
32. Shintaku M, Karlya M, Shime H, et al. Adenocarcinoma of the uterine cervix with choriocarcinomatous and hepatoid differentiation: report of a case. Int J Gynecol Pathol. 2000;19:174–8.
33. Kato K, Suzuka K, Osaki T, Itami M, Tanaka N. Primary hepatoid adenocarcinoma of the uterine cervix. Int J Gynecol Cancer. 2007;17:1150–4.
34. McCluggage WG. Immunohistochemistry as a diagnostic aid in cervical pathology. Pathology. 2007;39: 97–111.
35. Kong CS, Beck AH, Longacre TA. A panel of 3 markers including p16, ProExC, or HPV ISH is optimal for distinguishing between primary endometrial and endocervical adenocarcinomas. Am J Surg Pathol. 2010;34:915–26.
36. Castrillon DH, Lee KR, Nucci MR. Distinction between endometrial and endocervical adenocarcinoma: an immunohistochemical study. Int J Gynecol Pathol. 2002;21:4–10.
37. McCluggage WG, Sumathi VP, McBride HA, Patterson A. A panel of immunohistochemical stains, including carcinoembryonic antigen, vimentin, and estrogen receptor, aids the distinction between primary endometrial and endocervical adenocarcinomas. Int J Gynecol Pathol. 2002;21:11–5.
38. Dabbs DJ, Geisinger KR, Norris HT. Intermediate filaments in endometrial and endocervical carcinomas. The diagnostic utility of vimentin patterns. Am J Surg Pathol. 1986;10:568–76.
39. Savargaonkar PR, Hale RJ, Mutton A, Manning V, Buckley CH. Neuroendocrine differentiation in cervical carcinoma. J Clin Pathol. 1996;49:139–41.
40. Yemelyanova A, Vang R, Seidman JD, Gravitt PE, Ronnett BM. Endocervical adenocarcinomas with prominent endometrial or endomyometrial involvement simulating primary endometrial carcinomas: utility of HPV DNA detection and immunohistochemical expression of p16 and hormone receptors to confirm the cervical origin of the corpus tumor. Am J Surg Pathol. 2009;33:914–24.

41. Ronnett BM, Yemelyanova AV, Vang R, Gilks CB, Miller D, Gravitt PE, Kurman RJ. Endocervical adenocarcinomas with ovarian metastases: analysis of 29 cases with emphasis on minimally invasive cervical tumors and the ability of the metastases to simulate primary ovarian neoplasms. Am J Surg Pathol. 2008;32:1835–53.
42. Chang MC, Nevadunsky NS, Viswanathan AN, Crum CP, Feltmate CM. Endocervical adenocarcinoma in situ with ovarian metastases: a unique variant with potential for long-term survival. Int J Gynecol Pathol. 2010;29:88–92.
43. Eftekhar Z, Marsden D, Robertson G, et al. Prognostic factors and survival of adenocarcinoma of the cervix. Int J Gynecol Cancer. 2002;12:612.
44. Liu WX, Chen Y, Yang GM. Analysis of prognostic-related factors in patients with invasive cervical adenocarcinoma. Eur J Gynaecol Oncol. 2011;32:500–4.
45. Hart WR. Symposium part II: special types of adenocarcinoma of the uterine cervix. Int J Gynecol Pathol. 2002;21:327–46.
46. McCluggage WG, Shah R, Connolly LE, McBride HA. Intestinal-type cervical adenocarcinoma in situ and adenocarcinoma exhibit a partial immunophenotype with consistent expression of CDX2. Int J Gynecol Pathol. 2008;27:92–100.
47. Lee KR, Trainer TD. Adenocarcinoma of the uterine cervix of intestinal type containing numerous Paneth cells. Arch Pathol Lab Med. 1990;114:731–3.
48. Raspollini MR, Baroni G, Taddei A, et al. Primary cervical adenocarcinoma with intestinal differentiation and colonic carcinoma metastatic to cervix. An investigation using cdx-2 and a limited immunohistochemical panel. Arch Pathol Lab Med. 2003;127:1586–90.
49. Fox H, Wells M, Harris M, et al. Enteric tumors of the lower female genital tract: a report of three cases. Histopathology. 1988;12:167–76.
50. Zhang PJ, Shah M, Spiegel GW, Brooks JJ. Cytokeratin 7 immunoreactivity in rectal adenocarcinomas. Appl Immunohistochem Mol Morphol. 2003;11:306–10.
51. Savargaonkar PR, Hale RJ, Pope R, Fox H, Buckley CH. Enteric differentiation in cervical adenocarcinomas and its prognostic significance. Histopathology. 1993;23:275–7.
52. Suarez-Penaranda JM, Abdulkader I, Baron-Duarte FJ, Gonzalez Patino E, Novo-Dominguez A, Varela-Duran J. Signet-ring cell carcinoma presenting in the uterine cervix: report of a primary and 2 metastatic cases. Int J Gynecol Pathol. 2007;26:254–8.
53. Balci S, Saglam A, Usubutun A. Primary signet-ring cell carcinoma of the cervix: case report and review of the literature. Int J Gynecol Pathol. 2010;29:181–4.
54. Kupryjanczyk J, Kujawa M. Signet-ring cells in squamous cell carcinoma of the cervix and in non-neoplastic ectocervical epithelium. Int J Gynecol Pathol. 1992;2:152–6.
55. McKenna M, McCluggage WG. Signet ring cells of stromal derivation in the uterine cervix secondary to cauterisation: report of a previously undescribed phenomenon. J Clin Pathol. 2008;61:648–51.
56. Gilks CB, Young RH, Aguirre P, et al. Adenoma malignum (minimal deviation adenocarcinoma) of the uterine cervix. A clinicopathological and immunohistochemical analysis of 26 cases. Am J Surg Pathol. 1989;13:717–29.
57. Silverberg SG, Hurt WG. Minimal deviation adenocarcinoma ("adenoma malignum") of the cervix: a reappraisal. Am J Obstet Gynecol. 1975;121:971–5.
58. Menko FH. LKB1/SKT11. Peutz-Jeghers cancer syndrome and cancer. Fam Cancer. 2011;10:413–4.
59. Kuragaki C, Enomoto T, Ueno Y, et al. Mutations in the SKT11 gene characterize minimal deviation adenocarcinoma of the uterine cervix. Lab Invest. 2003;83:35–46.
60. Connolly DC, Katabuchi H, Cliby WA, Cho KR. Somatic mutations in the SKT11/LKB1 gene are uncommon in rare gynecologic tumor types associated with Peutz-Jegher's syndrome. Am J Pathol. 2000;156:339–45.
61. Toki T, Zhai YL, Park JS, Fujii S. Infrequent occurrence of high-risk human papillomavirus and of p53 mutation in minimal deviation adenocarcinoma of the cervix. Int J Gynecol Pathol. 1999;18:215–9.
62. Xu J, Hashi A, Kondo T, et al. Absence of human papillomavirus infection in minimal deviation adenocarcinoma and lobular endocervical glandular hyperplasia. Int J Gynecol Pathol. 2005;24:296–302.
63. Mikami Y, Kiyokawa T, Hata S, Fujiwara K, Moriya T, Sasano H, et al. Gastrointestinal immunophenotype in adenocarcinomas of the uterine cervix and related glandular lesions: a possible link between lobular endocervical glandular hyperplasia/pyloric gland metaplasia and 'adenoma malignum'. Mod Pathol. 2004;17:962–72.
64. Nucci MR, Clement PB, Young RH. Lobular endocervical glandular hyperplasia, not otherwise specified: a clinicopathologic analysis of thirteen cases of a distinctive pseudoneoplastic lesion and comparison with fourteen cases of adenoma malignum. Am J Surg Pathol. 1999;23:886–91.
65. Mikami Y, McCluggage WG. Endocervical glandular lesions exhibiting gastric differentiation: an emerging spectrum of benign, premalignant and malignant lesions. Adv Anat Pathol. 2013;20:227–37.
66. Tsuda H, Mikami Y, Kaku T, et al. Interobserver variation in the diagnosis of adenoma malignum (minimal deviation adenocarcinoma) of the uterine cervix. Pathol Int. 2003;53:440–9.
67. Kondo T, Hashi A, Murata SI, et al. Gastric mucin is expressed in a subset of endocervical tunnel clusters: type A tunnel clusters of gastric phenotype. Histopathology. 2007;50:843–50.
68. Ichimura T, Koizumi T, Tateiwa H, et al. Immunohistochemical expression of gastric mucin and p53 in minimal deviation adenocarcinoma of the uterine cervix. Int J Gynecol Pathol. 2001;20:220–6.
69. Toki T, Shiozawa T, Hosaka N, Ishii K, Nikaido T, Fujii S. Minimal deviation adenocarcinoma of the

uterine cervix has abnormal expression of sex steroid receptors, CA125, and gastric mucin. Int J Gynecol Pathol. 1997;16:111–6.
70. Utsugi K, Hirai Y, Takeshima N, et al. Utility of the monoclonal antibody HIK1083 in the diagnosis of adenoma malignum of the uterine cervix. Gynecol Oncol. 1999;75:345–8.
71. Michael H, Grawe L, Kraus FT. Minimal deviation endocervical adenocarcinoma: clinical and histologic features, immunohistochemical staining for carcinoembryonic antigen, and differentiation from confusing benign lesions. Int J Gynecol Pathol. 1984;3:261–76.
72. Mikami Y, Kiyokawa T, Moriya T, Sasano H. Immunophenotypic alteration of the stromal component in minimal deviation adenocarcinoma ('adenoma malignum') and endocervical glandular hyperplasia: a study using oestrogen receptor and alpha-smooth muscle actin double immunostaining. Histopathology. 2005;46:130–6.
73. Hayashi I, Tsuda H, Shimoda T. Reappraisal of orthodox histochemistry for the diagnosis of minimal deviation adenocarcinoma of the cervix. Am J Surg Pathol. 2000;24:559–62.
74. Seidman JD. Mucinous lesions of the fallopian tube. Am J Surg Pathol. 1994;18:1205–12.
75. Young RH, Scully RE. Mucinous tumors of the ovary associated with mucinous adenocarcinomas of the cervix. A clinicopathologic analysis of 16 cases. Int J Gynecol Pathol. 1988;7:99–111.
76. Kojima A, Mikami Y, Sudo T, et al. Gastric morphology and immunophenotype predict poor outcome in mucinous adenocarcinoma of the uterine cervix. Am J Surg Pathol. 2007;31:664–72.
77. Kusanagi Y, Kogima A, Mikami Y, et al. Absence of high-risk human papillomavirus (HPV) detection in endocervical adenocarcinoma with gastric morphology and phenotype. Am J Pathol. 2010;177:2169–75.
78. McCluggage WG, Harley I, Houghton JP, Geyer FC, McKay A, Reis-Filho JS. Composite cervical adenocarcinoma composed of adenoma malignum and gastric type adenocarcinoma (dedifferentiated adenoma malignum) in patient with Peutz-Jeghers syndrome. J Clin Pathol. 2010;63:935–41.
79. Jones MW, Silverberg SG, Kurman RJ. Well-differentiated villoglandular adenocarcinoma of the uterine cervix: a clinicopathological study of 24 cases. Int J Gynecol Pathol. 1993;12:1–7.
80. Young RH, Scully RE. Villoglandular papillary adenocarcinoma of the uterine cervix. A clinicopathologic analysis of 13 cases. Cancer. 1989;63:1773–9.
81. Macdonald RD, Kirwan J, Hayat K, et al. Villoglandular adenocarcinoma of the cervix: clarity is needed on the histological definition for this difficult diagnosis. Gynecol Oncol. 2006;100:192–4.
82. Jones MW, Kounelis S, Papadaki H, et al. Well-differentiated villoglandular adenocarcinoma of the uterine cervix: oncogene/tumor suppressor alterations and human papillomavirus genotyping. Int J Gynecol Pathol. 2000;19:110–7.
83. Heatley MK. Villoglandular adenocarcinoma of the uterine cervix-a systematic review of the literature. Histopathology. 2007;51:268–9.
84. Alfsen GC, Thoresen SO, Kristensen GB, et al. Histopathologic subtyping of cervical adenocarcinoma reveals increasing incidence rates of endometrioid tumors in all groups. Cancer. 2000;89:1291–9.
85. Zaino RJ. Glandular lesions of the uterine cervix. Mod Pathol. 2000;13:261–74.
86. Hirschowitz L, Sen C, Murdoch J. Primary endometrioid adenocarcinoma of the cervix with widespread squamous metaplasia–a potential diagnostic pitfall. Diagn Pathol. 2007;2:40.
87. Rahilly MA, Williams AR, Al-Nafussi A. Minimal deviation endometrioid adenocarcinoma of cervix: a clinicopathological and immunohistochemical study of two cases. Histopathology. 1992;20:351–4.
88. Young RH, Scully RE. Minimal-deviation endometrioid adenocarcinoma of the uterine cervix. A report of five cases of a distinctive neoplasm that may be misinterpreted as benign. Am J Surg Pathol. 1993;17:660–5.
89. Kamoi S, Al Juboury ML, Akin MR, et al. Immunohistochemical staining in the distinction between endometrial and endocervical adenocarcinomas: another viewpoint. Int J Gynecol Pathol. 2002;21:217–23.
90. Hanselaar A, van Loosbroek M, Schuurbiers O, Helmerhorst T, Bulten J, Bernhelm J. Clear cell adenocarcinoma of the vagina and cervix. An update of the central Netherlands registry showing twin age incidence peaks. Cancer. 1997;79:2229–36.
91. Herbst AL. Behaviour of estrogen-associated female genital tract cancer and its relation to neoplasia following intrauterine exposure to diethylstilbestrol (DES). Gynecol Oncol. 2000;76:147–56.
92. Kaminski PF, Maier RC. Clear cell adenocarcinoma of the cervix unrelated to diethylstilbestrol exposure. Obstet Gynecol. 1983;62:720–7.
93. Matias-Guiu X, Lerma E, Prat J. Clear cell tumors of the female genital tract. Semin Diagn Pathol. 1997;14:233–9.
94. Zhou C, Gilks CB, Hayes M, Clement PB. Papillary serous carcinoma of the uterine cervix: a clinicopathologic study of 17 cases. Am J Surg Pathol. 1998;22:113–20.
95. Nofech-Mozes S, Rasty G, Ismiil N, Covens A, Khalifa MA. Immunohistochemical characterization of endocervical papillary serous carcinoma. Int J Gynecol Cancer. 2006;16 Suppl 1:286–92.
96. Clement PB, Young RH, Keh P, Ostor AG, Scully RE. Malignant mesonephric neoplasms of the uterine cervix. A report of eight cases, including four with a malignant spindle cell component. Am J Surg Pathol. 1995;19:1158–71.
97. Bague S, Rodriquez IM, Prat J. Malignant mesonephric tumors of the female genital tract. A clinicopathologic study of 9 cases. Am J Surg Pathol. 2004;28:601–7.
98. Silver SA, Devouassoux-Shisheboran M, Mezzetti TP, Tavassoli FA. Mesonephric adenocarcinomas of the uterine cervix: a study of 11 cases with immunohistochemical findings. Am J Surg Pathol. 2001;25:379–87.

99. Kenny SL, McBride HA, Jamison J, McCluggage WG. Mesonephric adenocarcinomas of the uterine cervix and corpus: HPV-negative neoplasms that are commonly PAX8, CA125, and HMGA2 positive and that may be immunoreactive with TTF1 and Hepatocyte Nuclear Factor 1-β. Am J Surg Pathol. 2012;36: 799–807.
100. McCluggage WG, Oliva E, Herrington CS, McBride H, Young RH. CD10 and calretinin staining of endocervical glandular lesions, endocervical stroma and endometrioid adenocarcinomas of the uterine corpus: CD10 positivity is characteristic of, but not specific for, mesonephric lesions and is not specific for endometrial stroma. Histopathology. 2003;43:144–50.
101. Ordi J, Ramagosa C, Tavassoli FA. CD10 expression in epithelial tissues and tumors of the gynecologic tract. Am J Surg Pathol. 2003;27:178–86.
102. Seidman JD, Tavassoli FA. Mesonephric hyperplasia of the uterine cervix: a clinicopathologic study of 51 cases. Int J Gynecol Pathol. 1995;14:293–9.
103. Gallup DG, Harper RH, Stock RJ. Poor prognosis in patients with adenosquamous cell carcinoma of the cervix. Obstet Gynecol. 1985;65:416–22.
104. Lea JS, Coleman RL, Garner EO, et al. Adenosquamous histology predicts poor outcome in low-risk stage 1B1 cervical adenocarcinoma. Gynecol Oncol. 2003;91:558–62.
105. Fujiwara H, Mitchell MF, Arseneau J, et al. Clear cell adenosquamous carcinoma of the cervix. An aggressive tumor associated with human papillomavirus-18. Cancer. 1995;76:1591–600.
106. Shingleton HM, Bell MC, Fremgen A, et al. Is there really a difference in survival of women with squamous cell carcinoma, adenocarcinoma and adenosquamous carcinoma? Cancer. 1995;76:1948–55.
107. Farley JH, Hickey KW, Carlson JW, Rose GS, Kost ER, Harrison TA. Adenosquamous histology predicts a poor outcome for patients with advanced-stage, but not early-stage, cervical carcinoma. Cancer. 2003;97:2196–202.
108. Samlal RA, Ten Kate FJ, Hart AA, Lammes FB. Do mucin-secreting squamous cell carcinomas of the uterine cervix metastasize more frequently to pelvic lymph nodes? A case-control study? Int J Gynecol Pathol. 1988;17:201–4.
109. Lennerz JK, Perry A, Mills JC, Huettner PC, Pfeifer JD. Mucoepidermoid carcinoma of the cervix: another tumor with the t(11;19)-associated CRTC1-MAML2 gene fusion. Am J Surg Pathol. 2009;33:835–43.
110. Littman P, Clement PB, Henriksen B, Wang CC, Robboy SJ, Taft PD, et al. Glassy cell carcinoma of the cervix. Cancer. 1976;37:2238–46.
111. Kato N, Katayama Y, Kaimori M, Motoyama T. Glassy cell carcinoma of the uterine cervix: histochemical, immunohistochemical, and molecular genetic observations. Int J Gynecol Pathol. 2002;21: 134–40.
112. Gray HJ, Garcia R, Tamimi HK, et al. Glassy cell carcinoma of the cervix revisited. Gynecol Oncol. 2002;85:274–7.
113. Ferry JA, Scully RE. "Adenoid cystic" carcinoma and adenoid basal carcinoma of the uterine cervix. A study of 28 cases. Am J Surg Pathol. 1988;12: 134–44.
114. Grayson W, Taylor LF, Cooper K. Adenoid cystic and adenoid basal carcinoma of the uterine cervix: comparative morphologic, mucin, and immunohistochemical profile of two rare neoplasms of putative 'reserve cell' origin. Am J Surg Pathol. 1999;23:448–58.
115. Dominguez-Malagon HR, Flores-Flores G, Meneses Garcia A, et al. Adenoid cystic carcinoma of the uterine cervix. A tumor with myoepithelial cells and neuroendocrine differentiation. Int J Surg Pathol. 1996;4:77–82.
116. Grayson W, Taylor L, Cooper K. Detection of integrated high risk human papillomavirus in adenoid cystic carcinoma of the uterine cervix. J Clin Pathol. 1996;49:805–9.
117. Parwani AV, Smith Sehdev AE, Kurman RJ, Ronnett BM. Cervical adenoid basal tumors comprised of adenoid basal epithelioma associated with various types of invasive carcinoma: clinicopathologic features, human papillomavirus DNA detection, and p16 expression. Hum Pathol. 2005;36:82–90.
118. Albores-Saavedra J, Manivel C, Mora A, Vuitch F, Milchgrub S, Gould E. The solid variant of adenoid cystic carcinoma of the cervix. Int J Gynecol Pathol. 1992;11:2–10.
119. Grayson W, Cooper K. A reappraisal of "basaloid carcinoma" of the cervix, and the differential diagnosis of basaloid cervical neoplasms. Adv Anat Pathol. 2002;9:290–300.
120. Brainard JA, Hart WR. Adenoid basal epitheliomas of the uterine cervix: a reevaluation of distinctive cervical basaloid lesions currently classified as adenoid basal carcinoma and adenoid basal hyperplasia. Am J Surg Pathol. 1998;22:965–75.
121. Chen T-D, Chuang H-C, Lee L. Adenoid basal carcinoma of the uterine cervix: clinicopathologic features of 12 cases with reference to CD117 expression. Int J Gynecol Pathol. 2012;31:25–32.
122. Lemoine NR, Hall PA. Epithelial tumors metastatic to the uterine cervix. A study of 33 cases and review of the literature. Cancer. 1986;57:2002–5.
123. McCluggage WG, Hirschowitz L, Wilson GE, et al. Significant variation in the assessment of cervical involvement in endometrial carcinoma: an interobserver variation study. Am J Surg Pathol. 2011;35: 289–94.
124. Hoogduin KJ, Hopman AN, Ramaekers FC, McCluggage WG, Smedts F. BCL2 and keratin 5 define the uterine-cervix-isthmus junction, a transition between endocervical and tubal-like epithelium. Int J Gynecol Pathol. 2013;32:122–30.
125. Jordan LB, Al-Nafussi A. Clinicopathological study of the pattern and significance of cervical involve-

ment in cases of endometrial adenocarcinoma. Int J Gynecol Cancer. 2002;12:42–8.

126. Scott M, Lyness RW, McCluggage WG. Atypical reactive proliferation of endocervix: a common lesion associated with endometrial carcinoma and likely related to prior endometrial sampling. Mod Pathol. 2006;19:470–4.
127. Kalyanasundaram K, Ganesan R, Perunovic B, McCluggage WG. Diffusely infiltrating endometrial carcinomas with no stromal response: report of a series, including cases with cervical and ovarian involvement and emphasis on the potential for misdiagnosis. Int J Surg Pathol. 2010;18:138–43.
128. Tambouret R, Clement PB, Young RH. Endometrial endometrioid adenocarcinoma with a deceptive pattern of spread to the uterine cervix: a manifestation of stage IIb endometrial carcinoma liable to be misinterpreted as an independent carcinoma or a benign lesion. Am J Surg Pathol. 2003;27:1080–8.
129. McCluggage WG, Hurrell DP, Kennedy K. Metastatic carcinomas in the cervix mimicking primary cervical adenocarcinoma and adenocarcinoma in situ: report of a series of cases. Am J Surg Pathol. 2010;34:735–41.
130. Malpica A, Deavers MT. Ovarian low-grade serous carcinoma involving the cervix mimicking a cervical primary. Int J Gynecol Pathol. 2011;30:613–9.
131. Yemelyanova A, Ji H, Shih IM, Wang TL, Wu LS, Ronnett BM. Utility of p16 expression for distinction of uterine serous carcinomas from endometrial endometrioid and endocervical adenocarcinomas: immunohistochemical analysis of 201 cases. Am J Surg Pathol. 2009;33:1504–14.
132. Chiesa-Vottero AG, Malpica A, Deavers MT, Broaddus R, Nuovo GJ, Silva EG. Immunohistochemical overexpression of p16 and p53 in uterine serous carcinoma and ovarian high-grade serous carcinoma. Int J Gynecol Pathol. 2007;26:328–33.
133. McCluggage WG, Soslow RA, Gilks CB. Patterns of p53 immunoreactivity in endometrial carcinomas: "all or nothing" staining is of importance. Histopathology. 2011;59:786–8.
134. Kobel M, Reuss A, Du Bois A, et al. The biological and clinical value of p53 expression in pelvic high-grade serous carcinomas. J Pathol. 2010;222:191–8.

Other Neoplasms of the Cervix

5

W. Glenn McCluggage

Abstract

This chapter deals with uncommon primary cervical neoplasms. Tumours covered in this chapter include neuroendocrine neoplasms of which the most common are small cell and large cell neuroendocrine carcinoma. Transitional tumours and various mesenchymal, mixed epithelial and mesenchymal, melanocytic and haematopoetic neoplasms are also covered.

Keywords

Neuroendocrine carcinoma • Transitional cell carcinoma • Mesenchymal neoplasms • Malignant melanoma • Malignant lymphoma

Introduction

Apart from squamous carcinoma, adenocarcinoma and adenosquamous carcinoma, other primary cervical epithelial neoplasms are uncommon or rare. The most prevalent are neuroendocrine neoplasms, especially small cell and large cell neuroendocrine carcinoma. Mixed epithelial and mesenchymal neoplasms (mixed Mullerian tumours) occur in the cervix but much more uncommonly than in the uterine corpus. Pure mesenchymal neoplasms, especially smooth muscle tumours, also occur in the cervix, as do rarely lymphoid and melanocytic lesions and a variety of other uncommon neoplasms. These various neoplasms are discussed in this chapter.

Neuroendocrine Neoplasms

Definition and General Comments

The current 2003 World Health Organization (WHO) classifies cervical neuroendocrine neoplasms as carcinoid tumour, atypical carcinoid tumour, small cell carcinoma and large cell neuroendocrine carcinoma (LCNEC) [1]. The term small cell neuroendocrine carcinoma (SCNEC) is preferred rather than small cell carcinoma (see below). The WHO classification is identical to the classification currently employed for pulmonary neuroendocrine neoplasms but different than that used for gastrointestinal neuroendocrine tumours where the terms grade 1, 2

W.G. McCluggage et al., *Cellular Pathology of Glandular Lesions and Uncommon Neoplasms of the Cervix*, DOI 10.1007/978-1-4471-2210-4_5,

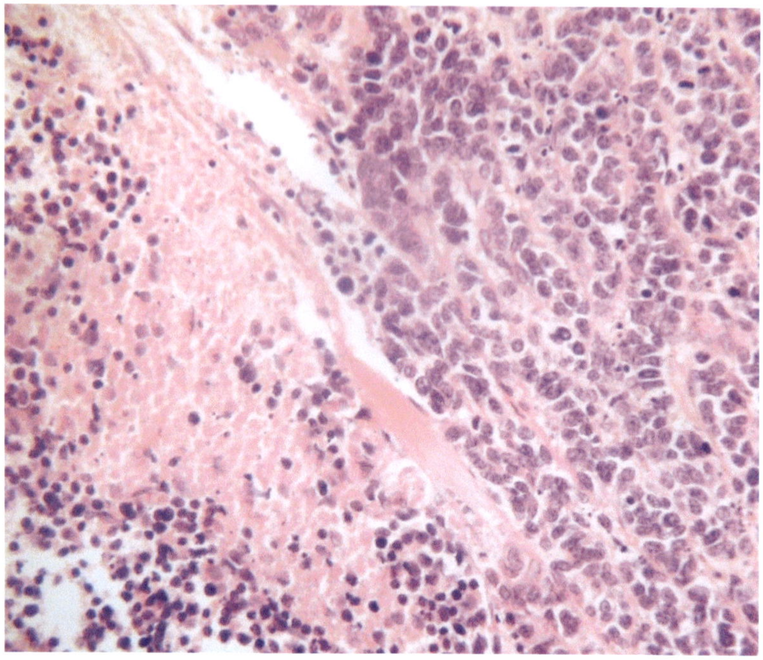

Fig. 5.1 Cervical small cell neuroendocrine carcinoma composed of cells with scant cytoplasm. There is nuclear moulding and necrosis

and 3 neuroendocrine tumour are used. In the cervix, SCNEC is the most common of these neoplasms followed by LCNEC; carcinoid and atypical carcinoid are extremely rare and are morphologically identical to the corresponding neoplasms in other organs [2–8]. It is recommended that the term SCNEC should be used rather than simply small cell carcinoma since a small cell variant of squamous carcinoma exists and use of the term small cell carcinoma can result in confusion. This is important since the management of SCNEC and LCNEC differs significantly from non-neuroendocrine carcinomas. For example, if a diagnosis of SCNEC or LCNEC is made on a biopsy specimen, surgical resection will generally not be undertaken even if the tumour is small and clinically and radiologically confined to the cervix. In addition, the chemotherapy regime will include specific agents which are active against neuroendocrine carcinomas and prophylactic cranial irradiation may be administered.

Cervical SCNEC and LCNEC are HPV-associated neoplasms, the most common HPV types being 16 and 18; in most studies, HPV18 has been more common than 16 [6, 8]. There is a definite association between cervical neuroendocrine carcinomas and premalignant or malignant endocervical glandular lesions; foci of CIN or squamous carcinoma are also occasionally present. Occasional neoplasms are composed of an admixture of SCNEC and LCNEC and in some cases, the morphological features are such that it may be difficult to categorise an individual neoplasm as SCNEC or LCNEC. LCNEC is likely underdiagnosed and may be misclassified as poorly differentiated squamous carcinoma or adenocarcinoma, since the pathologist may not think of the diagnosis and fail to perform appropriate immunohistochemical studies.

Morphological Features of SCNEC

SCNEC is characterised by the presence of a monotonous population of cells with ovoid or slightly spindled hyperchromatic nuclei, often exhibiting moulding, and scanty cytoplasm (Fig. 5.1). There is usually abundant mitotic and apoptotic activity. There may be extensive crush artefact, nuclear fragmentation and necrosis. The growth pattern is usually predominantly diffuse but nests, trabeculae, glandular and rosette-like structures are sometimes present. As discussed,

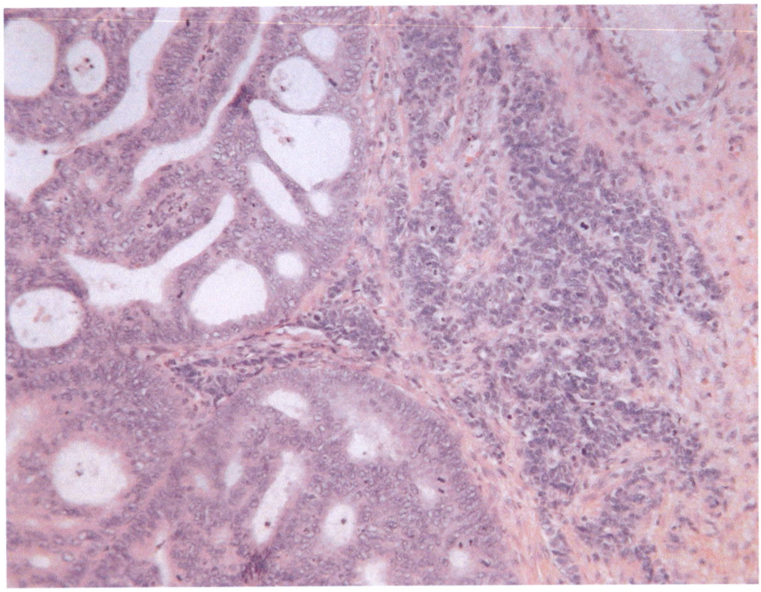

Fig. 5.2 Combined cervical small cell neuroendocrine carcinoma and adenocarcinoma

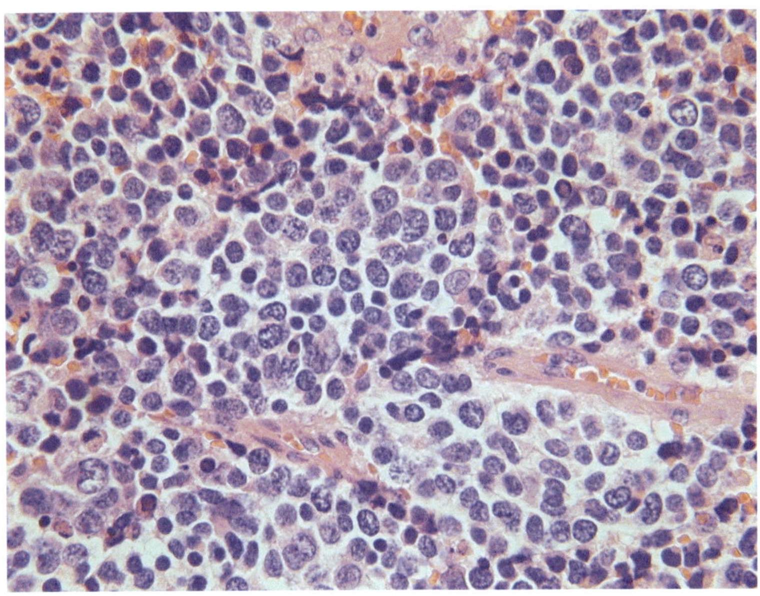

Fig. 5.3 Cervical large cell neuroendocrine carcinoma composed of cells with abundant cytoplasm and an organoid growth pattern

a premalignant or malignant endocervical glandular lesion may also be present (Fig. 5.2) and more uncommonly there is a component of CIN or squamous carcinoma.

Morphological Features of LCNEC

LCNEC, as defined by Travis et al. [9] for the corresponding pulmonary tumours, is characterised by:- (a) cells of large size, polygonal shape and low nuclear to cytoplasmic ratio, (b) nuclei with coarse chromatin and prominent nucleoli, (c) mitotic activity in excess of 10 per 10 high power fields, (d) immunohistochemical or ultrastructural evidence of neuroendocrine differentiation. Insular, nested, trabecular, glandular and solid growth patterns are often present, either alone or in combination (Fig. 5.3). There is often extensive geographic necrosis. Nuclear palisading

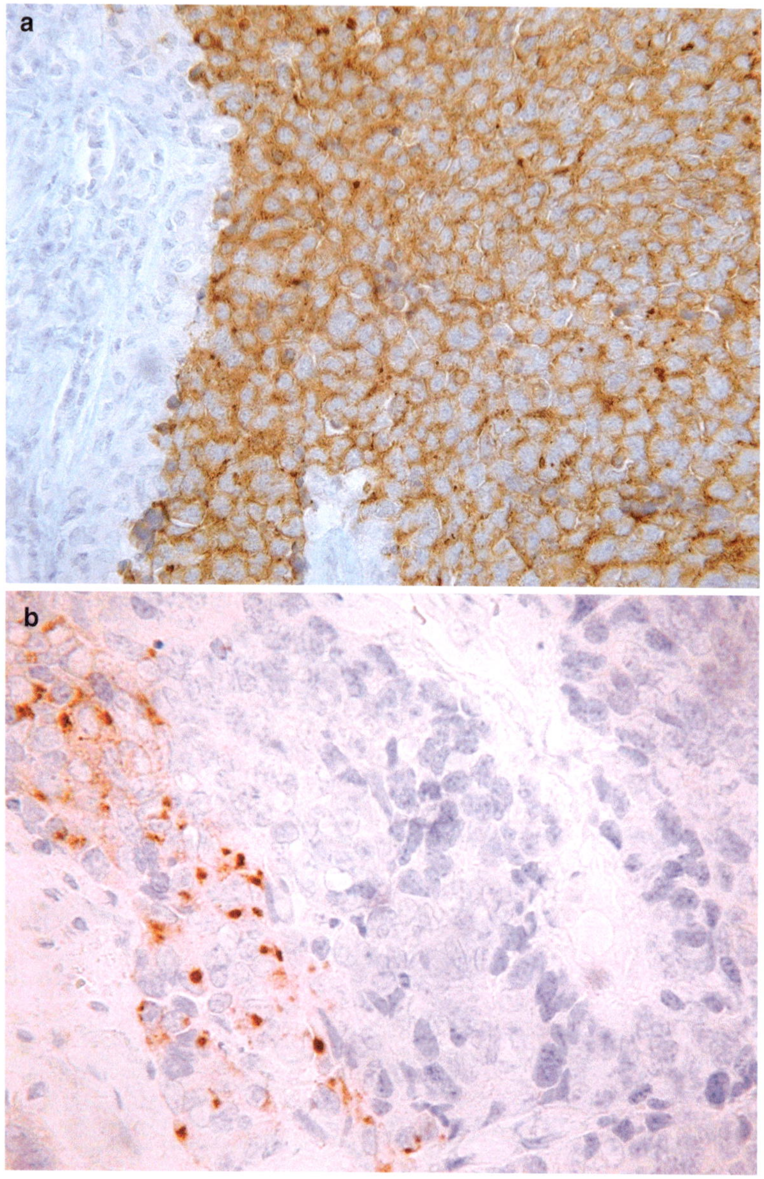

Fig. 5.4 Cervical small cell neuroendocrine carcinoma exhibiting diffuse cytoplasmic staining with synaptophysin (**a**) and focal punctuate cytoplasmic staining with chromogranin (**b**)

may be apparent around the periphery of cell nests and eosinophilic cytoplasmic granules are present in some cases. A premalignant or malignant squamous or glandular lesion may be present and occasionally there is a component of SCNEC. It should be noted that, analogous to the situation in other organs, small numbers of neuroendocrine cells, as demonstrated by immunohistochemistry, may be present in cervical squamous carcinomas and more commonly in adenocarcinomas, especially when poorly differentiated [10, 11], and this does not justify a diagnosis of LCNEC.

Immunohistochemistry

SCNEC is variably positive with the neuroendocrine markers chromogranin, CD56, synaptophysin and PGP9.5 (Fig. 5.4a). Of these, CD56 and synaptophysin are the most sensitive but CD56 lacks specificity. Chromogranin is the most

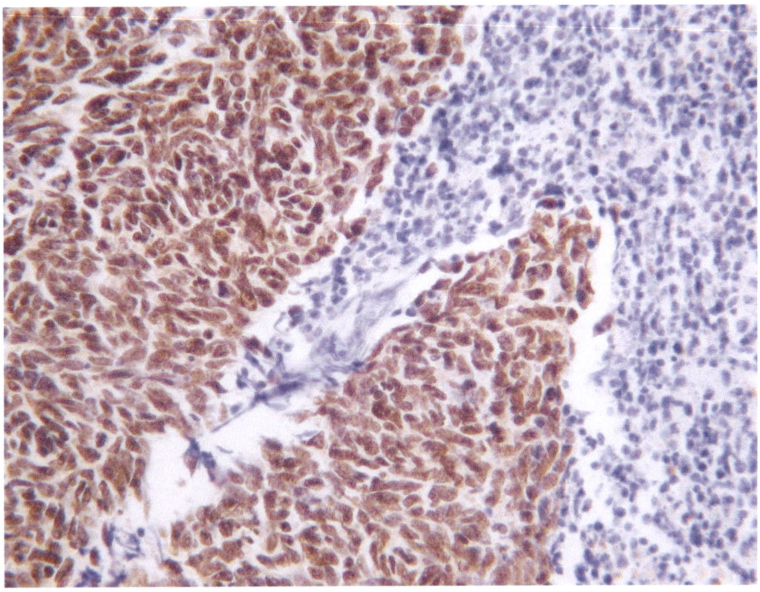

Fig. 5.5 Cervical small cell neuroendocrine carcinoma exhibiting diffuse nuclear staining with TTF1

specific neuroendocrine marker but lacks sensitivity with only about 50 % of these neoplasms being positive [12]. Chromomogranin positivity may be very focal with punctuate cytoplasmic immunoreactivity which is only visible on high power magnification (Fig. 5.4b). A diagnosis of SCNEC can be made in the absence of neuroendocrine marker positivity if the morphological appearances are typical. SCNEC may be only focally positive (often punctuate cytoplasmic staining) or even negative with broad spectrum cytokeratins. A diagnosis of LCNEC requires neuroendocrine marker positivity and most of these neoplasms are diffusely positive with broad spectrum cytokeratins.

A high percentage of primary cervical SCNEC and LCNEC are TTF1 positive, including some with diffuse immunoreactivity (Fig. 5.5), and this marker is of no value in distinction from a pulmonary metastasis [12, 13]. Most SCNEC and LCNEC are diffusely positive with p16 secondary to the presence of high risk HPV [12]. Diffuse p63 nuclear positivity is useful in confirming a small cell variant of squamous carcinoma rather than SCNEC [14, 15]. However, occasional SCNEC and LCNEC exhibit p63 nuclear immunoreactivity [12]. Some SCNEC and LCNEC are positive with CK7, CK20, neurofilament or CD99; such aberrant staining reactions may result in misdiagnosis as a Merkel cell carcinoma or a tumour in the Ewing family [12]. Peptide hormones, including ACTH, serotonin, somatostatin, calcitonin, glucagon and gastrin, have been demonstrated in some of these neoplasms [7].

Prognosis

Cervical neuroendocrine carcinomas of small cell and large cell type are highly aggressive neoplasms with a propensity for widespread systemic metastasis; even neoplasms with a minor component of SCNEC or LCNEC may behave aggressively. The overall prognosis is poor with survival rates of 25–35 % [2–8]. Involvement of regional and distant lymph nodes, lung, liver, bone and brain is common.

Transitional Neoplasms

Occasional cervical neoplasms morphologically resemble transitional cell tumours of the urological tract. These usually take the form of papillary neoplasms which are similar to papillary transitional cell carcinomas of the urological tract [16–18]. These have been variously termed

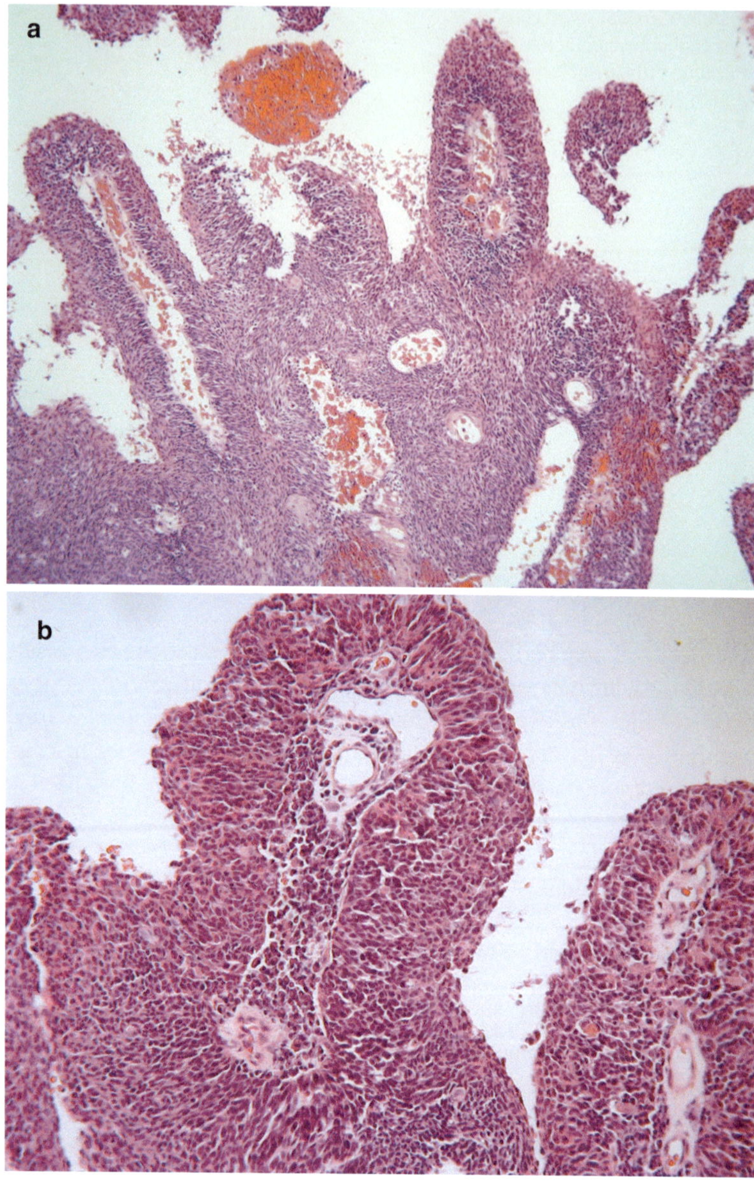

Fig. 5.6 Papillary transitional carcinoma of cervix with broad papillary arrangements of epithelial cells (**a**). On higher power examination, the nuclear features are relatively bland (**b**)

papillary transitional cell carcinoma or papillary squamotransitional carcinoma. Morphologically they are composed of broad papillary arrangements of stratified epithelium (Fig. 5.6a) sometimes, but not always, with relatively bland nuclear features (Fig. 5.6b). Nuclear grooves may be present and there can be evidence of squamous differentiation in the form of keratinisation. Rare neoplasms have also exhibited glandular differentiation [19]. Often these neoplasms are entirely located on the mucosal surface with no underlying stromal invasion, although this is not always the case. These are usually HPV related neoplasms, most commonly type 16. Given the close morphological overlap between transitional and squamous epithelium, it is likely that these are related to papillary squamous carcinomas and in some cases the distinction between a papillary variant of squamous carcinoma, squamotransitional carcinoma and transitional carcinoma will be subjective. Occasional invasive cervical carcinomas with transitional features

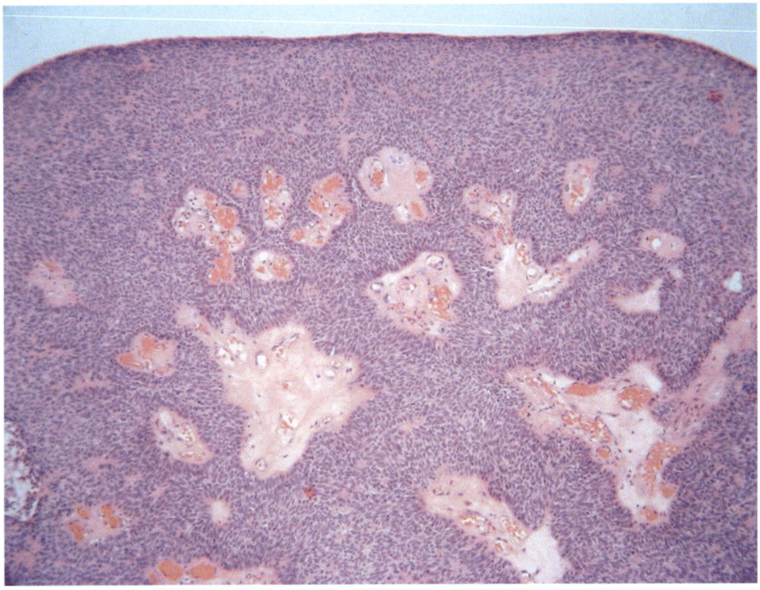

Fig. 5.7 Cervical neoplasm resembling inverted transitional papilloma of urinary tract

and high grade cytology have been reported but these may simply be unusual variants of squamous carcinoma [17]. A cervical neoplasm morphologically resembling inverted transitional papilloma of the urinary bladder has been reported (Fig. 5.7); both this neoplasm and a similar vaginal lesion contained HPV 42 [20].

Mesenchymal Neoplasms

Mesenchymal neoplasms are much more uncommon in the cervix than in the uterine corpus and some involve the cervix by direct spread from the corpus.

Smooth Muscle Neoplasms

Leiomyomas are by far the most common mesenchymal neoplasm to occur within the cervix but are much more uncommon than in the uterine corpus. The morphological features are usually those of a typical leiomyoma but compared to their counterparts in the corpus, cervical leiomyomas are more likely to exhibit nuclear palisading, reminiscent of a neurilemmoma ("neurilemmoma-like" leiomyoma or "schwannoma-like" leiomyoma) (Fig. 5.8). Leiomyoma variants, similar to those occurring in the corpus, also occur in the cervix. Leiomyosarcomas, including epithelioid and myxoid variants, occasionally occur as primary cervical neoplasms.

Embryonal Rhabdomyosarcoma

Embryonal rhabdomyosarcoma (sarcoma botryoides) occurs as a primary cervical neoplasm, most commonly in the late teens and early twenties (mean age 18 years), although the age range is relatively wide [21–25]. The usual presentation is vaginal bleeding or a mass protruding from the introitus. There is a rare association between cervical embryonal rhabdomyosarcoma, ovarian Sertoli-Leydig cell tumour and pleuropulmonary blastoma and this is thought to be due to underlying DICER1 mutation [24, 26].

Grossly, cervical embryonal rhabdomyosarcoma usually takes the form of a polypoid mass or multiple polyps which may be totally removed by polypectomy. Occasionally, there is an infiltrative growth pattern without a polypoid architecture but this is uncommon. The cut surface may be myxoid with areas of necrosis and some neoplasms have an overtly botryoid (grape-like) gross appearance.

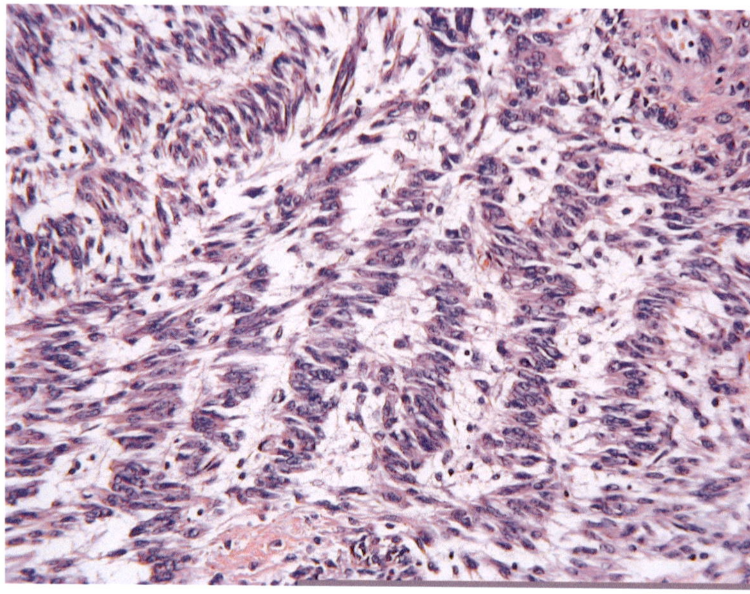

Fig. 5.8 Leiomyoma of cervix exhibiting nuclear palisading, in keeping with "neurilemmoma-like" leiomyoma

Histological examination characteristically shows a polypoid lesion covered by a variety of types of benign glandular Mullerian type epithelium, sometimes with focal squamous differentiation (Fig. 5.9a). Glands may also be present quite deep within the core of the neoplasm. The features of malignancy may be subtle in that, in large part, the stroma can be hypocellular and myxoid or oedematous. However, tightly packed hypercellular foci are also present which sometimes coalesce to form large cellular aggregates. There is usually mitotic and apoptotic activity within the cellular foci (Fig. 5.9b). Characteristically there is increased cellularity around the glandular elements, resulting in a cambium layer and here mitotic figures and apoptotic bodies are usually apparent. Most of the stromal cells have small hyperchromatic nuclei with scant cytoplasm and delicate cytoplasmic processes but cells with larger nuclei and an almost epithelioid appearance may be present. Cells with more abundant eosinophilic cytoplasm and cytoplasmic cross striations may also be identified (Fig. 5.9c) but these are typically difficult to find, are not present in all cases and are not necessary for the diagnosis. Islands of hyaline or cellular, but benign, cartilage are a common feature being found in approximately 50 % of these neoplasms (Fig. 5.9d), a much higher incidence than in embryonal rhabdomyosarcoma arising at other sites [21–25]. In occasional cases, there are foci resembling alveolar rhabdomyosarcoma or collections of pleomorphic cells with multilobated nuclei are present; the clinical significance of these features is uncertain [24, 27]. Hyaline globules may be present in association with the pleomorphic cells. There are commonly areas of haemorrhage with extravasated erythrocytes or necrosis. Positive nuclear staining with the skeletal muscle markers myogenin and myoD1 assists in diagnosis but typically only a minor proportion of the nuclei are immunoreactive (Fig. 5.10). Desmin is usually positive but it should be noted that normal cervical stroma is also desmin positive. Hormone receptors (ER and PR) are generally negative.

Given the polypoid nature of the lesion and the presence of a cambium layer, one of the main differential diagnoses is adenosarcoma with heterologous stromal elements, especially in those cases where glands are present deep within the core of the neoplasm. An absence of the typical phyllodes-like (club-like or leaf-like) architecture of adenosarcoma is helpful, as is the usual relative paucity of glands deep within the stroma. Adenosarcomas usually occur in an older age group. However, in some cases the distinction between embryonal rhabdomyosarcoma and adenosarcoma may be arbitrary and it is possible that some cervical embryonal rhabdomyosarcomas represent a form of adenosarcoma with heterologous stromal elements and stromal overgrowth. Given the hypocellular background, an unusual benign endocervical or endometrial polyp or endometriosis may also be considered in the differential diagnosis but these are usually easily excluded given the morphological features described above.

Most cervical embryonal rhabdomyosarcomas are treated by a combination of surgery (which may be radical or comprise local conservative excision) and chemotherapy and the overall prognosis is good with an 80 % overall survival [21, 24, 25]. The main adverse prognostic feature is deep invasion of the cervical stroma but this is uncommon.

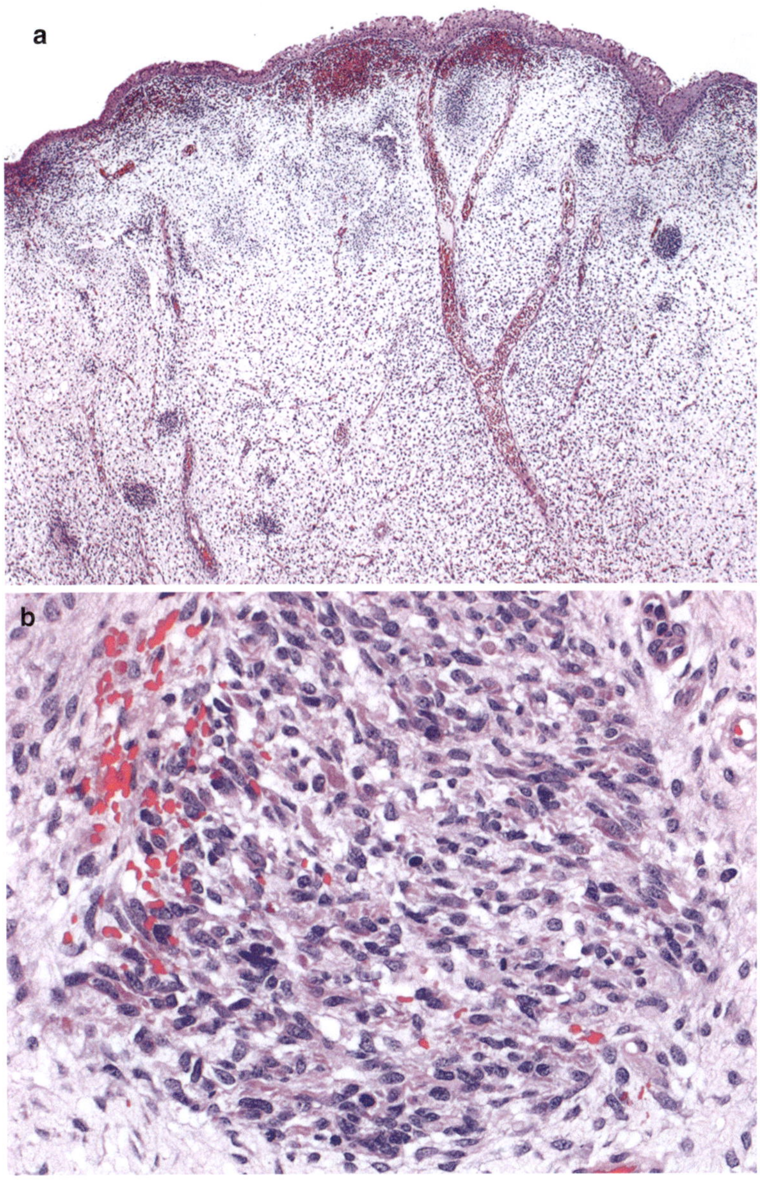

Fig. 5.9 Embryonal rhabdomyosarcoma of cervix with low power polypoid architecture. The lesion is covered by squamous epithelium and the underlying stroma is somewhat oedematous with cellular foci (**a**). Cellular aggregates exhibiting mitotic activity (**b**). Collections of cells with more abundant eosinophilic cytoplasm are present in some cases (**c**). Islands of cellular cartilage are present in some cases (**d**)

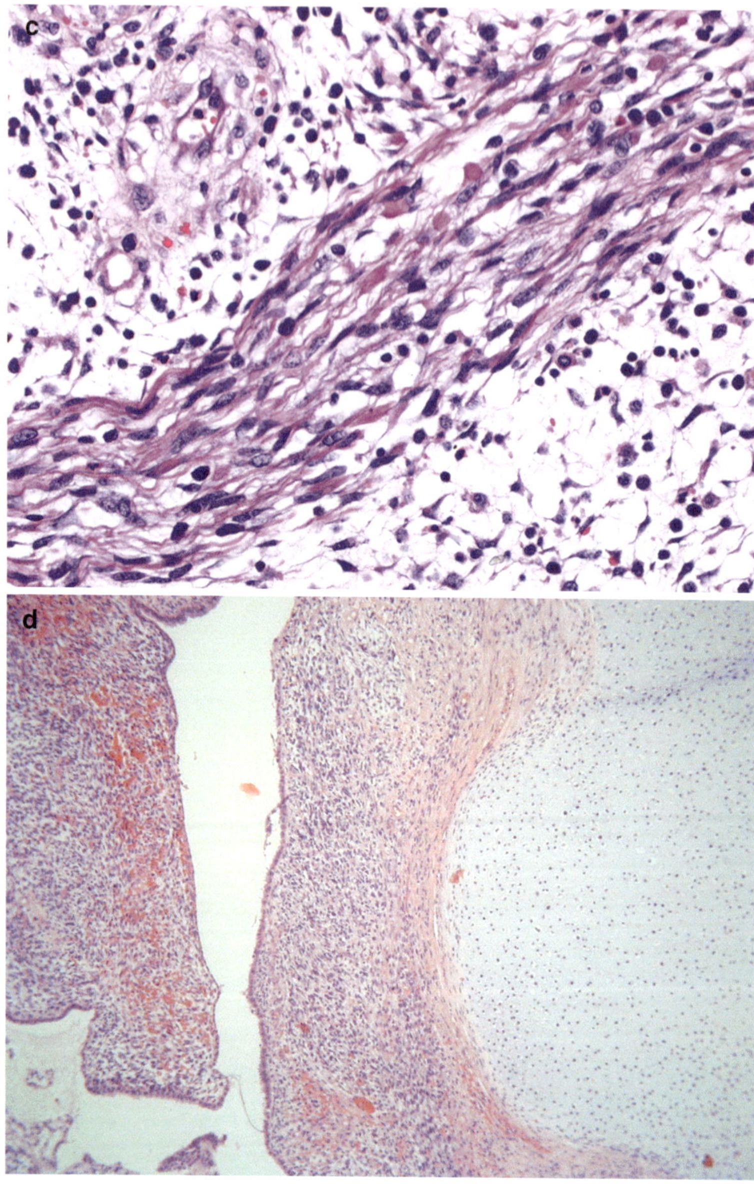

Fig. 5.9 (continued)

Myofibroblastoma of the Lower Female Genital Tract

Myofibroblastoma of the lower female genital (also referred to as superficial cervicovaginal myofibroblastoma) is an uncommon mesenchymal neoplasm most commonly occurring in the vagina but also arising more uncommonly in the cervix [28–30].

This lesion was first described by Laskin et al. who reported a distinctive mesenchymal tumour arising in the superficial lamina propria of the cervix and vagina [28]. The term superficial cervicovaginal myofibroblastoma was proposed to encompass the superficial location in the cervix or vagina and presumed myofibroblastic differentiation. A subsequent series of cases involved the vagina and the vulva and the term superficial myofibroblastoma of the lower female genital tract was proposed since some neoplasms have a vulval location [29].

These neoplasms occur in premenopausal or postmenopausal women and usually present as

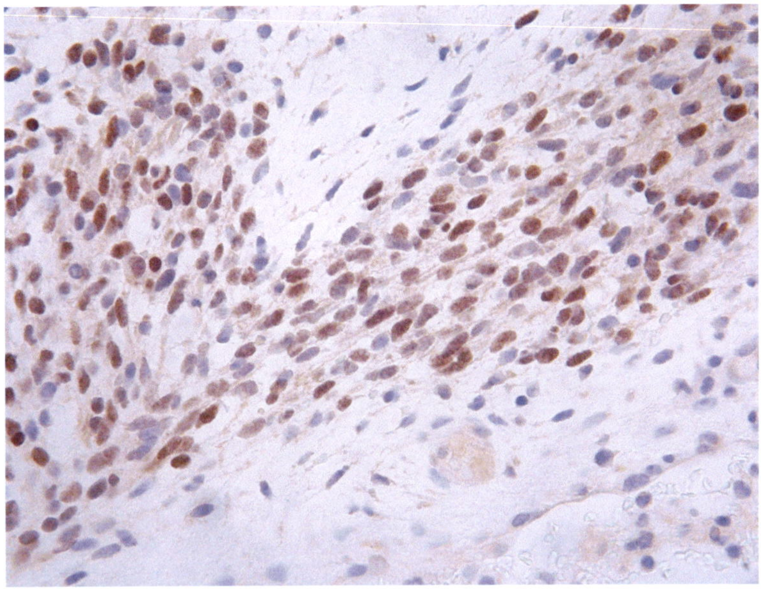

Fig. 5.10 Cervical embryonal rhabdomyosarcoma exhibiting nuclear staining with myogenin

polypoid lesions. Some patients have been taking tamoxifen, raising the possibility of an association with this medication [28–30]. Based on the morphology and follow up, superficial myofibroblastoma of the lower female genital tract is a benign lesion, although there is uncommonly local recurrence following excision [28–30]. Metastasis or malignant transformation has not been reported.

Grossly these are well circumscribed and are often, but not always, polypoid in appearance. Histological examination shows a well-circumscribed but unencapsulated lesion covered by unremarkable squamous or glandular epithelium. Deep to the surface epithelium, there is usually an uninvolved Grenz zone, although sometimes the lesion extends up to the epithelial-stromal junction. There are typically areas of varying cellularity, the constituent cells having bland ovoid, spindled or stellate nuclei, sometimes with a somewhat wavy appearance, embedded in a finely collagenous stroma, sometimes with thicker collagen bundles (Fig. 5.11a). Multiple architectural patterns, including lace-like, sieve-like and fascicular, which result in a heterogeneous appearance, are a characteristic feature, as are myxoid or oedematous foci. Few or no mitoses are present.

The cells are positive with vimentin and usually with desmin [28–30]. CD34 and smooth muscle actin (SMA) are positive in some cases and most are ER and PR positive. S100, EMA, h-caldesmon, HMGA2 and cytokeratins are negative. Desmin staining typically highlights the ramifying dendritic processes of many of the tumour cells (Fig. 5.11b) [28–30]. The immunophenotype is nonspecific and identical to that of many of the other site specific mesenchymal lesions which involve the lower female genital tract, especially the vulva and vagina.

The main differential diagnosis in the cervix is likely to be an unusual endocervical polyp and focally the stroma of endocervical polyps may resemble myofibroblastoma of the lower female genital tract. However, mucinous glands are usually present throughout endocervical polyps while more than an occasional entrapped gland is unusual in myofibroblastoma of the lower female genital tract. A fibroepithelial polyp may also enter into the differential diagnosis. The Grenz zone which is typical of superficial myofibroblastoma of the lower female genital tract is not a feature of fibroepithelial polyp and the former is characterised by a more heterogenous appearance with a variety of architectural patterns. Negative staining with S100 helps to exclude a neural lesion since some of the morphological features, such as the presence of wavy nuclei, may raise this possibility.

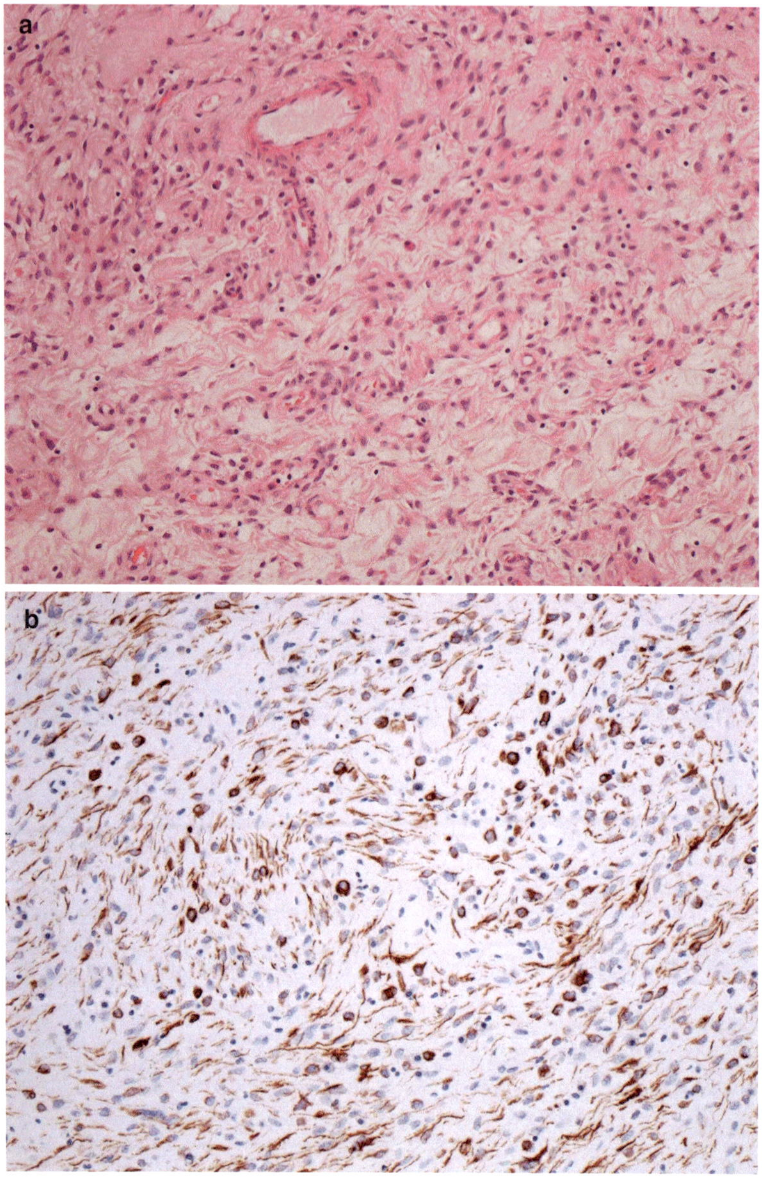

Fig. 5.11 Superficial myofibroblastoma of the lower female genital tract with bland spindle shaped cells in an oedematous stroma (**a**). There is diffuse staining with desmin which highlights dendritic cell processes (**b**)

Other Mesenchymal Neoplasms

Other mesenchymal tumours reported as primary neoplasms in the cervix include endometrial stromal neoplasms, uterine tumour resembling ovarian sex cord tumour (UTROSCT), alveolar soft part sarcoma (more common in cervix than uterine corpus), inflammatory myofibroblastic tumour, epithelioid sarcoma, perivascular epithelioid cell tumour (PEComa), malignant rhabdoid tumour, schwannoma, neurofibroma, haemangioma, liposarcoma, tumours in the Ewing family and malignant peripheral nerve sheath tumour (malignant schwannoma) [31–38-reviewed in 38]. The morphological features are identical to when these tumours occur at more usual sites but the pathologist may not think of the diagnosis given the rarity of these neoplasms in the cervix. Three cases of an S100 and CD34 positive cervical sarcoma which the authors termed fibroblastic malignant peripheral nerve sheath tumour (neurofibrosarcoma) have been

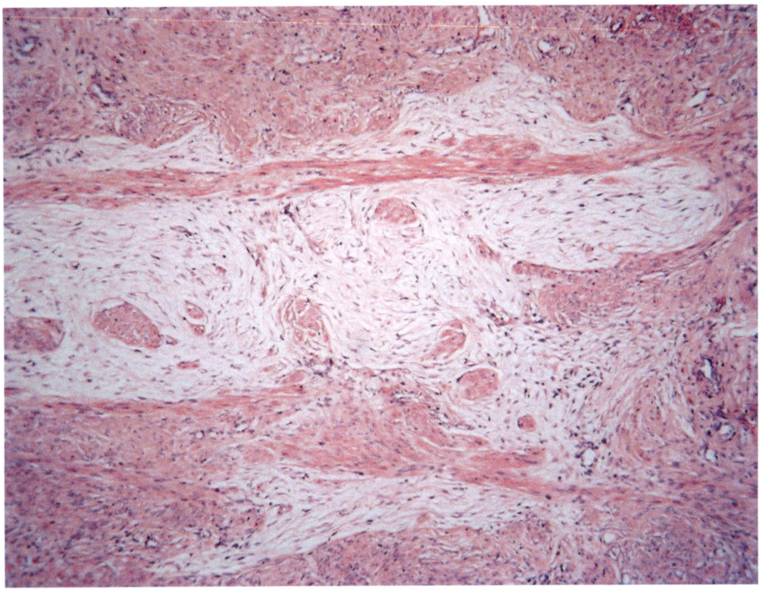

Fig. 5.12 Pseudoneoplastic myxoid change of cervical stroma

reported [39]. Rare cases of pseudoneoplastic myxoid change of the cervical stroma have been reported (Fig. 5.12) [40]. Fibroepithelial polyps, similar to those occurring in the vulva or vagina, rarely arise within the cervix and may contain a population of atypical stromal fibroblasts.

Mixed Epithelial and Mesenchymal Neoplasms

The same variety of mixed epithelial and mesenchymal neoplasms (mixed Mullerian tumours) that affect the uterine corpus, namely carcinosarcoma, adenofibroma and adenosarcoma, occur more uncommonly in the cervix. It is doubtful whether the entity of carcinofibroma exists and a primary cervical example has never been reported.

Carcinosarcoma

Carcinosarcomas of the cervix are much more uncommon than their counterpart within the uterine corpus [41]. Morphologically they are characterized by a malignant epithelial and mesenchymal component, both of which are typically high grade and sharply demarcated from one another. The epithelial component may be squamous, glandular of various types or undifferentiated. Compared to carcinosarcomas of the uterine corpus, the epithelial component is more likely to be squamous, adenoid cystic, adenoid cystic-like or adenoid basal in type (Fig. 5.13). The mesenchymal component may comprise undifferentiated sarcoma, fibrosarcoma, leiomyosarcoma or heterologous elements such as chondrosarcoma or rhabdomyosarcoma may be present. Before making a diagnosis of a primary carcinosarcoma of the cervix, spread from a neoplasm in the uterine corpus should be excluded. Carcinosarcoma of the cervix with a squamous element should be distinguished from squamous carcinoma with a spindle cell component (spindle cell squamous carcinoma); positive staining with cytokeratins or p63 in the spindle cell elements may assist in diagnosing spindle cell squamous carcinoma, although expression of these markers is often absent or markedly reduced in the spindle cells.

Adenofibroma and Adenosarcoma

Adenofibroma and adenosarcoma are rare primary cervical neoplasms and are much more uncommon than their counterparts in the uterine

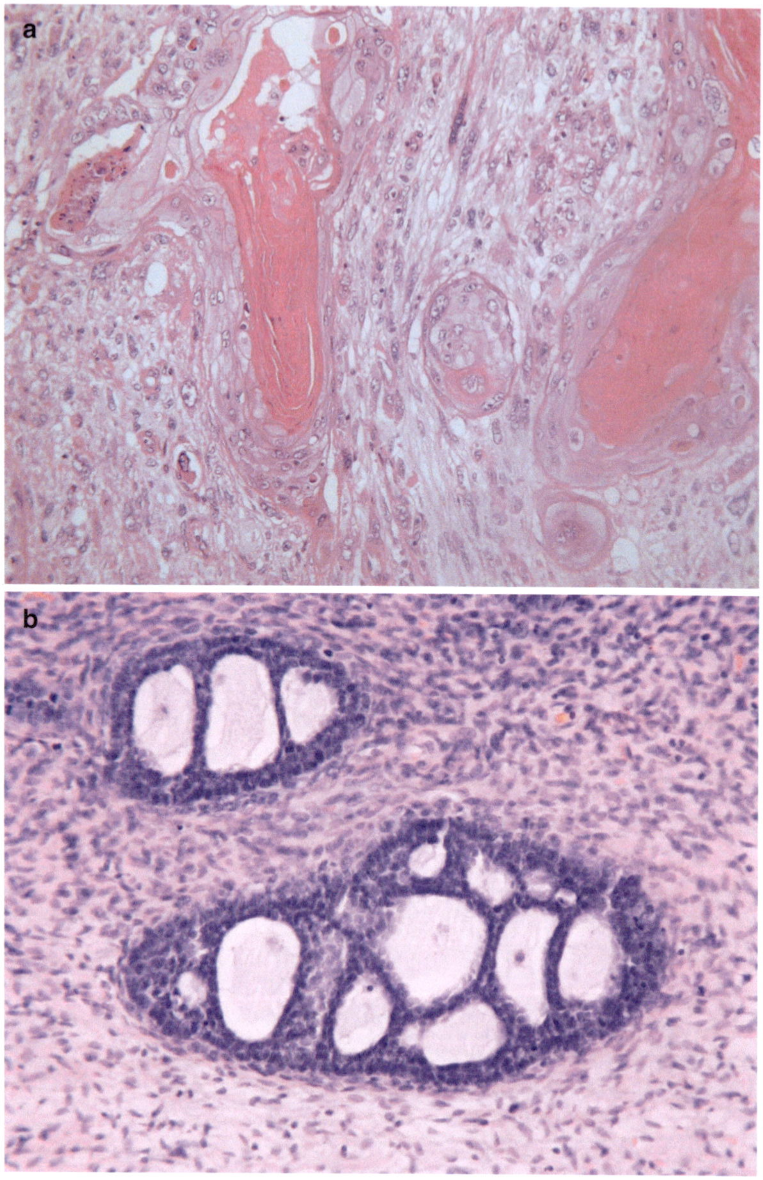

Fig. 5.13 Carcinosarcoma of cervix composed of malignant epithelial and mesenchymal components. The epithelial element is squamous in type (**a**). In (**b**) the epithelial component is adenoid cystic-like

corpus which may involve the cervix [42, 43]. They are composed of a benign epithelial component and a stromal component which is benign (adenofibroma) or malignant (adenosarcoma). Adenofibroma is more uncommon than adenosarcoma and some doubt the existence of the former [42, 44]. Grossly these are usually polypoid lesions, sometimes with a lobulated architecture or a "spongy" appearance on cut surface, which project into the cervical canal (Fig. 5.14a). Morphologically, the low power architecture is "club-like", "leaf-like" or "phyllodes-like" (Fig. 5.14b). The surface is covered by benign glandular epithelium of a variety of Mullerian types; there may be foci of squamous epithelium. The stromal component is usually morphologically quite bland and non-descript fibrous or endometrial stromal-like. According to the WHO, adenosarcoma is distinguished from adenofibroma by increased cellularity surrounding the epithelial elements (cambium layer) and stromal atypia and mitotic activity in excess of 2 per 10 high power fields (Fig. 5.14c) [42–44]. However, in practice, a diagnosis of adenosarcoma is usually made in the absence of this degree of mitotic activity if the characteristic low power architecture and cambium layer are present [42]. Sometimes, there is focal "sex cord-like" differentiation within the stromal component where the stromal cells have an epithelioid appearance and are arranged in nests, cords and trabeculae, resembling ovarian sex cord cells (Fig. 5.14d). Rarely there are heterologous elements in the form of rhabdomyoblasts or cartilage.

The treatment of choice of these neoplasms is hysterectomy given the risk of recurrence following polypectomy. Even adenofibromas may recur. The main adverse prognostic features with adenosarcoma are deep stromal invasion and sarcomatous overgrowth, both of which are uncommon [42]. Sarcomatous overgrowth is defined as areas of pure sarcoma without epithelium involving greater than 25 % of the neoplasm.

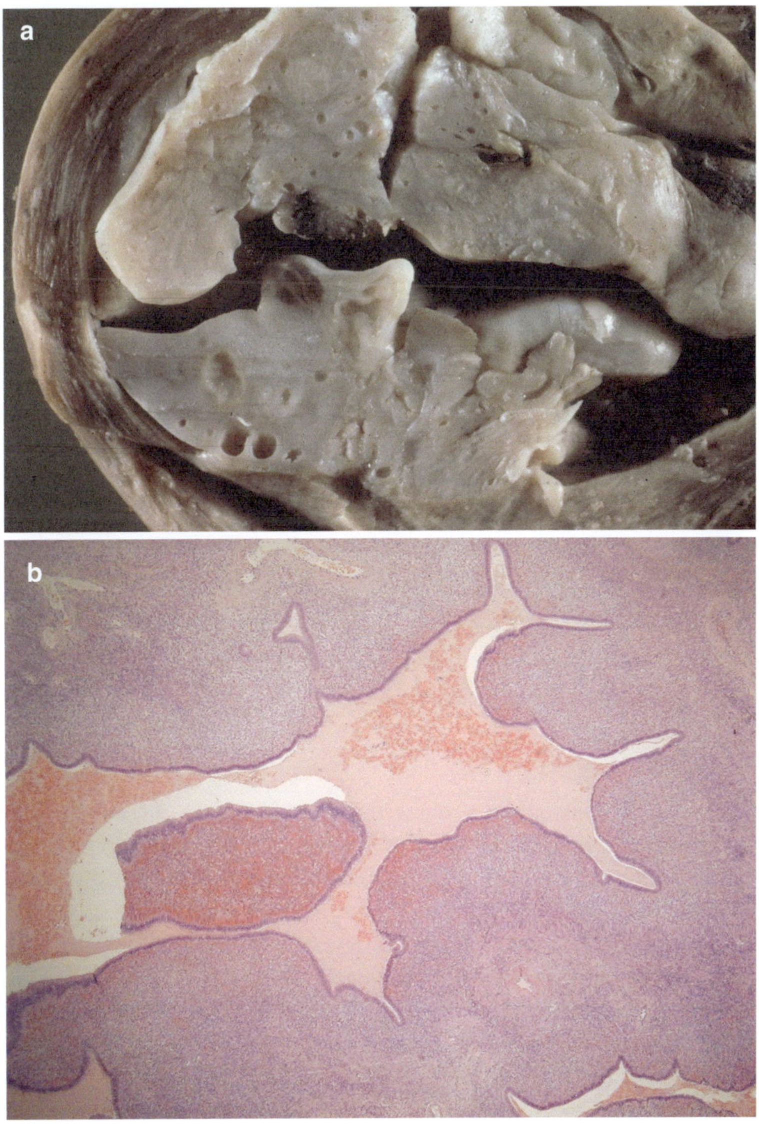

Fig. 5.14 Adenosarcoma of cervix exhibiting gross lobulated architecture (**a**). On low power there is a "phyllodes-like" architecture with increased cellularity around glands (cambium layer) (**b**). There is mitotic activity within the cambium layer (**c**). Adenosarcoma exhibiting sex cord-like foci within the stromal component (**d**)

Fig. 5.14 (continued)

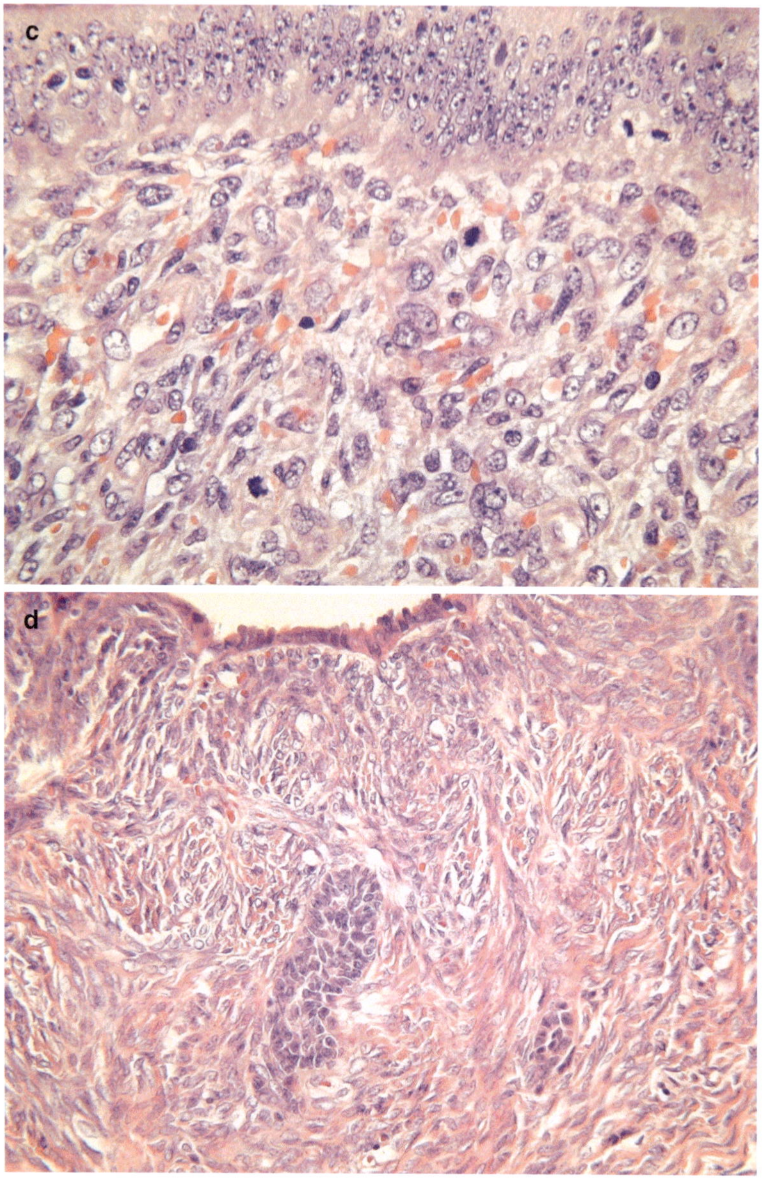

The areas of sarcomatous overgrowth, which often comprise much more than 25 % of the neoplasm such that residual benign epithelium may be identified only focally, are usually composed of poorly differentiated sarcoma, resembling undifferentiated sarcoma, with much more atypia and mitotic activity than in the sarcomatous element of the residual adenosarcoma. As such, this can be regarded as dedifferentiation of the low grade stromal component. Heterologous elements, most commonly rhabdomyosarcoma, may be present in the areas of sarcomatous overgrowth.

Previously, there was no staging system for uterine adenosarcoma but FIGO staging systems for uterine sarcomas were published in 2009 [45]. Adenosarcomas have a separate staging system to leiomyosarcomas and endometrial stromal sarcomas. Stage 1 adenosarcomas are confined to the uterus (corpus and cervix) with substages of 1A, 1B and 1C (tumour limited to endometrium/endocervix with no myometrial invasion, less than or equal to half myometrial invasion, more than half myometrial invasion respectively) [45].

It has been proposed to combine adenofibroma and adenosarcoma into a single category of mixed epithelial and stromal neoplasm and recognise that these are a spectrum of tumours composed of a benign epithelial component and a stromal element which is an integral part of the neoplasm and which is generally of low grade malignancy [42, 44]. One reason for this is that it has been shown that occasional tumours which would be categorised as adenofibroma on the basis of mitotic count can recur or even metastasise [45]. Additionally, there are multiple problems in counting mitotic figures with significant interobserver variation amongst pathologists.

Occasional benign endocervical (or endometrial) polyps contain focal areas which raise the possibility of a lesion in the adenofibroma/adenosarcoma category. For example, focally there may be a "phyllodes-like" architecture and/or increased cellularity surrounding the glands. Such cases are best reported as benign endocervical polyps with unusual features and follow up in such cases is usually uneventful [46]. The differential diagnosis between adenosarcoma and embryonal rhabdomyosarcoma is discussed in the section on "Embryonal rhabdomyosarcoma".

Haematopoietic Lesions

Lymphomas and Leukaemias

Lymphomas and leukaemias uncommonly involve the cervix, usually as part of a systemic process [47, 48]. Rare primary cervical lymphomas occur but strict criteria should be used to exclude spread from elsewhere. Primary cervical lymphomas are most commonly of diffuse large B cell or follicular type but a variety of rarer types have also been reported. In primary cervical lymphomas, there is often a subepithelial zone of uninvolved stroma with entrapmenent of endocervical glands and intact surface epithelium. There is usually deep stromal invasion with a nodular pattern. One peculiar feature is the tendency for primary cervical lymphomas to exhibit marked sclerosis which can result in "epithelial" patterns, including single cells, groups and cords; this may to some extent obscure the underlying lymphoid nature of the lesion [49] (Fig. 5.15). Cytoplasmic clearing may also be present. Immunohistochemistry and/or molecular studies are necessary for diagnosis and precise classification. Primary cervical lymphomas are not uncommonly misdiagnosed by the pathologist since lymphomas are rare at this site and the morphological features may be

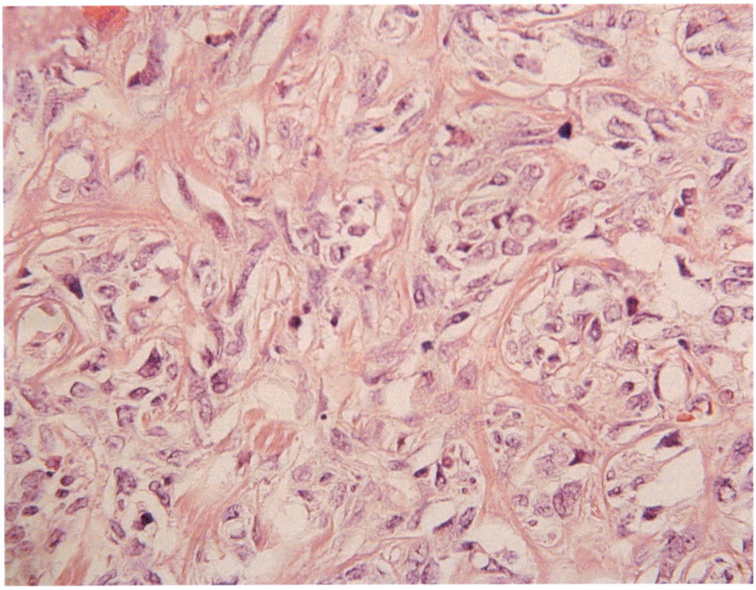

Fig. 5.15 Diffuse large B cell lymphoma of the cervix exhibiting cytoplasmic clearing and marked sclerosis which may obscure the underlying lymphoid nature of the lesion

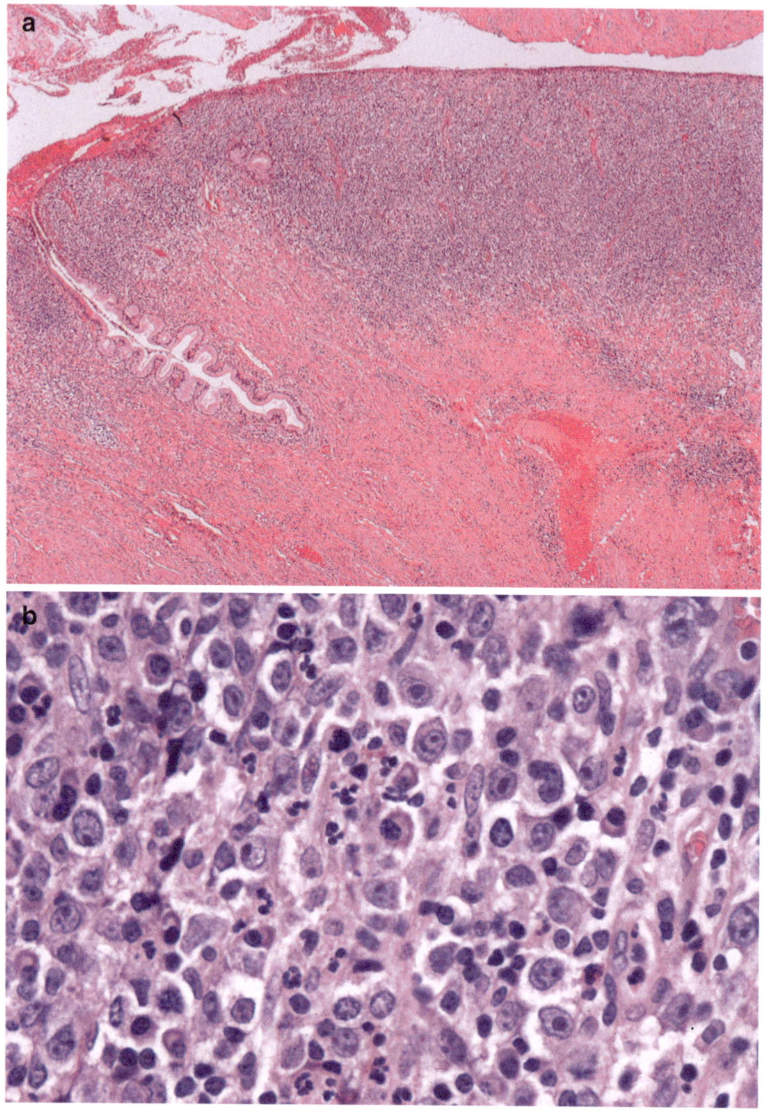

Fig. 5.16 Lymphoma-like lesion with dense band of lymphoid cells involving the mucosal surface of the cervix which is ulcerated (**a**). On high power, there is a polymorphous population of cells with significant numbers of blasts (**b**)

confused with another neoplasm or even an inflammatory process.

Lymphoma-Like Lesion

This uncommon lesion usually occurs in women in the reproductive years [50, 51]. It is most common in the cervix but may also involve the endometrium. Rare cases have been associated with cytomegalovirus or Epstein Barr virus. It has also been suggested that a prior surgical procedure may be an aetiological factor [52]. Although there may be surface ulceration, lymphoma-like lesion is usually an incidental microscopic finding, in contrast to lymphoma which typically forms a mass and this may be useful in the distinction. Lymphoma-like lesion is morphologically composed of a dense infiltrate of lymphoid cells which may result in consideration of a lymphoma. The lymphoid infiltrate is usually band-like and is situated just deep to the surface mucosa which, as stated, may be ulcerated (Fig. 5.16a). There is no deep extension. The lymphoid population is polymorphic but significant numbers of large blasts exhibiting mitotic activity can be present (Fig. 5.16b).

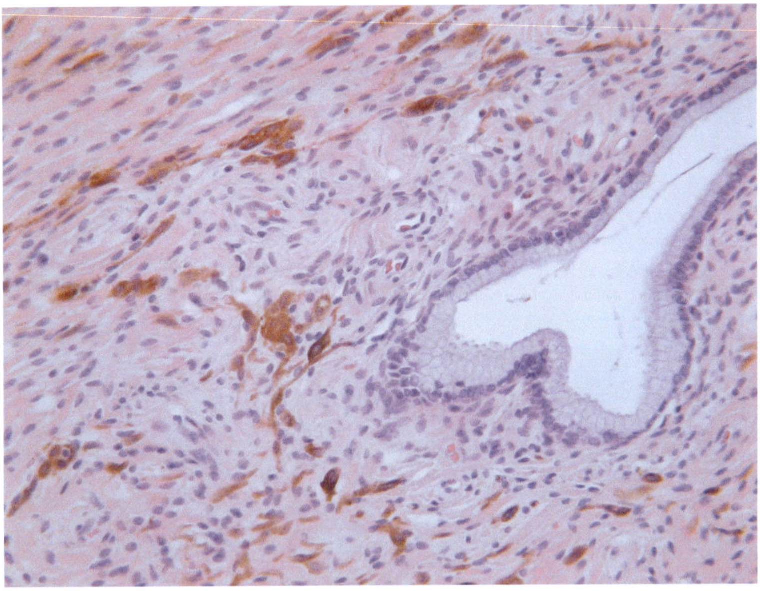

Fig. 5.17 Blue naevus of cervix composed of spindle shaped cells with melanin pigment

Plasma cells, lymphocytes and polymorphs are often admixed. Immunohistochemical studies show a mixture of B and T lymphoid cells without evidence of light chain restriction. Occasional cases exhibit clonal immunoglobulin heavy chain gene rearrangement which does not warrant a diagnosis of lymphoma [50].

Melanocytic Neoplasms

Primary melanocytic neoplasms are rare within the cervix but benign and malignant variants occasionally occur. They may arise from melanin containing cells (melanocytes) which have been identified in cervical epithelium. The most common benign melanocytic lesion in the cervix is a blue naevus [53]. This is usually an incidental microscopic finding but occasionally is visible grossly as an area of pigmentation. Blue naevus consists of S100 positive polygonal and spindle cells containing melanin pigment within the superficial cervical stroma (Fig. 5.17). Melanosis is characterized by an area of mucosal pigmentation on gross examination. Histology shows pigmentation of the basal layers of the squamous epithelium with or without the presence of basal melanocytes [54].

Malignant melanomas also occur rarely within the cervix and are morphologically similar to melanomas elsewhere [55]. They are usually composed of polygonal or spindle cells or a combination with intracytoplasmic pigment, although some can be amelanotic. Before diagnosing a primary cervical malignant melanoma, a metastasis or direct spread from elsewhere, for example the vagina, should be excluded. Adjacent in situ melanoma is useful in helping to confirm a primary cervical neoplasm. However, occasionally secondary melanomas in the cervix can exhibit an intraepidermal growth pattern which can mimic in situ melanoma. As in other sites, primary cervical malignant melanomas can mimic a variety of other neoplasms and the pathologist should always suspect this diagnosis, especially with a poorly differentiated tumour. Positive staining with melanocytic markers (S100, HMB45, melan-A) assists in establishing the diagnosis.

Miscellaneous Neoplasms

Miscellanous neoplasms which rarely arise in the cervix include trophoblastic tumours, yolk sac tumour, teratomas and extramammary Paget's disease [56, 57].

References

1. Tavassoli FA, Devilee P, editors. World Health Organization classification of tumours. Pathology and genetics. Tumours of the breast and female genital organs. Lyon: IARC Press; 2003.
2. Gilks CB, Young RH, Gersell DJ, Clement PB. Large cell neuroendocrine carcinoma of the uterine cervix: a clinicopathologic study of 12 cases. Am J Surg Pathol. 1997;21:905–14.
3. Albores-Saavedra J, Martinez-Benitez B, Luevano E. Small cell carcinomas and large cell neuroendocrine carcinomas of the endometrium and cervix: polypoid tumors and those arising in polyps may have a favourable prognosis. Int J Gynecol Pathol. 2008;27:333–9.
4. Sato Y, Shimamoto T, Amada S, et al. Large cell neuroendocrine carcinoma of the uterine cervix: a clinicopathological study of six cases. Int J Gynecol Pathol. 2003;22:226–30.
5. Conner MG, Richter H, Moran CA, et al. Small cell carcinoma of the cervix: a clinicopathologic and immunohistochemical study of 23 cases. Ann Diagn Pathol. 2002;6:345–8.
6. Grayson W, Rhemtula HA, Taylor LF, et al. Detection of human papillomavirus in large cell neuroendocrine carcinoma of the uterine cervix: a study of 12 cases. J Clin Pathol. 2002;55:108–14.
7. Ishida GM, Kato N, Hayasaka T, et al. Small cell neuroendocrine carcinomas of the uterine cervix: a histological, immunohistochemical and molecular genetic study. Int J Gynecol Pathol. 2004;23: 366–72.
8. Stoler MH, Mills SE, Gersell DJ, Walker AN. Small-cell neuroendocrine carcinoma of the cervix. A human papillomavirus type 18-associated cancer. Am J Surg Pathol. 1991;15:28–32.
9. Travis WD, Linnoila RI, Tsokos MG, et al. Neuroendocrine tumors of the lung with proposed criteria for large-cell neuroendocrine carcinoma. An ultrastructural, immunohistochemical and flow cytometric study of 35 cases. Am J Surg Pathol. 1991;15: 529–53.
10. Chavez-Blanco A, Taja-Chayeb L, Cetina L, et al. Neuroendocrine marker expression in cervical carcinomas of non-small cell type. Int J Gynecol Pathol. 2002;21:368–74.
11. Savargaonkar PR, Hale RJ, Mutton A, Manning V, Buckley CH. Neuroendocrine differentiation in cervical carcinoma. J Clin Pathol. 1996;49:139–41.
12. McCluggage WG, Kennedy K, Busam KJ. An immunohistochemical study of cervical neuroendocrine carcinomas: neoplasms that are commonly TTF1 positive and which may express CK20 and P63. Am J Surg Pathol. 2010;34:525–32.
13. Li JD, Zhuang Y, Li YF, et al. A clinicopathological aspect of primary small-cell carcinoma of the uterine cervix: a single-centre study of 25 cases. J Clin Pathol. 2011;64:1102–7.
14. Wang TY, Chen BF, Yang YC, et al. Histologic and immunophenotypic classification of cervical carcinomas by expression of the p53 homologue p63: a study of 250 cases. Hum Pathol. 2001;32:479–86.
15. Houghton O, McCluggage WG. The expression and diagnostic utility of p63 in the female genital tract. Adv Anat Pathol. 2009;16:316–21.
16. Koenig C, Turnicky RP, Knakam CF, et al. Papillary squamotransitional cell carcinoma of the cervix. Report of 32 cases. Am J Surg Pathol. 1997;21:915–21.
17. Albores-Saavadra J, Young RH. Transitional cell neoplasms (carcinomas and inverted papillomas) of the uterine cervix. A report of five cases. Am J Surg Pathol. 1995;19:1138–45.
18. Lininger RA, Wistuba I, Gazdar A, et al. Human papillomavirus type 16 is detected in transitional cell carcinomas and squamotransitional cell carcinomas of the cervix and endometrium. Cancer. 1998;83:521–7.
19. Robinson CE, Sarode VR, Albores-Saavadra J. Mixed papillary transitional cell carcinoma and adenocarcinoma of the uterine cervix: a clinicopathologic study of three cases. Int J Gynecol Pathol. 2003;22:220–5.
20. Hennell C, Jamison J, Wells M, McCluggage WG. Inverted papilloma of the cervix and vagina: report of 2 cases of a rare lesion associated with human papillomavirus 42. Hum Pathol. 2012;43:435–9.
21. Daya D, Scully RE. Sarcoma botryoides of the uterine cervix in young women: a clinicopathological analysis of 13 cases. Gynecol Oncol. 1998;29:290–304.
22. McClean GE, Kurian S, Walter N, Kekre A, McCluggage WG. Cervical embryonal rhabdomyosarcoma and ovarian Sertoli-Leydig cell tumour: a more than coincidental association of two rare neoplasms? J Clin Pathol. 2007;60:326–8.
23. Golbang P, Khan A, Scurry J, MacIsaac I, Planner R. Cervical sarcoma botryoides and ovarian Sertoli-Leydig cell tumor. Gynecol Oncol. 1997;67:102–6.
24. Dehner LP, Jarzembowski JA, Hill DA. Embryonal rhabdomyosarcoma of the uterine cervix: a report of 14 cases and a discussion of its unusual clinicopathological associations. Mod Pathol. 2012;25:602–14.
25. Li FL, Gupta M, McCluggage WG, Ronnett BM. Embryonal rhabdomyosarcoma (botryoid type) of the uterine corpus and cervix in adult women: report of a case series and review of the literature. Am J Surg Pathol. 2013;37:344–55.
26. Foulkes WD, Bahubeshi A, Hamel N, et al. Expanding the phenotypes associated with DICER1 mutations. Hum Mutat. 2011;32:1381–4.
27. Houghton JP, McCluggage WG. Embryonal rhabdomyosarcoma of the cervix with focal pleomorphic areas. J Clin Pathol. 2007;60:88–9.
28. Laskin WB, Fetsch JF, Tavassoli FA. Superficial cervicovaginal myofibroblastoma: fourteen cases of a distinctive mesenchymal tumor arising from the specialized subepithelial stroma of the lower female genital tract. Hum Pathol. 2001;32:715–25.
29. Ganesan R, McCluggage WG, Hirschowitz L, Rollason TP. Superficial myofibroblastoma of the lower female genital tract: report of a series including tumours with a vulval location. Histopathology. 2005;46:137–43.

30. Stewart CJ, Amanuel B, Brennan BA, et al. Superficial cervicovaginal myofibroblastoma: a report of five cases. Pathology. 2005;37:144–8.
31. Nielsen GP, Oliva E, Young RH, et al. Alveolar soft-part sarcoma of the female genital tract. Int J Gynecol Pathol. 1995;24:131–5.
32. Rabban JT, Zaloudek CJ, Shekitka KM, Tavassoli FA. Inflammatory myofibroblastic tumor of the uterus: a clinicopathologic study of 6 cases emphasizing distinction from aggressive mesenchymal tumors. Am J Surg Pathol. 2005,29:1348–55.
33. Kabbani W, Deavers MT, Malpica A, et al. Uterine tumor resembling ovarian sex-cord tumor: report of a case mimicking cervical adenocarcinoma. Int J Gynecol Pathol. 2003;22:297–302.
34. Wei EX, Albores-Saavedra J, Fowler MR. Plexiform neurofibroma of the uterine cervix: a case report and review of the literature. Arch Pathol Lab Med. 2005;129:783–6.
35. Wang YC, Chen CH, Su HY, et al. Huge spindle cell hemangioma of the cervix mimicking a pelvic tumor. Gynecol Obstet Invest. 2005;60:98–101.
36. Keel SB, Clement PB, Prat J, Young RH. Malignant schwannoma of the uterine cervix: a study of three cases. Int J Gynecol Pathol. 1998;17:223–30.
37. Cenacchi G, Pasquinelli G, Montanaro L, et al. Primary endocervical extraosseous Ewing's sarcoma/PNET. Int J Gynecol Pathol. 1998;17:83–8.
38. Fadare O. Uncommon sarcomas of the uterine cervix: a review of selected entities. Diagn Pathol. 2006;1:30.
39. Mills AM, Karamchandani JR, Vogel H, Longacre TA. Endocervical fibroblastic malignant peripheral nerve sheath tumor (neurofibrosarcoma): report of a novel entity possibly related to endocervical CD34 fibrocytes. Am J Surg Pathol. 2011;35:404–12.
40. McCluggage WG, Young RH. Myxoid change of the myometrium and cervical stroma: description of a hitherto unreported non-neoplastic phenomenon with discussion of myxoid uterine lesions. Int J Gynecol Pathol. 2010;29:351–7.
41. Clement PB, Zubovits JT, Young RH, Scully RE. Malignant mullerian mixed tumors of the uterine cervix: a report of nine cases of a neoplasm with morphology often different from its counterpart in the corpus. Int J Gynecol Pathol. 1998;17:211–22.
42. McCluggage WG. Mullerian adenosarcoma of the female genital tract. Adv Anat Pathol. 2010;17:122–9.
43. Clement PB, Scully RE. Mullerian adenosarcoma of the uterus: a clinicopathologic analysis of 100 cases with a review of the literature. Hum Pathol. 1990;21:363–81.
44. Gallardo A, Prat J. Mullerian adenosarcoma: a clinicopathologic and immunohistochemical study of 55 cases challenging the existence of adenofibroma. Am J Surg Pathol. 2009;33:278–88.
45. Prat J. FIGO staging for uterine sarcomas. Int J Gynecol Obstet. 2009;104:177–8.
46. Howitt BE, Quade BJ, Nucci MR. Atypical uterine polyps sub-diagnostic of Mullerian adenosarcoma: a clinicopathologic analysis of 28 cases with long term follow-up. Mod Pathol. 2012;25(supp 2):1159.
47. Ferry JA, Young RH. Malignant lymphoma of the genitourinary tract. Curr Diagn Pathol. 1997;4:145–69.
48. Kosari F, Daneshbod Y, Parwaresch R, et al. Lymphomas of the female genital tract. A study of 186 cases and review of the literature. Am J Surg Pathol. 2005;29:1512–20.
49. Harris NL, Scully RE. Malignant lymphoma and granulocytic sarcoma of the uterus and vagina. A clinicopathologic analysis of 27 cases. Cancer. 1984;53:2530–5.
50. Geyer JT, Ferry JA, Harris NL, Young RH, Longtine JA, Zukerberg LR. Florid reactive lymphoid hyperplasia of the lower female genital tract (lymphoma-like lesion): a benign condition that frequently harbors clonal immunoglobulin heavy chain gene rearrangements. Am J Surg Pathol. 2010;34:161–8.
51. Young RH, Harris NL, Scully RE. Lymphoma-like lesions of the lower female genital tract: a report of 16 cases. Int J Gynecol Pathol. 1985;4:289–99.
52. Ramalingam P, Zoroquiain P, Valbuena JR, et al. Florid reactive lymphoid hyperplasia (lymphoma-like lesion) of the uterine cervix. Ann Diagn Pathol. 2012;16:21–8.
53. Patel DS, Bhagavan BS. Blue nevus of the uterine cervix. Hum Pathol. 1985;16:79–86.
54. Yilmaz AJ, Chandler P, Hahm GK, et al. Melanosis of the uterine cervix: a report of two cases and discussion of pigmented cervical lesions. Int J Gynecol Pathol. 1999;18:73–6.
55. Chan KC, Butz WR, Hapke MR. Primary malignant melanoma of the uterine cervix: case report with world literature review. Int J Gynecol Pathol. 1999;18:265–73.
56. Lloyd J, Evans DJ, Flanagan A. Extension of extramammary Paget disease of the vulva to the cervix. J Clin Pathol. 1999;52:538–40.
57. Copeland LJ, Sneige N, Ordonez NG, et al. Endodermal sinus tumor of the vagina and cervix. Cancer. 1985;55:2558–65.

Cytology of Glandular Lesions

6

John H.F. Smith

Abstract

In this chapter the appearance of in situ and invasive glandular neoplasms of the cervix and their cytological mimics will be described.

Keywords

Endocervix • Adenocarcinoma in situ • Cervical glandular intraepithelial neoplasia • AIS • CGIN • Adenocarcinoma of the cervix

Introduction

Although the histological appearance of adenocarcinoma in situ of the endocervix (AIS) was described by Friedel and McKay in 1953, it was not until nearly 20 years later that Barter and Waters provided the first description of the cytological manifestations of AIS in conventional cervical cytology preparations, which were subsequently expanded and refined by other workers, and the cytological appearances suggestive of invasive cervical adenocarcinoma described [1–7]. More recently, defining criteria to separate normal or metaplastic from neoplastic endocervical cells and the cytological appearances in the two most commonly used liquid based cytology systems have also been described [8–14].

Cervical Glandular Intraepithelial Neoplasia (CGIN)/Adenocarcinoma In Situ (AIS)

The cytological appearance of CGIN/AIS in both conventional and liquid-based cervical cytology preparations reflects the histological appearances described in Chap. 3 and it is often the abnormal microarchitecture of crowded cellular groups that first draws attention at routine screening magnification.

Sheets of exfoliated cells from CGIN present as variable sized groups of crowded cells with frequent overlapping nuclei of uniform size and loss of the "honeycomb" pattern of normal endocervical cells (Fig. 6.1). At the margin of the cell groups there may be disrupted crypt openings

W.G. McCluggage et al., *Cellular Pathology of Glandular Lesions and Uncommon Neoplasms of the Cervix*, DOI 10.1007/978-1-4471-2210-4_6, © Springer-Verlag London 2014

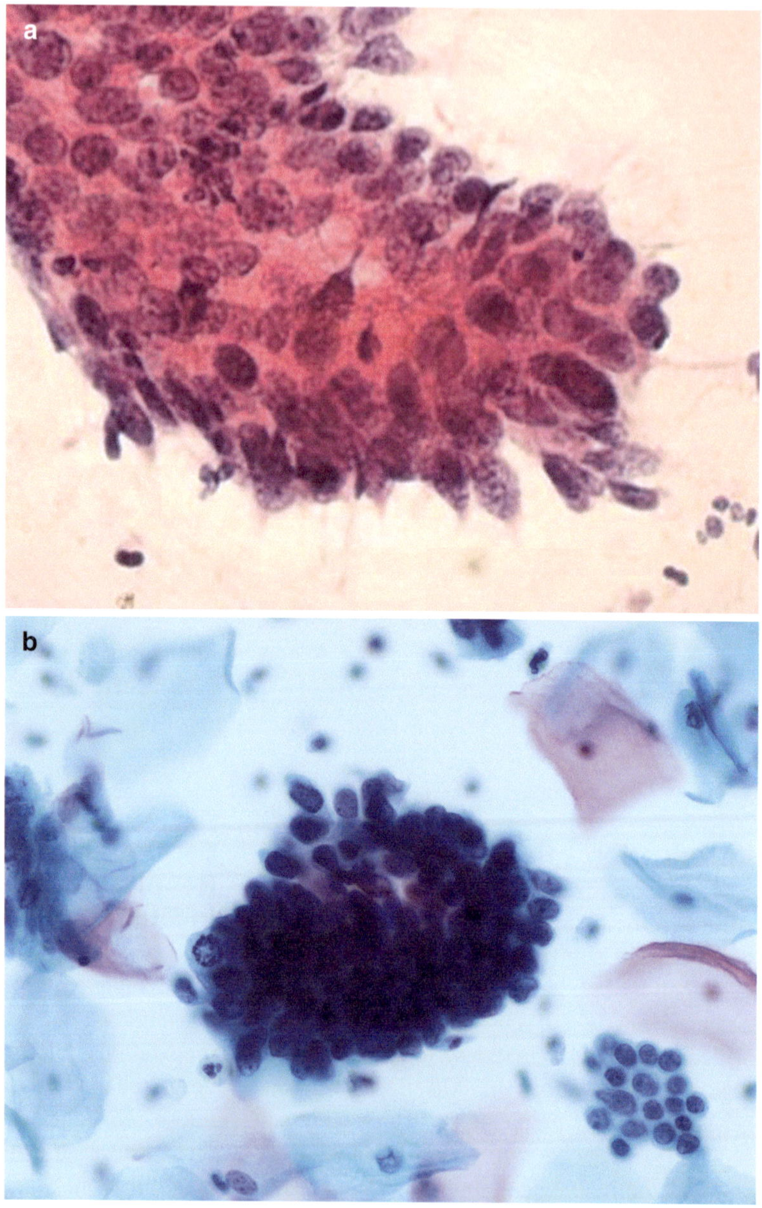

Fig. 6.1 A group of crowded disorganised atypical endocervical cells derived from adenocarcinoma in situ in a conventional cervical smear (**a**) and a SurePath LBC preparation (**b**)

and within the cell groups rosette formation, representing abortive attempts at glandular differentiation. Isolated rosettes may also be present (Fig. 6.2). In addition, at the margin of the cell groups, the nuclei of the constituent cells may lie at different levels (pseudostratification) and as a result of partial or complete loss of cytoplasm, bare nuclei or nuclei with tapering delicate cytoplasmic tags project from the crowded cell groups: an appearance first described as "feathering" by Pacey and colleagues in conventional cervical smears (Fig. 6.3). Although this appearance is less common and may be more subtle in liquid based cervical cytology preparations, it may still be a useful criteria to distinguish neoplastic glandular from squamous lesions in hyperchromatic crowded cell groups.

Cells derived from CGIN may also present as short strips with a straight or slightly curved contour in which there is pseudostratification of nuclei with a common cytoplasmic border (Fig. 6.4). Especially in SurePath liquid based cytology preparations the dyskaryotic nuclei tend to fan out resulting in an appearance resembling a bird's tail or fish tail (Fig. 6.5).

Isolated or loosely cohesive small groups of neoplastic glandular cells may also be present in the background and as described above frequently have delicate cytoplasm which tends to taper from the nucleus resulting in a so-called "snake and egg" effect (Fig. 6.6).

Cell nuclei, whether in individual cells or groups of cells, are usually of similar size to that of normal endocervical cell nuclei, show minimal anisonucleosis, and are oval in shape with smooth nuclear membranes of variable thickness. Nuclear chromatin is of even distribution but varies from fine to coarse granularity resulting in a

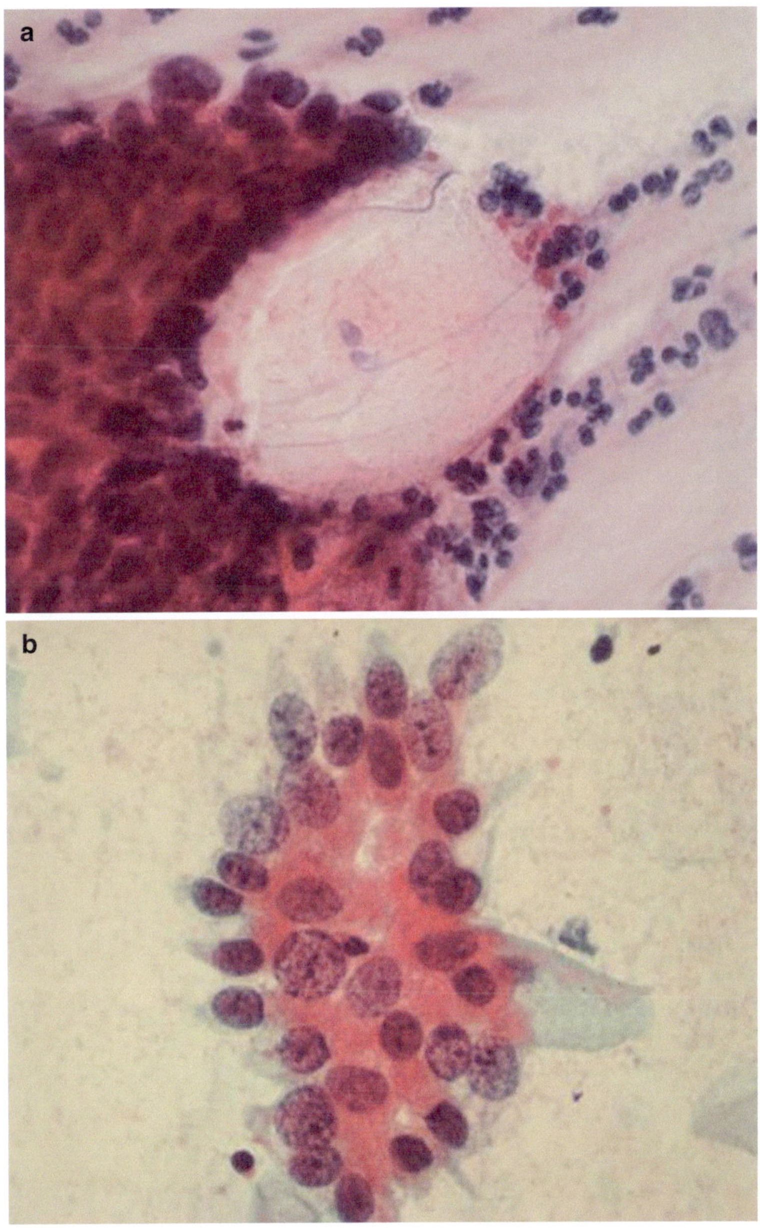

Fig. 6.2 Disrupted crypt opening ('torn open gland') at the edge of a group of cells derived from adenocarcinoma in situ in a conventional cervical smear (**a**) and rosette formation in a conventional cervical smear (**b**) and a SurePath LBC preparation (**c**)

Fig. 6.2 (continued)

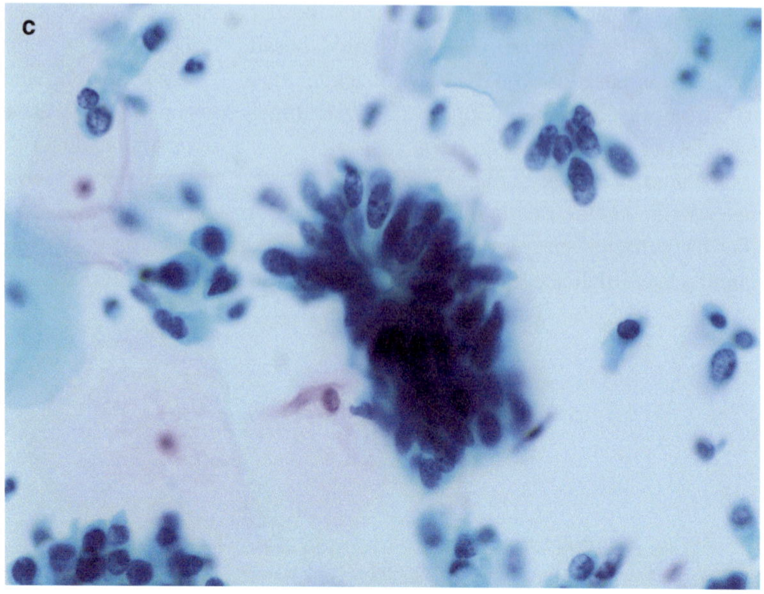

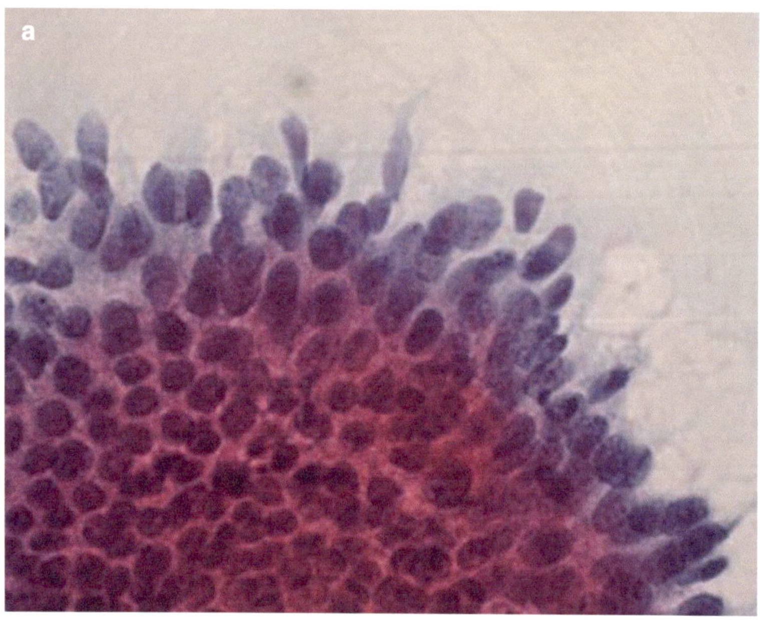

Fig. 6.3 "Feathering" in adenocarcinoma in situ in a conventional cervical smear (**a**) and a SurePath LBC preparation (**b**). Note the bare nuclei and nuclei with tapering delicate cytoplasmic tags projecting from the cell group

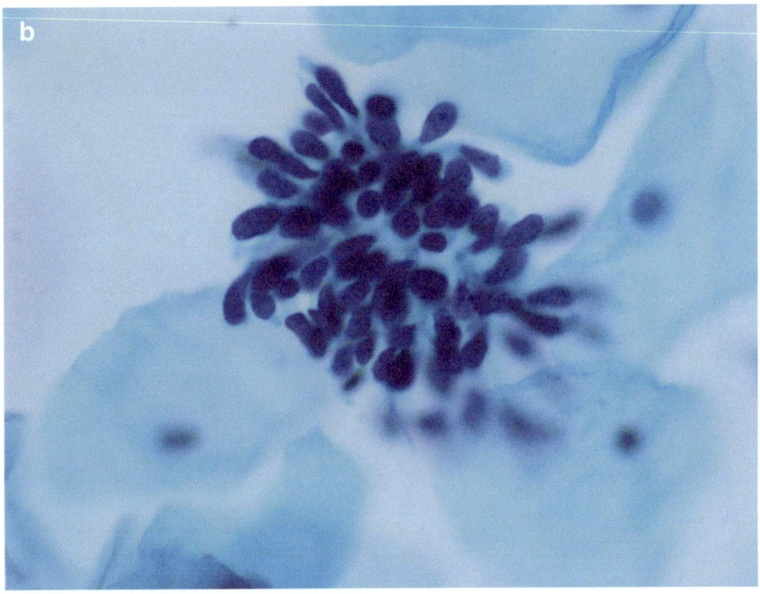

Fig. 6.3 (continued)

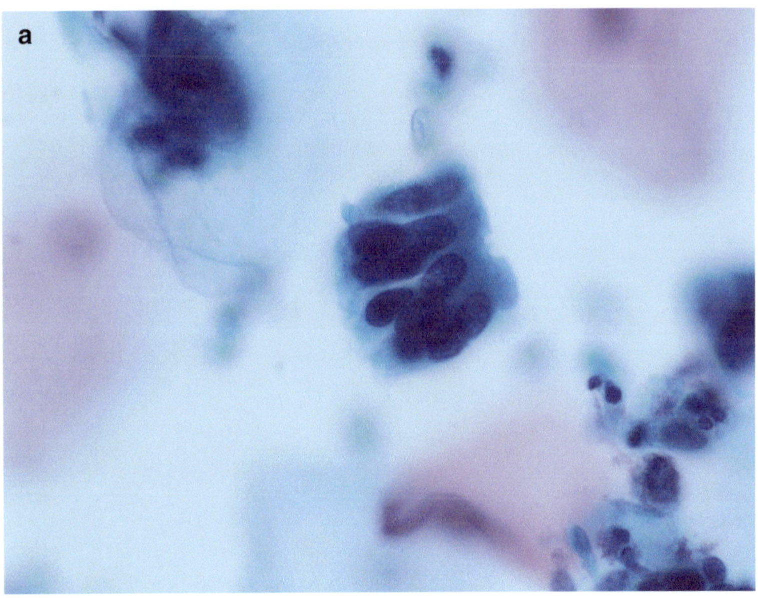

Fig. 6.4 Strips of cells from adenocarcinoma in situ with characteristic nuclear pseudostratification and a common cytoplasmic border (**a**, **b**). SurePath LBC

Fig. 6.4 (continued)

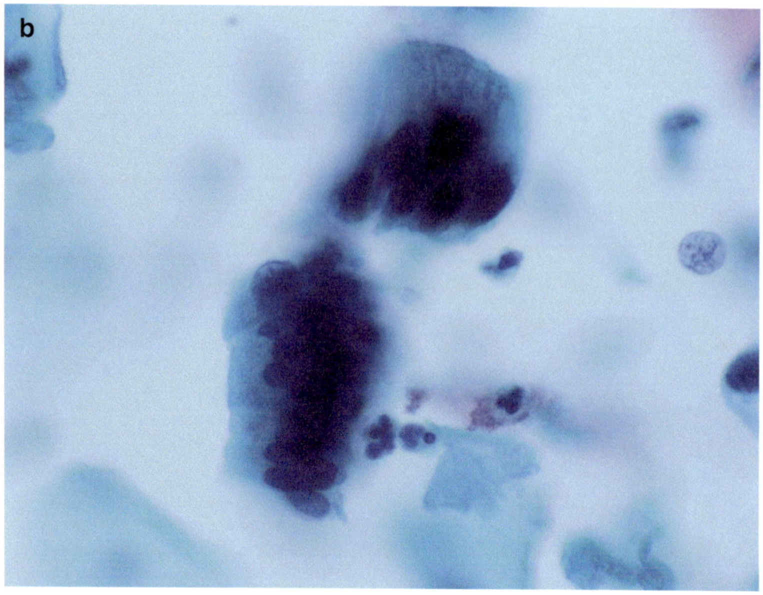

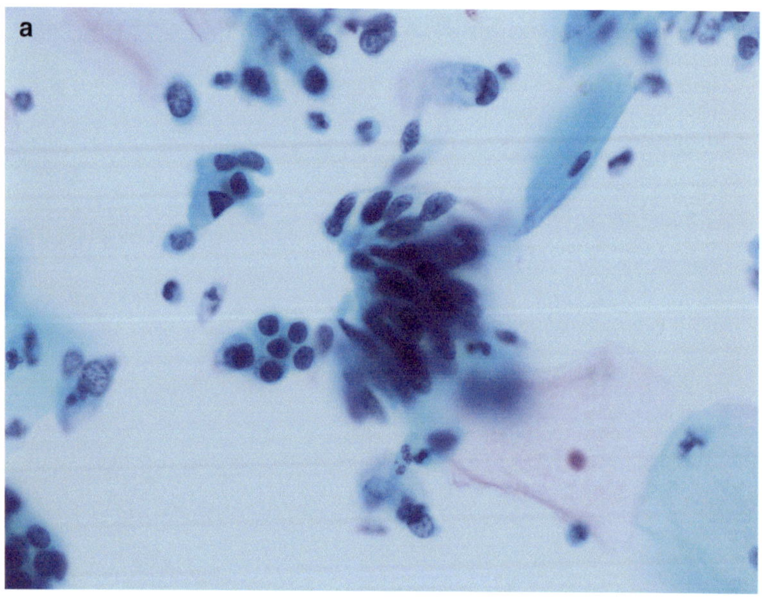

Fig. 6.5 Slightly curved pesudostratified strips of cells from adenocarcinoma in situ resembling a bird's tail or fish tail (**a**, **b**). SurePath LBC

Fig. 6.5 (continued)

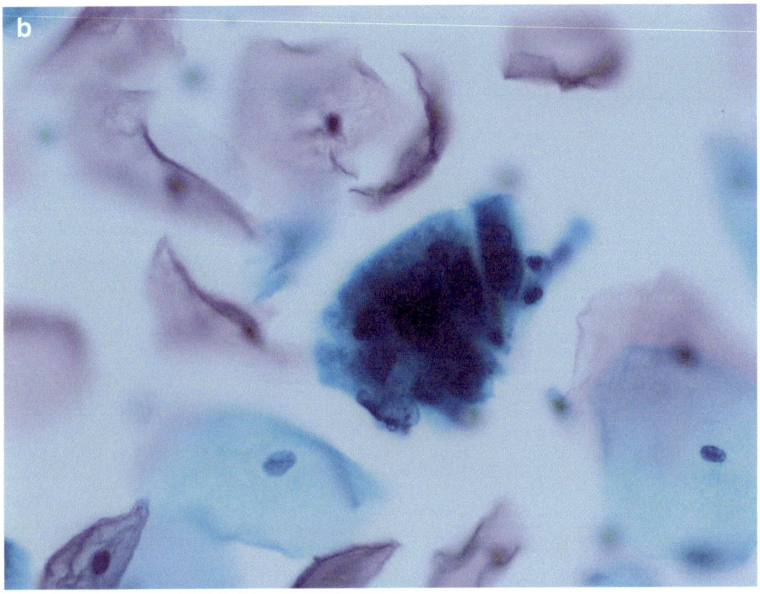

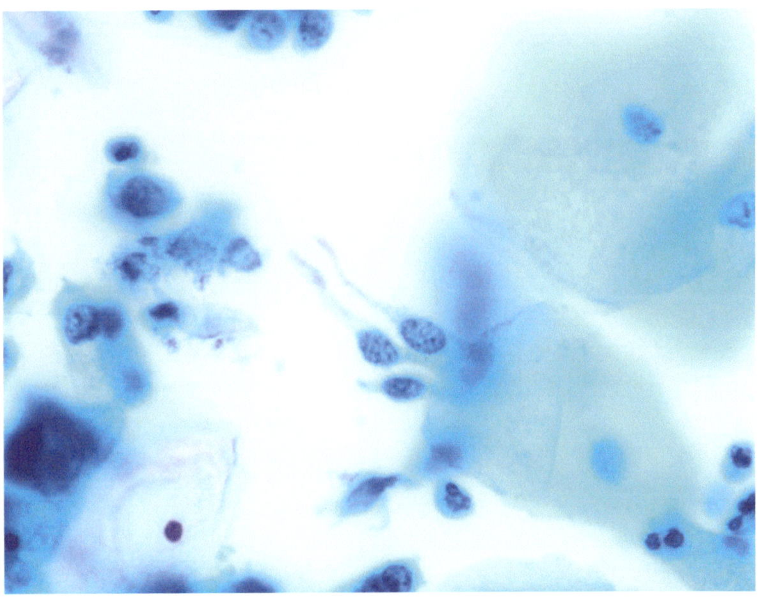

Fig. 6.6 Neoplastic glandular cells with tapering delicate cytoplasm – "snake and egg" appearance. Note the characteristic fine and coarse granular nuclear chromatin. SurePath LBC

"salt-and-pepper" appearance. Mitoses and apoptotic bodies are frequently identified in crowded cell groups and may be present in exfoliated strips of neoplastic endocervical cells.

The appearances described above relate to the usual or endocervical type of CGIN. In intestinal type CGIN individual cells with prominent solitary cytoplasmic vacuoles (goblet cells) are present and an extremely useful clue as to the neoplastic nature of the process (see Chap. 3) (Fig. 6.7). In endometrioid type CGIN the overall microarchitectural and cytomorphological features are similar to those of usual type CGIN but the individual cells have small even sized nuclei which are rounded rather than oval [15] (Fig. 6.8).

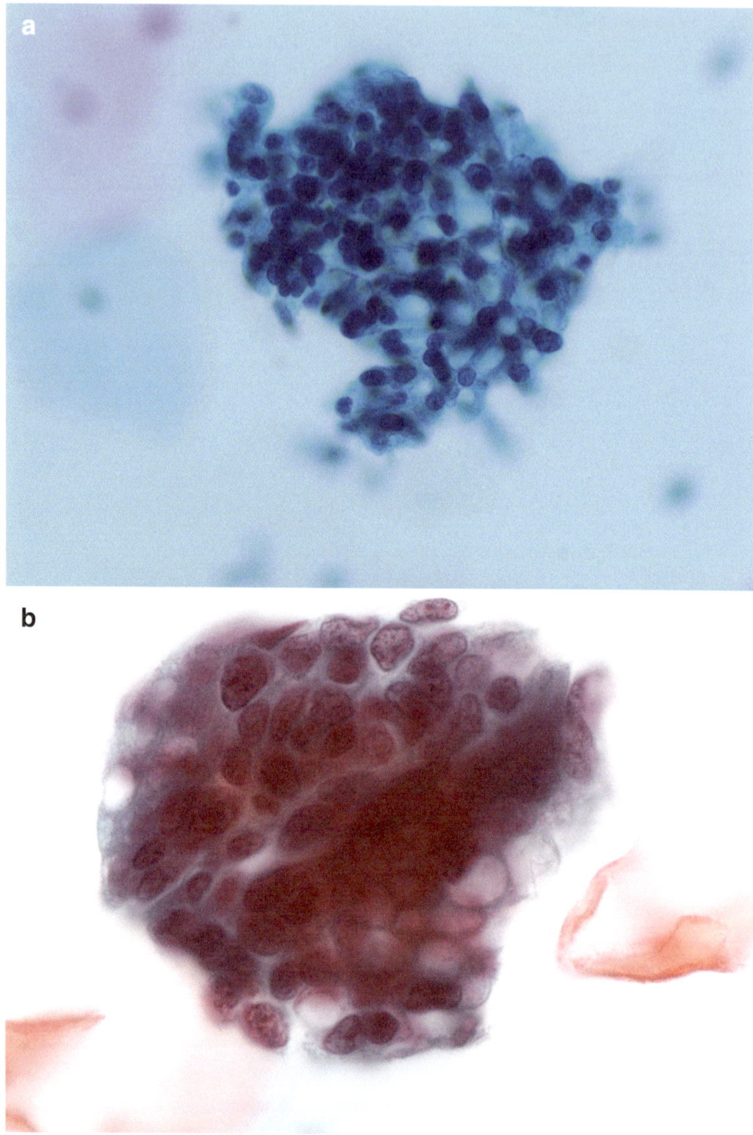

Fig. 6.7 Intestinal type adenocarcinoma in situ with characteristic goblet cell formation (**a**, **b**). SurePath LBC

Mimics of CGIN

There are a number of conditions which may in part cytologically mimic CGIN and cause diagnostic confusion, reflected in the generally reduced sensitivity and specificity of cytological detection of CGIN compared with CIN [16–21]. Furthermore, CGIN and CIN may coexist resulting in a mixed cytological pattern in cervical cytology preparations [16].

Endocervical Crypt Involvement by High Grade CIN (CIN 2/3) (HSIL)

The cytological appearance of endocervical crypt involvement by high grade CIN has been described by Selvaggi and is similar in both conventional and liquid-based cervical cytology preparations [22, 23].

Exfoliated cells from crypts involved by high grade CIN may present one of two patterns. The

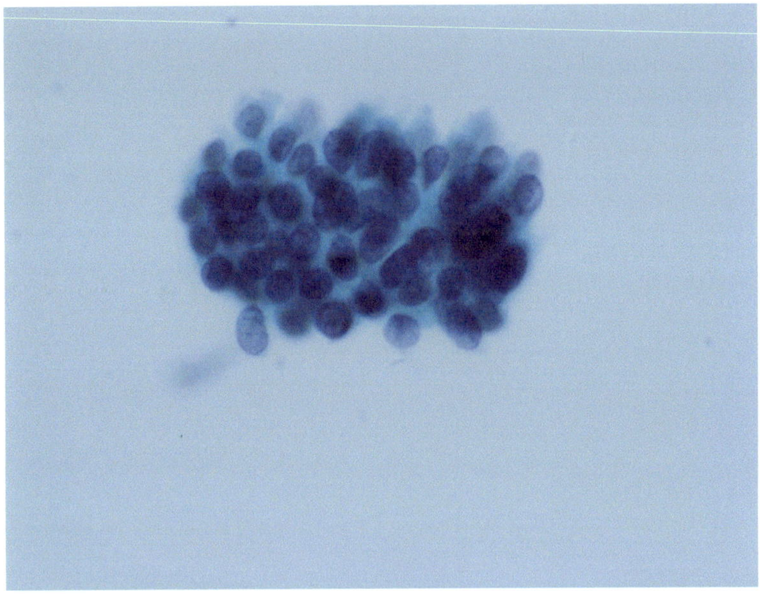

Fig. 6.8 Endometrioid type adenocarcinoma in situ. A disorganised crowded group of small glandular cells with even sized rounded nuclei. SurePath LBC

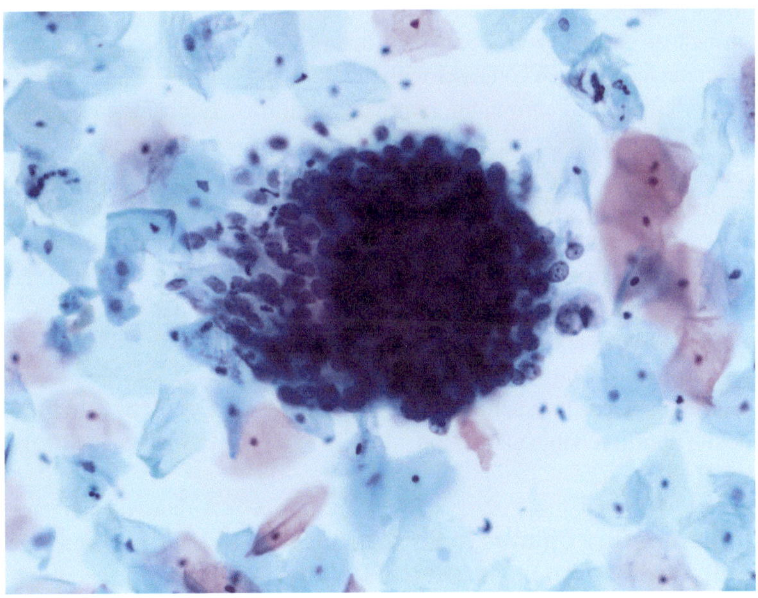

Fig. 6.9 High grade CIN involving an endocervical crypt. An oval cluster of abnormal cells with smooth cell borders. Note the transition from totally disorganised cells in the centre, lacking any honeycomb pattern, to flattened disorganised cells at the periphery. SurePath LBC

type A pattern designated by Selvaggi consists of oval clusters of abnormal cells with smooth cell or slightly irregular borders in which the cells at the periphery are flattened or disorganised and those within the centre totally disorganised often with a spindling or whirling arrangement, in contrast to the residual honeycomb pattern of CGIN; the constituent cells show an increased nuclear/cytoplasmic ratio and hyperchromatic nuclei with granular chromatin (Fig. 6.9). The type B pattern consists of sheets of columnar cells with peripheral palisading and nuclear pseudostratification, suggestive of CGIN, but with nuclear features of squamous differentiation. The latter is characterised by evenly distributed chromatin or chromatin clumping and clearing, variation in

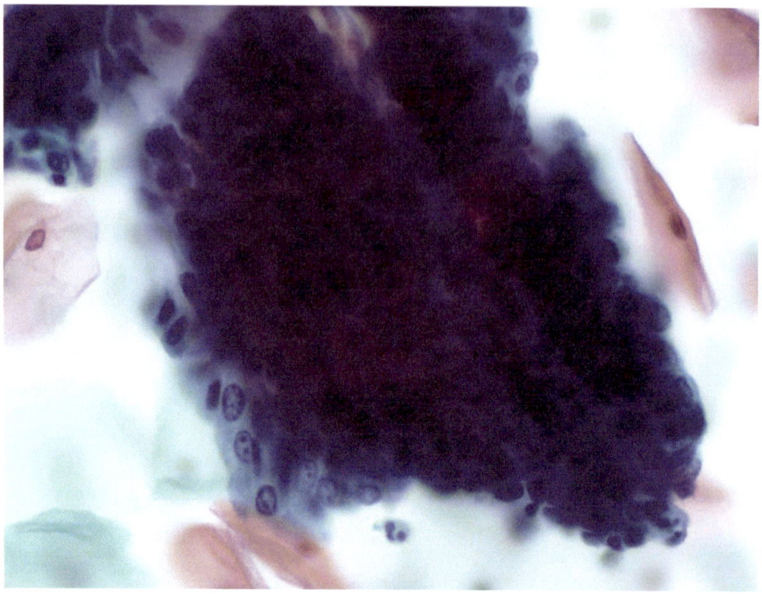

Fig. 6.10 High grade CIN involving an endocervical crypt. Sheets of columnar cells with peripheral palisading and nuclear pseudostratification, suggestive of CGIN, but nuclear features of squamous differentiation, no feathering and intact cytoplasm. SurePath LBC

size and shape of peripheral nuclei, irregularity of nuclear outlines with occasional notches and micronucleoli, which contrasts with the "salt and pepper" pattern of chromatin, relatively uniform nuclear size, shape and outline, and prominent nucleoli in neoplastic endocervical cells. Furthermore if palisaded or pseudo-stratified cells are present at the periphery of groups of cells derived from crypts involved by CIN, the cytoplasm is usually intact and dense with smooth edges and does not show the wispy cytoplasmic tags typical of CGIN (Fig. 6.10). Apoptosis and mitoses are clearly visualized in both entities and do not permit reliable distinction.

Inflammatory Change in Endocervical Cells and Benign Endocervical Polyps

In many women with cervicitis or a benign endocervical polyp, cytology samples are entirely normal but in some cases endocervical cells may show reactive changes consisting of crowded cell groups with dense cyanophilic or eosinophilic cytoplasm, maintenance of internuclear spacing, anisonucleosis in round or ovoid nuclei, hyperchromasia and prominent nucleoli [12, 24, 25] (Fig. 6.11).

Occasionally polypoid tissue fragments from endocervical polyps appear in cervical cytology samples, comprising an inner core of numerous small dark stromal cells, covered by a layer of columnar cells with basal nuclei and tissue fragments from lower uterine segment polyps, which typically have a low gland to stroma ratio, present as small vessels running in various directions connected by thin sheets of small ovoid cells with indistinct cytoplasm [26].

Microglandular hyperplasia, as described below, is sometimes seen in cytology samples from a polyp.

Cervical Endometriosis and Lower Uterine Segment Sampling

Although spontaneous endometriosis of the cervix has been described, it is uncommon unless there has been a previous operative procedure such as a loop or cone biopsy or trachelectomy, superficial endometriosis then resulting from direct implantation at the site of injury during a subsequent menstrual period; alternatively endocervical brush samplers or spatulae with elongated tips may directly sample the lower uterine segment and harvest endometrial glands and stroma as intact tissue fragments [24, 27–35].

In conventional and liquid based cervical cytology samples, endometrial cells from the cervix are well preserved and are arranged in large sheets or strips showing gland openings and nuclear

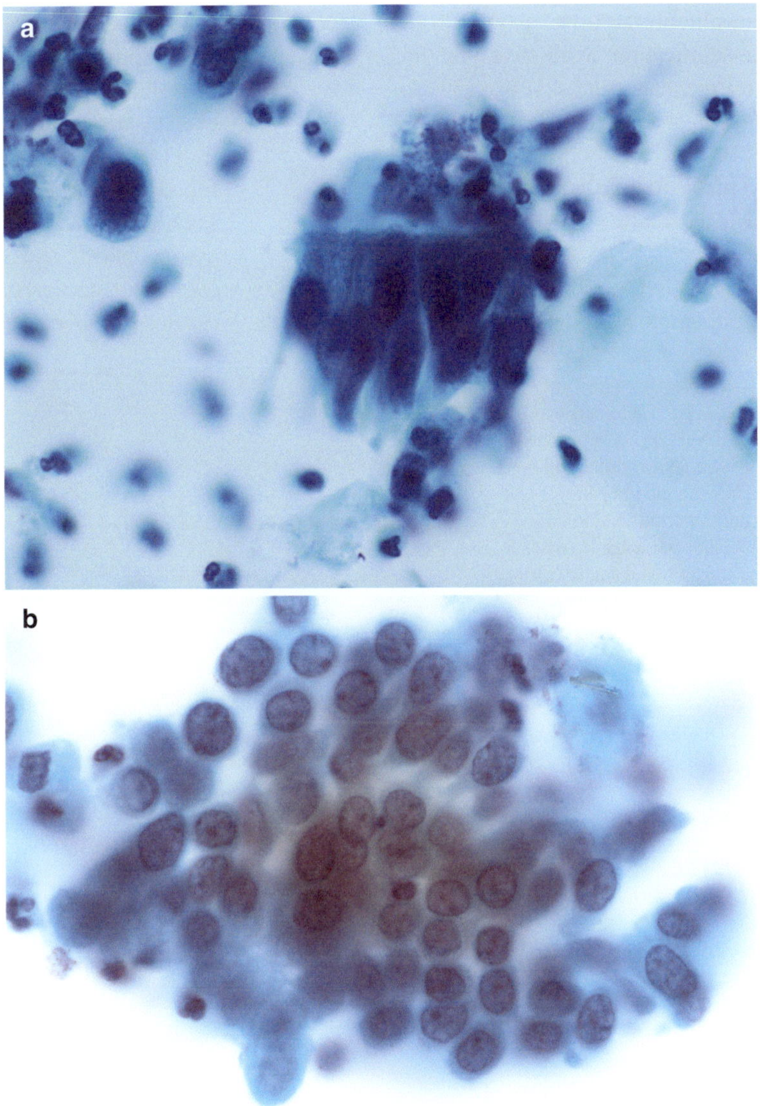

Fig. 6.11 Reactive changes in endocervical cells viewed in strips (**a**) and sheets (**b**)

stratification respectively composed of cuboidal cells with a high nuclear/cytoplasmic ratio, relatively hyperchromatic nuclei with irregular contours and coarse chromatin; prominent nucleoli and mitoses may be found (Fig. 6.12). These features, together with the exfoliation pattern described, carry the risk that the cells may be mistaken for dyskaryotic endocervical cells. The latter cells, however, typically present as sheets of monotonous cells with crowded overlapping nuclei and the sheets have more striking architectural abnormalities.

Endometrial stromal cells may also be present, either in loose groups with ragged edges or admixed with the epithelial cells. Stromal cells are oval or round with rounded or reniform nuclei and scanty ill-defined cytoplasm, which is more abundant during the secretory phase of the cycle. The presence of stromal cells enables the diagnosis of endometriosis to be made [24, 28]. In conventional smears in particular the specimen may also be heavily blood stained. Directly sampled tissue from the lower uterine segment consists of tubular structures with well demarcated outlines composed of small uniform cuboidal cells with a peripheral rim of elongated delicate stromal cells orientated along the long axis of the tubular structure; these characteristic features are readily identified at low power routine screening magnification. Such structures are often likened to "elephant trunks" (Fig. 6.13).

Tubal and Tuboendometrioid Metaplasia

Tubal metaplasia refers to replacement of epithelium at Mullerian-derived sites, such as the endometrial cavity or endocervix, by benign epithelium resembling that of the fallopian tube; in addition, tubal metaplasia frequently includes cells of endometrial type, so-called tuboendometrioid metaplasia. Tubal metaplasia has been found in between 31 and 100 % of adequately sampled cervices removed for both neoplastic and non-neoplastic reasons and tubal or tuboendometrioid metaplasia has been reported in 26 % of cervices removed after cone biopsy [27, 36–38].

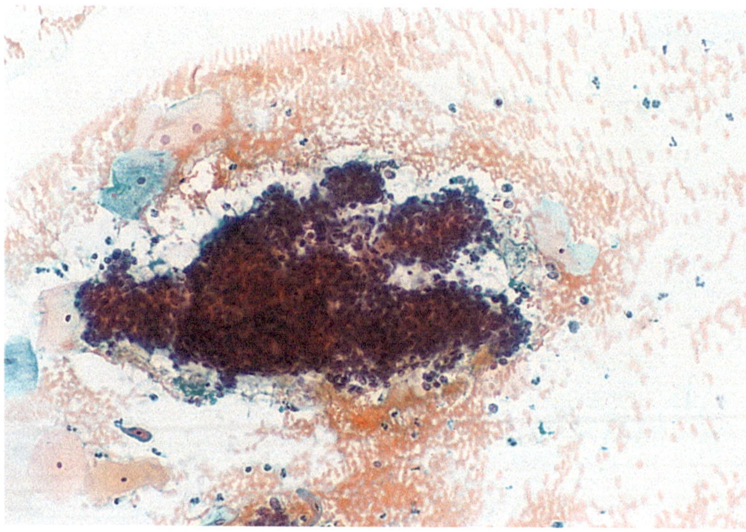

Fig. 6.12 Endometriosis of the cervix. A large sheet of cuboidal endometrial cells showing gland openings and nuclear stratification on a haemorrhagic background in a conventional smear (From Smith [84] with permission)

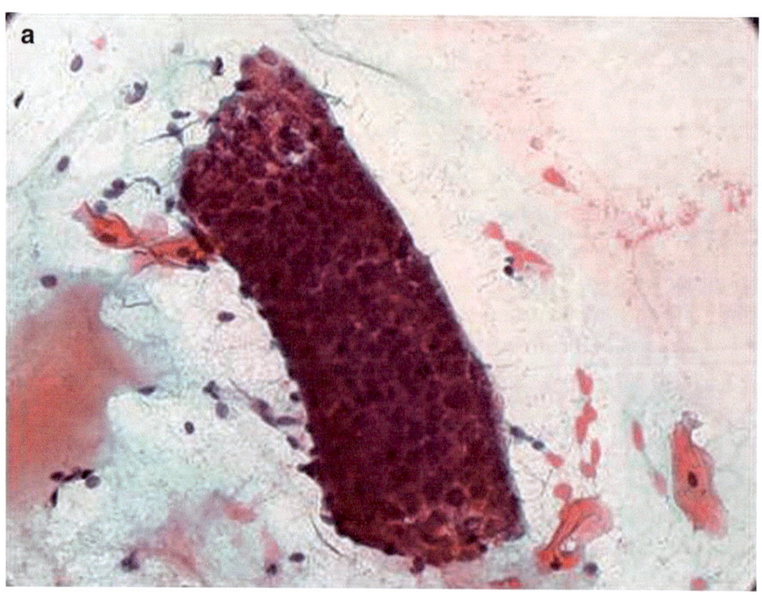

Fig. 6.13 Directly sampled tissue from the lower uterine segment in a conventional cervical smear (**a**) and SurePath LBC preparation (**b**)

Fig. 6.13 (continued)

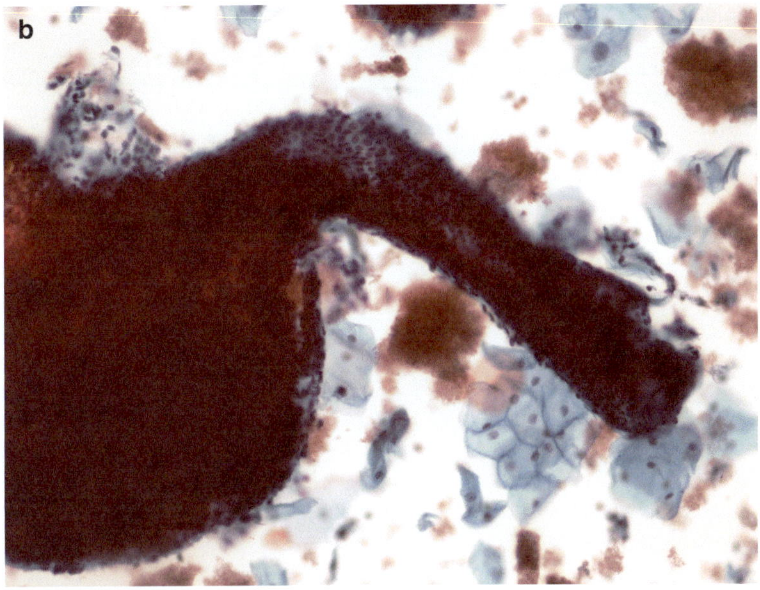

Tubal and tuboendometrioid metaplasia tends to be multifocal and involve upper endocervical crypts rather than the lower endocervix and surface epithelium. Therefore it is more likely to be encountered in cervical cytology specimens following the use of brush devices for liquid based cytology sampling [38, 39]. Endometriosis may also occur in the same group of patients, as already described, although it is a less frequent event.

Although not thought to be preneoplastic, it is important that the cytological appearances are recognized and not misinterpreted as indicating endocervical glandular dysplasia: in one study tubal metaplasia accounted for the smear appearances in 76 % of cases in which endocervical glandular dysplasia had been suggested [40].

The cytological appearances in both conventional smears and liquid based preparations have been described in detail [39, 41–43]. All three cell types found in normal fallopian tube epithelium should be present, namely ciliated cells, secretory non-ciliated cells and intercalary cells. Although the proportion of these cells varies greatly between individual samples, ciliated columnar cells with apical terminal bars are necessary for the diagnosis and typically present as aligned groups of cells with well demarcated cytoplasm, which contrasts with the pseudostratified edge, bare nuclei and tapering cytoplasm of AIS (Fig. 6.14).

The cells, which are smaller than endocervical cells, may be arranged in flat sheets, three-dimensional clusters, small poorly cohesive groups or occur singly. Their nuclei, which are oval, round or elongated and are usually basal in position, tend to be larger than those of endocervical cells and evenly spaced with finely granular nuclear chromatin which is slightly darker than that of endocervical cell nuclei. Nucleoli are more often visible in LBC preparations and are small and single.

Intercalary cells, exclusive to tubal metaplasia but less readily identified in cytology samples, have triangular dark staining nuclei and little cytoplasm, in contrast to the other cells which have varying amounts of granular or vacuolated cytoplasm. Mitoses are rare.

The differential diagnosis includes cervical endometriosis, endometrial cells from the lower uterine segment, microglandular and reserve cell hyperplasia, 'reactive' endocervical cells, and dyskaryotic cells from CIN 3 involving endocervical glands. Cilia are usually a feature of benign endocervical cells although a solitary case has been reported of histologically confirmed ciliated adenocarcinoma of the cervix with prior

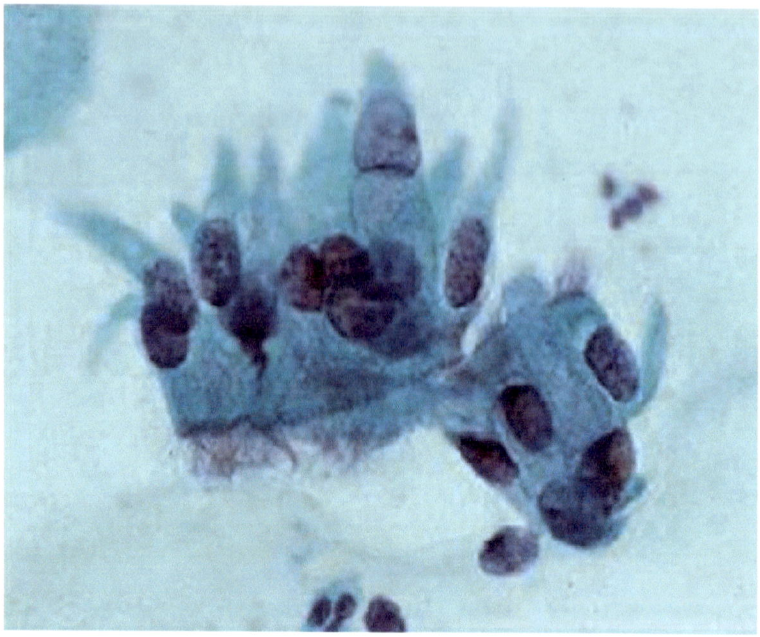

Fig. 6.14 Tuboendometrioid metaplasia in a SurePath LBC preparation. Note the cellular alignment, terminal bars and cilia

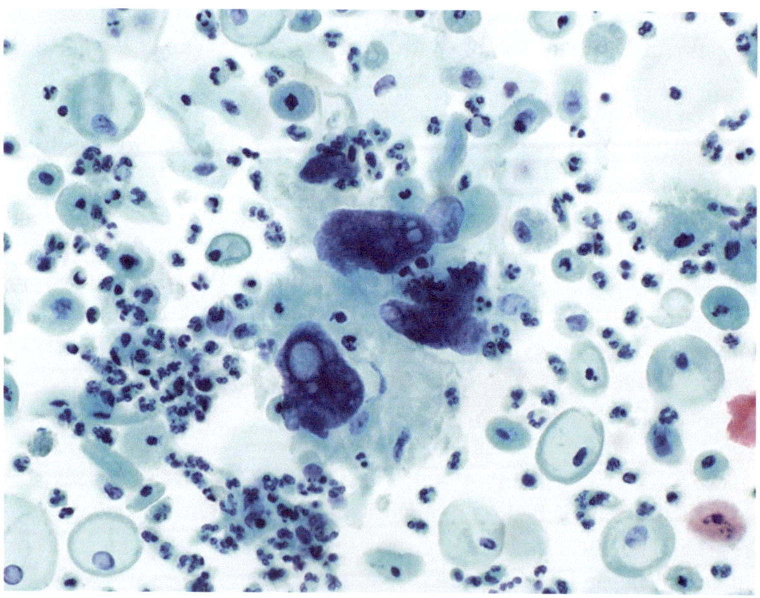

Fig. 6.15 Microglandular hyperplasia of the cervix in a SurePath LBC preparation. Small groups of glandular cells of variable size with bland nuclear features and abundant focally vacuolated cytoplasm (Courtesy of Dr C Waddell, Birmingham Cytology Training Centre)

liquid-based cervical cytology showing atypical, ciliated glandular cells that initially raised the diagnostic consideration of tubal metaplasia [44].

Microglandular Hyperplasia

The cytological appearances of microglandular hyperplasia reflect the histological appearances described in Chap. 2 and are characterised by bidimensional or tridimensional cellular clusters made up of cubic or cylindrical glandular cells with vacuolated cytoplasm; basaloid cells with dense cytoplasm, corresponding to immature squamous metaplasia; and subcylindrical reserve cells with small, round nuclei and scant cytoplasm. The clusters also show microlumina or fenestrated spaces, preserved polarity and absence of nuclear peripheral dispersion [45] (Fig. 6.15). Microglandular hyperplasia is a very common condition but is only likely to cause cytological confusion with endocervical or

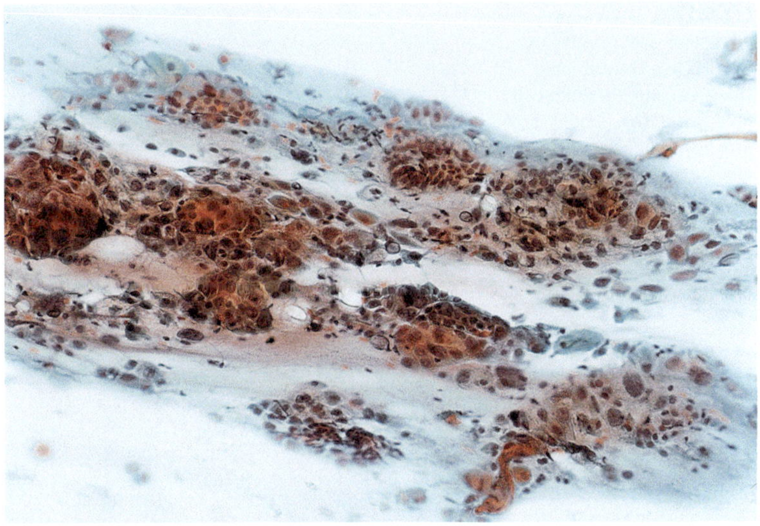

Fig. 6.16 Radiation change in endocervical cells in a conventional smear. Disorganised clusters of cells with loss of the normal honeycomb pattern, anisonucleosis, nucleolar enlargement, occasional multinucleation and abundant cytoplasm (From Waddell and Chandra [85] with permission)

endometrial neoplasia in the most florid papillary forms [39, 46–48].

Arias-Stella Change

Interpretative problems may arise during pregnancy if the endocervical glandular epithelium undergoes the type of extreme hypersecretory activity known as Arias–Stella change; it can also occur in other hyperprogestational states such as gestational trophoblastic disease and with high dose progestogen or ovulation inducing therapy [49].

The cytological features have been described in single case reports, and in one of these the cervical Arias-Stella reaction was associated with a cervical pregnancy [50, 51]. The atypical glandular cells occur singly, in syncytial clusters and cohesive sheets and are characterised by cyto- and karyomegaly, a high nuclear to cytoplasmic ratio, round to oval nuclei with finely granular or smudgy chromatin imparting a ground glass appearance, frequent intranuclear inclusions, and vacuolated or dense variable staining cytoplasm. Arias-Stella cells may be misinterpreted as malignant glandular cells if the history of pregnancy is not known [52].

Radiation Associated Changes

Although the cytological changes in cervical squamous cells after radiation therapy have been well described, the literature on the alterations in endocervical cells in response to radiation therapy is very limited. Frierson et al. studied the effect of radiation therapy for cervical cancer on endocervical cells in brush specimens at various times following treatment. Endocervical cells appeared as single cells or clusters lacking the honeycomb appearance of normal endocervical cells with lavender, mucin-filled cytoplasm. In samples taken within 6 months of treatment, the majority of endocervical cells were enlarged but usually had a normal nuclear/cytoplasmic ratio although the nuclei varied in size and had coarse chromatin, large nucleoli and were frequently multinucleated. Repair cells and multinucleated histiocytes were seen in 83 and 61 % of samples, respectively. Each of these cytological findings was less apparent in follow-up smears taken more than 6 months after the completion of radiotherapy. Awareness of these cytological changes in endocervical cells after radiation therapy should prevent the overdiagnosis of cancer in follow-up endocervical brush specimens [53] (Fig. 6.16).

Stratified Mucin Producing Intraepithelial Lesion (SMILE)

To date there are no published accounts of the appearance of this entity in cervical cytology preparations, but a personal review of conventional and SurePath liquid based cervical cytology specimens that preceded the diagnosis of

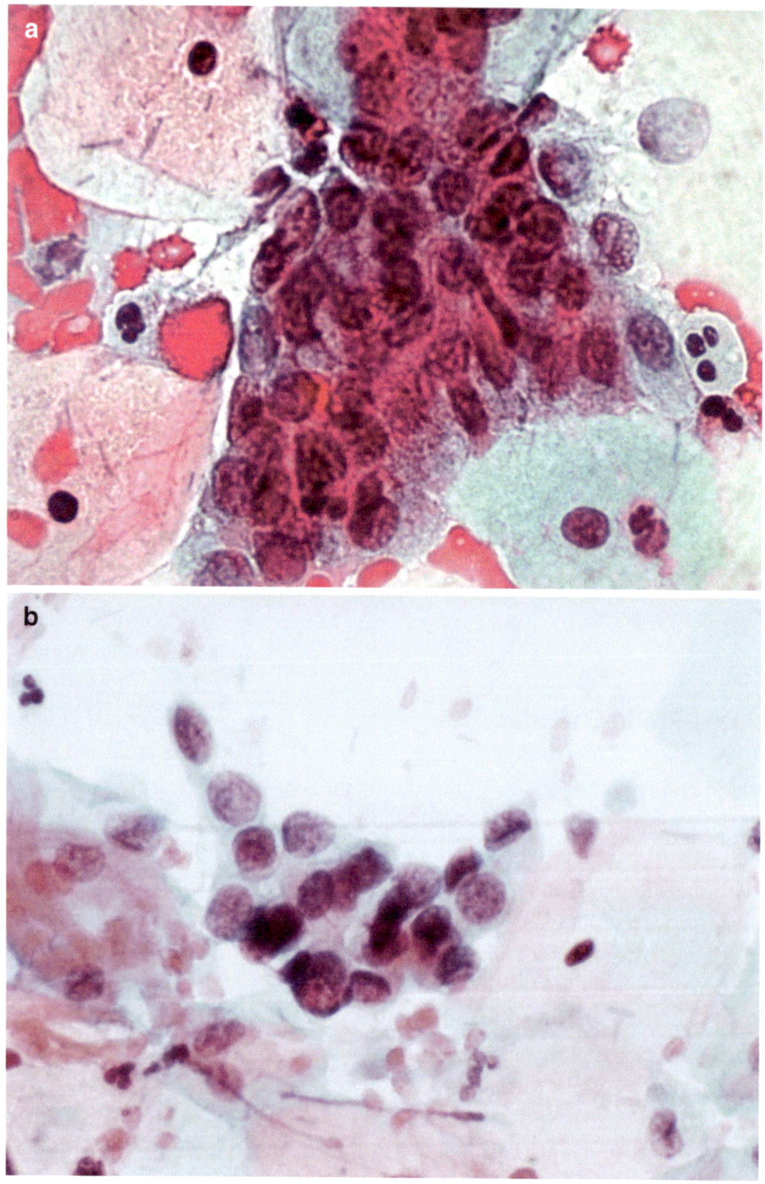

Fig. 6.17 Features consistent with origin from SMILE in a conventional smear (**a**) and SurePath LBC preparation (**b**). Crowded groups of neoplastic glandular cells with fine vacuolated cytoplasm

SMILE has identified hyperchromatic crowded groups of glandular cells with focal fine cytoplasmic vacuolation consistent with origin from SMILE (Fig. 6.17). These groups of cells were often associated with neoplastic squamous or endocervical glandular cells consistent with origin from CIN and CGIN respectively, which is frequently found in association with SMILE [54].

Invasive Adenocarcinoma

Endocervical Type Cervical Adenocarcinoma

A definitive diagnosis of endocervical adenocarcinoma cannot be made on cervical cytological preparations because the cytological features of adenocarcinoma in situ and invasive

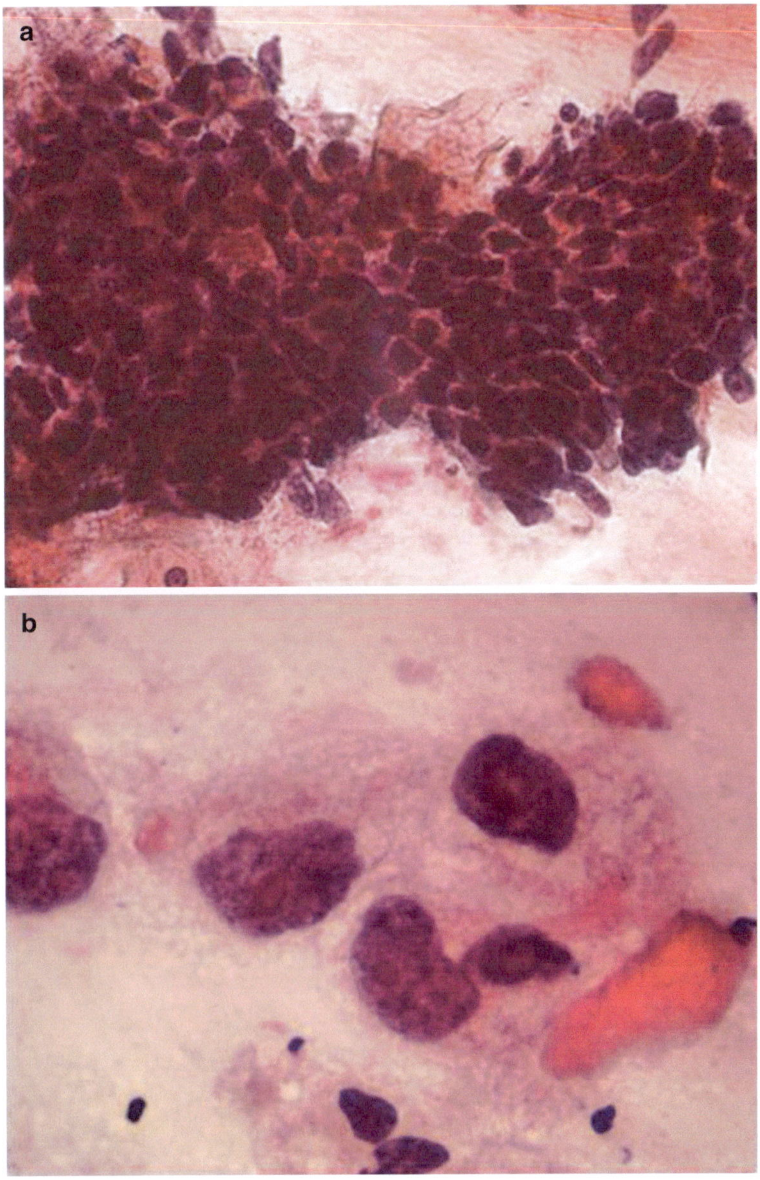

Fig. 6.18 Endocervical adenocarcinoma of the cervix in a conventional smear. Syncytial masses of large pleomorphic glandular cells (**a**) and dissociated neoplastic glandular cells with prominent irregular eosinophilic nucleoli (**b**)

adenocarcinoma overlap. However detailed analysis of conventional cervical smears from histologically confirmed cases of endocervical adenocarcinoma led Pacey and colleagues to suggest that syncytial masses of large pleomorphic glandular cells, small cells in very crowded sheets and papillary groupings of cells, when seen in conjunction with AIS, are suggestive of invasion. Dissociation of cells, variable nuclear pleomorphism dependent of the degree of differentiation of the tumour, an irregular chromatin pattern and inconspicuous-to-prominent nucleoli are also frequently present and in some cases a tumour diathesis in the smear background [4, 6] (Fig. 6.18). However although extreme nuclear crowding has been recognised as a feature suggestive of invasion in endocervical adenocarcinoma, other subtypes of cervical adenocarcinoma such as mucinous, endometrioid and serous or clear cell and glassy cell carcinoma have moderate or abundant cytoplasm respectively, and nuclear crowding is therefore not a reliable

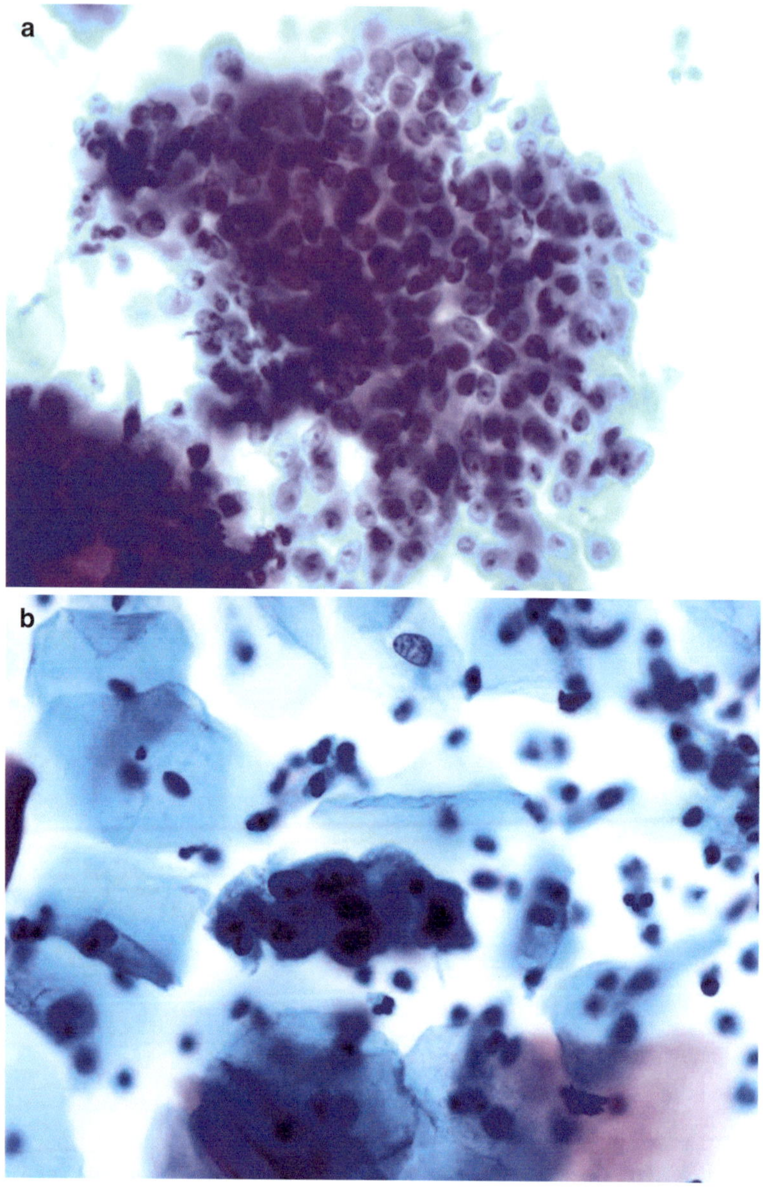

Fig. 6.19 Endocervical adenocarcinoma of the cervix in a SurePath LBC preparation. Syncytial masses of large pleomorphic glandular cells (**a**) and dissociated neoplastic glandular cells with prominent irregular nucleoli (**b**). Note the absence of tumour diathesis

morphological criteria for the diagnosis of these entities (see below).

The cytological features of endocervical adenocarcinoma in LBC preparations are similar to those in conventional smears except that nuclear morphology is better preserved and mitoses are more obvious, while tumour diathesis is less evident and if present corresponds to that seen in invasive squamous lesions: in SurePath preparations it tends to be bluish grey in colour and often closely associated with the malignant cells, so-called 'clinging diathesis', whilst in ThinPrep specimens lysed blood, a universal component of diathesis, is located at the periphery of the cell deposit and appears red in colour [10, 14] (Fig. 6.19).

Endometrioid Adenocarcinoma of the Cervix

The cytological appearances of this rare subtype of cervical adenocarcinoma, which some believe

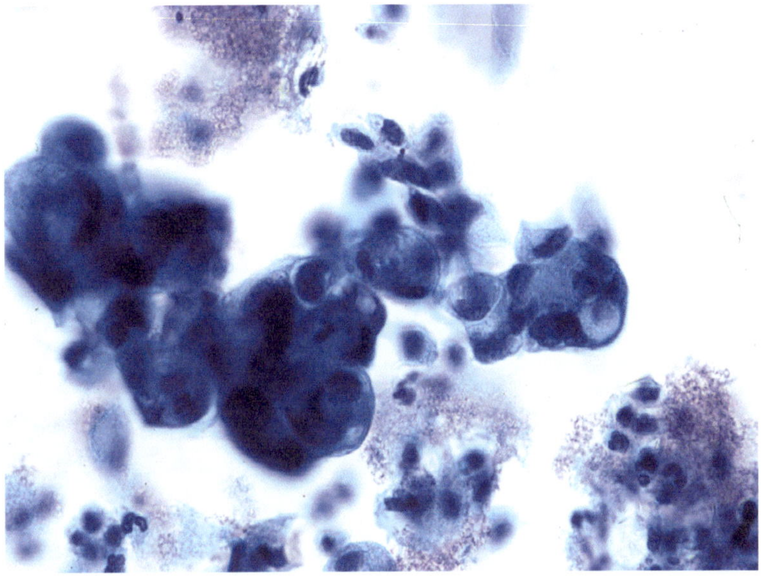

Fig. 6.20 Endometrioid adenocarcinoma of the cervix in a SurePath LBC preparation. Note the cuboidal or columnar cells with eccentric nuclei and occasional vacuolated cytoplasm, small nucleoli and dense cyanophilic cytoplasm. Compare with Fig. 6.17

is simply a variant of endocervical type cervical adenocarcinoma (see Chap. 5), are very similar to those of endometrioid adenocarcinoma of the endometrium being characterised by cuboidal or columnar cells with eccentric nuclei and occasional vacuolated cytoplasm, small nucleoli and dense cyanophilic cytoplasm (Fig. 6.20).

In tumours arising from the cervix, as opposed to the endometrium, there may be a tumour diathesis [55, 56].

Minimal Deviation Adenocarcinoma

The diagnosis of minimal deviation adenocarcinoma (MDA), and its putative precursor lesion lobular endocervical glandular hyperplasia (LEGH), is difficult and rarely made in cervical cytology preparations, reflecting the minimal and often focal cytological atypia seen in histological sections. In the majority of reported cases, the diagnosis has been made in retrospect on review of conventional cervical smears that preceded the biopsy diagnosis; to date the appearance in liquid based cytology preparations has not been described. In conventional cervical smears an abundance of glandular material consisting of flat honeycomb sheets with focal disorganisation, abundant lacy or vacuolated cytoplasm and nuclei enlarged up to twice normal size with fine or coarsely granular chromatin and occasional conspicuous nucleoli are features suggestive of origin from minimal deviation adenocarcinoma [57, 58]. In addition cytoplasmic mucin of cells derived from MDA and LEGH shows golden-yellow Papanicolaou staining in contrast to normal endocervical mucin which stains pink, and the cells themselves are immunoreactive to HIK1083 in keeping with their gastric pyloric phenotype [59, 60] (Fig. 6.21). Cells derived from LEGH may be distinguished from cells derived from MDA by the presence of intranuclear cytoplasmic inclusions [61].

Villoglandular Cervical Adenocarcinoma (VGA)

The cytological features of this uncommon type of cervical adenocarcinoma in conventional cervical smears were first described in 1996 and subsequently confirmed in other small series [62–65].

Characteristic cytological features include many large cohesive groups and sheets of endocervical glandular cells showing nuclear crowding and loss of the normal honeycomb pattern; the presence of long villous fronds and papillae

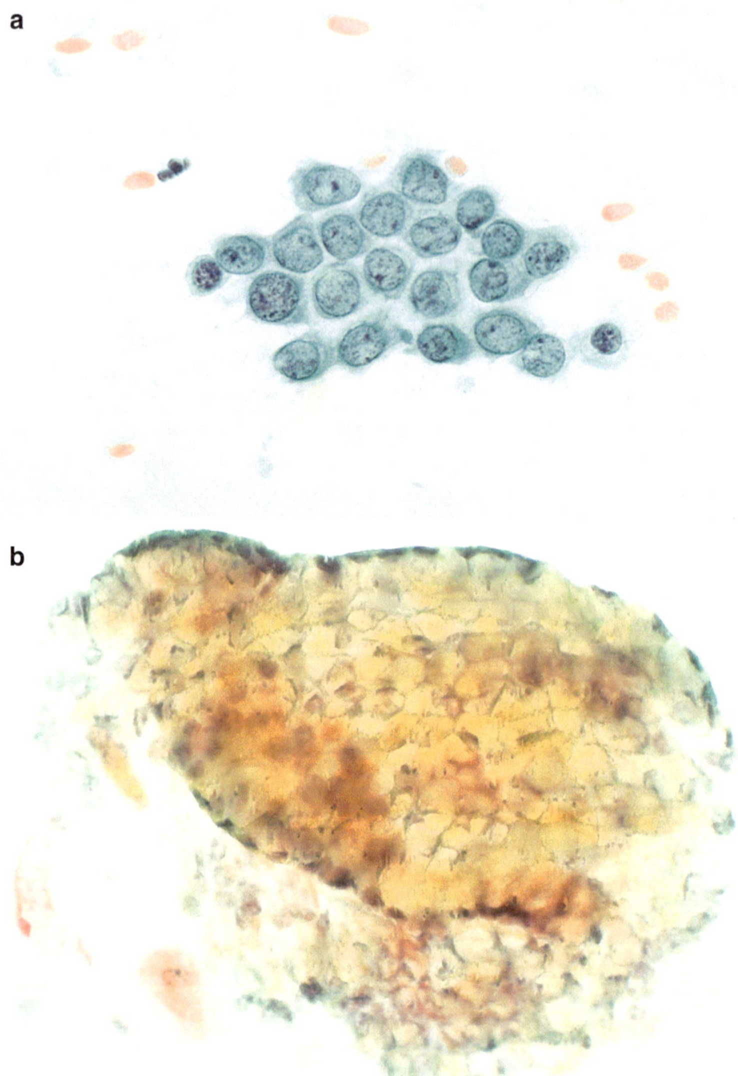

Fig. 6.21 Minimal deviation adenocarcinoma of the cervix in a conventional cervical smear. Endocervical cells retain the honeycomb pattern but show focal disorganisation, nuclear enlargement with minor variation in shape, fine or coarse granular chromatin, and finely vacuolated cytoplasm (**a**). Yellow stained cytoplasmic mucin in a flat sheet of endocervical cells with subtle disorganisation of the honeycomb pattern (**b**) (From Waddell and Chandra [85] with permission)

lined by columnar cells with intact smooth cytoplasmic borders and minimal to moderate cytological atypia; and strips and three-dimensional ball-like clusters of cells with smooth, intact communal cytoplasmic rims and flattened cells at the periphery. Cell nuclei are small, ovoid and hyperchromatic with granular evenly distributed chromatin and absent or inconspicuous nucleoli. Apoptotic bodies and scattered mitoses are present.

Similar appearances are seen in liquid based cytology preparations but nuclear membrane irregularity and nucleoli are more often identified as a result of better cell preservation [66]. The differential diagnosis of VGA includes adenocarcinoma in situ, papillary CIN 3 and CIN 3 involving endocervical glands, papillary squamous and squamotransitional neoplasms, directly sampled endometrial cells and reactive endocervical cells. However, the above constellation of features, and in particular the branching papillary fronds with smooth as opposed to "feathered" borders and characteristic architectural and nuclear features should permit an accurate diagnosis (Fig. 6.22).

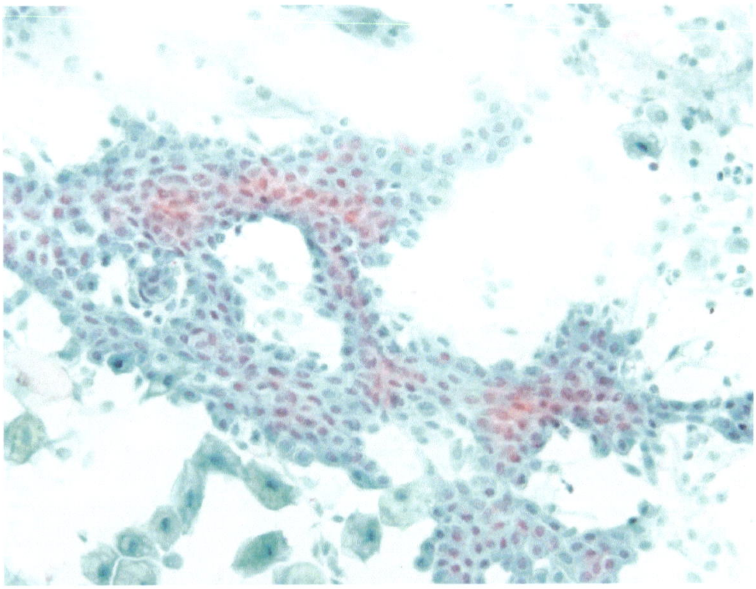

Fig. 6.22 Villoglandular adenocarcinoma of the cervix in a cystoscopy urine sample from a patient with tumour directly infiltrating the bladder. Note the branching papillary fronds composed of glandular cells showing only minor atypia (From Waddell and Chandra [85] with permission)

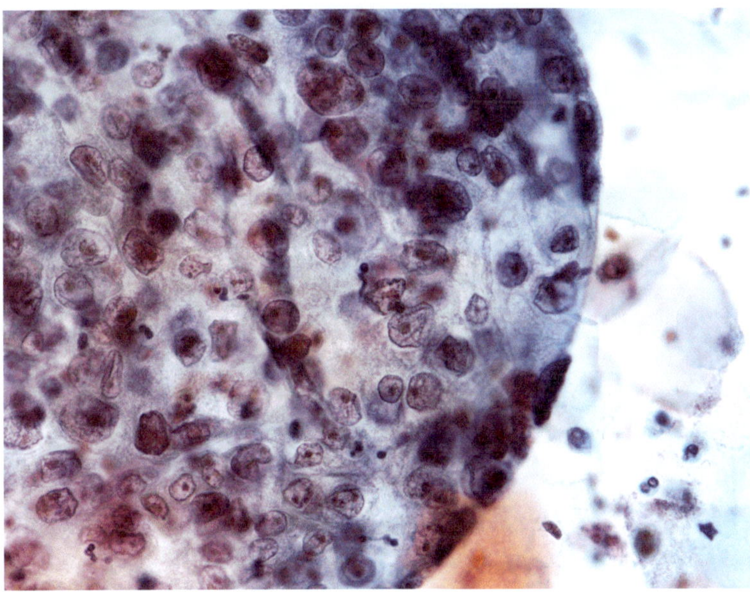

Fig. 6.23 Clear cell carcinoma of the cervix. A sheet of pleomorphic glandular cells with prominent nucleoli, sharply defined nuclear borders, prominent nucleoli and finely granular or clear cytoplasm. SurePath LBC

Clear Cell Carcinoma

Clear cell carcinoma of the cervix in young women was previously associated with prenatal exposure to diethylstilboestrol but following discontinuance of the use of this drug for the management of miscarriage in the early 1970s, this rare cervical tumour now tends to be seen more often in elderly women (see Chap. 4). The cytological appearance in cervical smears was first described in 1978 and more recently the appearance in liquid based cytology preparations [67–70]. Tumour cells present as single or clusters of cells showing anisonucleosis with variable amounts of finely granular or near optically clear cytoplasm and round or ovoid nuclei with delicate nuclear borders, finely granular chromatin and prominent, sometimes multiple, eosinophilic nucleoli (Fig. 6.23).

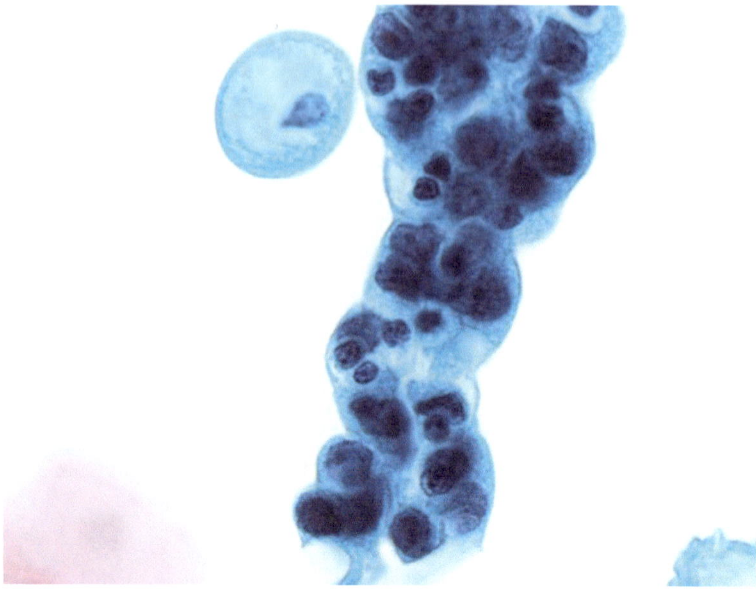

Fig. 6.24 Serous carcinoma of the cervix. Three-dimensional papillary group of cells showing nuclear pleomorphism, prominent nucleoli and cytoplasmic vacuolation. SurePath LBC (Courtesy of Manchester Cytology Training Centre)

Serous Carcinoma

Primary serous carcinoma of the cervix is very rare and most cases of cervical serous carcinoma represent either direct spread from a primary tumour of the endometrium or metastasis from the ovary or fallopian tube [71]. Cytomorphologically primary serous carcinoma of the cervix is of similar appearance to serous carcinoma of the ovary consisting of multilayered sheets of pleomorphic glandular cells, papillary fragments, tight balls and dissociated markedly atypical cells with vacuolated cytoplasm, prominent nucleoli and occasional associated psammoma bodies. Abundant tumour diathesis is usually found in primary serous carcinoma of the cervix but is scanty in cases of serous ovarian carcinoma metastatic to the cervix [72, 73] (Fig. 6.24).

Adenosquamous Carcinoma

Cervical cytology preparations from adenosquamous carcinoma of the cervix reflect the histological appearances and consist of dissociated or syncytial aggregates of atypical malignant epithelial cells showing features of both squamous and glandular differentiation associated with tumour diathesis; in some cases only one type differentiation may be apparent or predominate [16, 74–76].

Glassy Cell Carcinoma

Glassy cell carcinoma is considered to be a variant of adenosquamous carcinoma since ultrastructurally there is evidence of both glandular and squamous differentiation [77]. The cytological features in both conventional smears and liquid based preparations have been described [78, 79]. The tumour cells tend to be numerous and arranged in groups with a syncytial appearance or in sheets and clusters. A few single tumour cells may also be present. They are larger than severely dyskaryotic squamous cells and show marked anisokaryosis. The nuclei are large and hyperchromatic, the chromatin having a finely granular appearance. Large irregular nucleoli are often present. A moderate amount of cytoplasm is present which may have a finely granular appearance (Fig. 6.25). Inflammatory cells, including eosinophils, may be conspicuous in the background and may be seen closely associated with tumour cells.

The cytological features can be confused with poorly-differentiated large cell non-keratinizing squamous carcinoma, the nuclei of which tend to

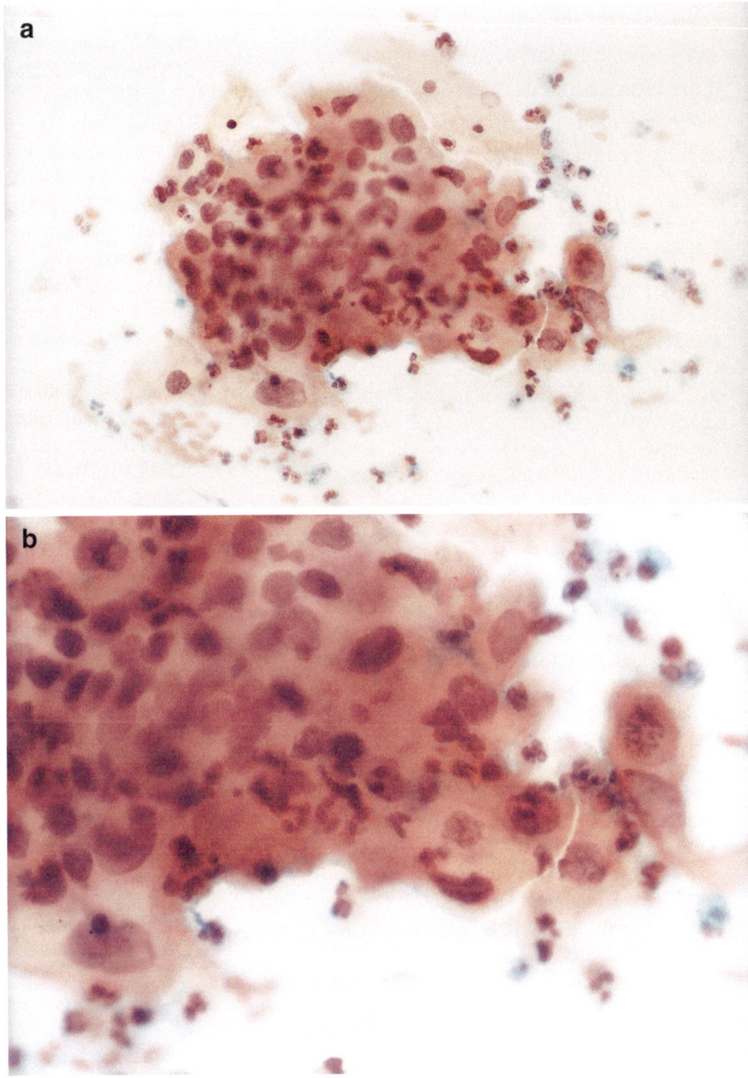

Fig. 6.25 Glassy cell carcinoma of the cervix. Medium (**a**) and high power (**b**) views of a conventional smear. A syncytial sheet of tumour cells, larger than severely dyskaryotic squamous cells, showing marked anisokaryosis and moderate amounts of finely granular cytoplasm (From Smith [84] with permission)

have coarser chromatin and less nucleolar abnormality, and with atypical reparative cells which do not full the nuclear criteria of malignancy. Misdiagnosis as a low-grade squamous abnormality can occur if the sheets of cells have bland nuclear features, leading to delay in diagnosis [80].

Adenoid Cystic Carcinoma and Adenoid Basal Carcinoma

These tumours are rarely diagnosed in cervical cytology samples, either because no tumour cells are present reflecting the fact that the overlying mucosa is usually intact or because the tumour cells present are misinterpreted as benign or abnormal endometrial cells. The cells are small, tend to be arranged in irregularly shaped three-dimensional groups and sheets, and have small uniform hyperchromatic nuclei, occasional small nucleoli and scanty cytoplasm. They may also form cords and acini, some of which contain globules of hyaline material if derived from an adenoid cystic carcinoma.

The differential diagnosis includes endocervical adenocarcinoma, endometrial adenocarcinoma, small cell neuroendocrine carcinoma, in which nuclear moulding and frequent mitoses are seen, and severe squamous dyskaryosis, in which the cells tend to be larger and less uniform.

If the tumours occur in association with in situ or invasive squamous neoplasia both tumour cell types may be present in the same smear [81–83].

References

1. Friedell GH, McKAY DG. Adenocarcinoma in situ of the endocervix. Cancer. 1953;6(5):887–97.
2. Barter RA, Waters ED. Cyto- and histo-morphology of cervical adenocarcinoma in situ. Pathology. 1970; 2(1):33–40.
3. Krumins I, Young Q, Pacey F, Bousfield L, Mulhearn L. The cytologic diagnosis of adenocarcinoma in situ of the cervix uteri. Acta Cytol. 1977; 21(2):320–9.
4. Bousfield L, Pacey F, Young Q, Krumins I, Osborn R. Expanded cytologic criteria for the diagnosis of adenocarcinoma in situ of the cervix and related lesions. Acta Cytol. 1980;24(4):283–96.
5. Ayer B, Pacey F, Greenberg M, Bousfield L. The cytologic diagnosis of adenocarcinoma in situ of the cervix uteri and related lesions. I. Adenocarcinoma in situ. Acta Cytol. 1987;31(4):397–411.
6. Ayer B, Pacey F, Greenberg M. The cytologic diagnosis of adenocarcinoma in situ of the cervix uteri and related lesions. II. Microinvasive adenocarcinoma. Acta Cytol. 1988;32(3):318–24.
7. Pacey F, Ayer B, Greenberg M. The cytologic diagnosis of adenocarcinoma in situ of the cervix uteri and related lesions. III. Pitfalls in diagnosis. Acta Cytol. 1988;32(3):325–30.
8. Raab SS, Isacson C, Layfield LJ, et al. Atypical glandular cells of undetermined significance. Cytologic criteria to separate clinically significant from benign lesions. Am J Clin Pathol. 1995;104(5):574–82.
9. Solomon D, Frable WJ, Vooijs GP, et al. ASCUS and AGUS criteria. International Academy of Cytology Task Force summary. Diagnostic Cytology Towards the 21st Century: an International Expert Conference and Tutorial. Acta Cytol. 1998;42(1):16–24.
10. Ozkan F, Ramzy I, Mody DR. Glandular lesions of the cervix on thin-layer Pap tests. Validity of cytologic criteria used in identifying significant lesions. Acta Cytol. 2004;48(3):372–9.
11. Solomon D, Nayar R. The Bethesda system for reporting cervical cytology. 2nd ed. New York: Springer; 2004.
12. Torres JC, Derchain SF, Gontijo RC, et al. Atypical glandular cells: criteria to discriminate benign from neoplastic lesions and squamous from glandular neoplasia. Cytopathology. 2005;16(6):295–302.
13. Belsley NA, Tambouret RH, Misdraji J, et al. Cytologic features of endocervical glandular lesions: comparison of SurePath, ThinPrep, and conventional smear specimen preparations. Diagn Cytopathol. 2008;36(4): 232–7.
14. Denton KJ, Herbert A, Turnbull LS, et al. The revised BSCC terminology for abnormal cervical cytology. Cytopathology. 2008;19(3):137–57.
15. Lee KR. Adenocarcinoma in situ with a small cell (endometrioid) pattern in cervical smears: a test of the distinction from benign mimics using specific criteria. Cancer. 1999;87(5):254–8.
16. van Aspert-van Erp AJ, Smedts FM, Vooijs GP. Severe cervical glandular cell lesions and severe cervical combined lesions: predictive value of the papanicolaou smear. Cancer. 2004;102(4):210–7.
17. Mathers ME, Johnson SJ, Wadehra V. How predictive is a cervical smear suggesting glandular neoplasia? Cytopathology. 2002;13(2):83–91.
18. Pisal NV, Sindos M, Desai S, Mansell E, Singer A. How significant is a cervical smear showing glandular dyskaryosis? Eur J Obstet Gynecol Reprod Biol. 2003;108(2):209–12.
19. Segal A, Frost FA, Miranda A, Fletcher C, Sterrett GF. Predictive value of diagnoses of endocervical glandular abnormalities in cervical smears. Pathology. 2003;35(3):198–203.
20. Kirwan JM, Herrington CS, Smith PA, Turnbull LS, Herod JJ. A retrospective clinical audit of cervical smears reported as 'glandular neoplasia'. Cytopathology. 2004;15(4):188–94.
21. Finall AI, Olafsdottir R. Outcomes of cervical liquid-based cytology suggesting a glandular abnormality. Cytopathology. 2009;20(6):367–74.
22. Selvaggi SM. Cytologic features of squamous cell carcinoma in situ involving endocervical glands in endocervical cytobrush specimens. Acta Cytol. 1994; 38(5):687–92.
23. Selvaggi SM. Cytologic features of high-grade squamous intraepithelial lesions involving endocervical glands on ThinPrep cytology. Diagn Cytopathol. 2002; 26(3):181–5.
24. Wood MD, Horst JA, Bibbo M. Weeding atypical glandular cell look-alikes from the true atypical lesions in liquid-based Pap tests: a review. Diagn Cytopathol. 2007;35(1):12–7.
25. Ghorab Z, Mahmood S, Schinella R. Endocervical reactive atypia: a histologic-cytologic study. Diagn Cytopathol. 2000;22(6):342–6.
26. Ngadiman S, Yang GC. Adenomyomatous, lower uterine segment and endocervical polyps in cervicovaginal smears. Acta Cytol. 1995;39(4): 643–7.
27. Ismail SM. Cone biopsy causes cervical endometriosis and tubo-endometrioid metaplasia. Histopathology. 1991;18(2):107–14.
28. Szyfelbein WM, Baker PM, Bell DA. Superficial endometriosis of the cervix: a source of abnormal glandular cells on cervicovaginal smears. Diagn Cytopathol. 2004;30(2):88–91.
29. Heaton Jr RB, Harris TF, Larson DM, Henry MR. Glandular cells derived from direct sampling of the lower uterine segment in patients status post-cervical cone biopsy. A diagnostic dilemma. Am J Clin Pathol. 1996;106(4):511–6.

30. Singh N, Titmuss E, Chin AJ, et al. A review of post-trachelectomy isthmic and vaginal smear cytology. Cytopathology. 2004;15(2):97–103.
31. Feratovic R, Lewin SN, Sonoda Y, et al. Cytologic findings after fertility-sparing radical trachelectomy. Cancer. 2008;114(1):1–6.
32. Ghorab Z, Ismiil N, Covens A, et al. Postradical vaginal trachelectomy follow-up by isthmic-vaginal smear cytology: a 13-year audit. Diagn Cytopathol. 2009; 37(9):641–6.
33. Edey K, Denton K, Murdoch J. The role of cytological follow-up after radical vaginal trachelectomy for early-stage cervical cancer. Cytopathology. 2014;25(2): 95–100.
34. de Peralta-Venturino MN, Purslow MJ, Kini SR. Endometrial cells of the "lower uterine segment" (LUS) in cervical smears obtained by endocervical brushings: a source of potential diagnostic pitfall. Diagn Cytopathol. 1995;12(3):263–8.
35. Lee KR, Genest DR, Minter LJ, Granter SR, Cibas ES. Adenocarcinoma in situ in cervical smears with a small cell (endometrioid) pattern: distinction from cells directly sampled from the upper endocervical canal or lower segment of the endometrium. Am J Clin Pathol. 1998;109(6):738–42.
36. Jonasson JG, Wang HH, Antonioli DA, Ducatman BS. Tubal metaplasia of the uterine cervix: a prevalence study in patients with gynecologic pathologic findings. Int J Gynecol Pathol. 1992;11(2):89–95.
37. Al-Nafussi A, Rahilly M. The prevalence of tubo-endometrial metaplasia and adenomatoid proliferation. Histopathology. 1993;22(2):177–9.
38. Babkowski RC, Wilbur DC, Rutkowski MA, Facik MS, Bonfiglio TA. The effects of endocervical canal topography, tubal metaplasia, and high canal sampling on the cytologic presentation of nonneoplastic endocervical cells. Am J Clin Pathol. 1996;105(4): 403–10.
39. Selvaggi SM, Haefner HK. Microglandular endocervical hyperplasia and tubal metaplasia: pitfalls in the diagnosis of adenocarcinoma on cervical smears. Diagn Cytopathol. 1997;16(2):168–73.
40. Novotny DB, Maygarden SJ, Johnson DE, Frable WJ. Tubal metaplasia. A frequent potential pitfall in the cytologic diagnosis of endocervical glandular dysplasia on cervical smears. Acta Cytol. 1992;36(1): 1–10.
41. Ducatman BS, Wang HH, Jonasson JG, Hogan CL, Antonioli DA. Tubal metaplasia: a cytologic study with comparison to other neoplastic and non-neoplastic conditions of the endocervix. Diagn Cytopathol. 1993;9(1):98–103.
42. Hirschowitz L, Eckford SD, Phillpotts B, Midwinter A. Cytological changes associated with tubo-endometrioid metaplasia of the uterine cervix. Cytopathology. 1994;5(1):1–8.
43. Johnson JE, Rahemtulla A. Endocervical glandular neoplasia and its mimics in ThinPrep Pap tests. A descriptive study. Acta Cytol. 1999;43(3): 369–75.
44. O'Connell F, Cibas ES. Cytologic features of ciliated adenocarcinoma of the cervix: a case report. Acta Cytol. 2005;49(2):187–90.
45. Alvarez-Santin C, Sica A, Rodriguez M, Feijo A, Garrido G. Microglandular hyperplasia of the uterine cervix. Cytologic diagnosis in cervical smears. Acta Cytol. 1999;43(2):110–3.
46. Valente PT, Schantz HD, Schultz M. Cytologic atypia associated with microglandular hyperplasia. Diagn Cytopathol. 1994;10(4):326–31.
47. Yahr LJ, Lee KR. Cytologic findings in microglandular hyperplasia of the cervix. Diagn Cytopathol. 1991; 7(3):248–51.
48. Selvaggi SM. Microglandular hyperplasia of the uterine cervix: cytologic diagnosis in cervical smears. Acta Cytol. 2000;44(3):480–1.
49. Lui M, Boerner S. Arias-Stella reaction in a cervicovaginal smear of a woman undergoing infertility treatment: a case report. Diagn Cytopathol. 2005;32(2): 94–6.
50. Yates WA, Persad RV, Stanbridge CM. The Arias-Stella reaction in the cervix: a case report with cervical cytology. Cytopathology. 1997;8(1):40–4.
51. Mulvany NJ, Khan A, Ostor A. Arias-Stella reaction associated with cervical pregnancy. Report of a case with a cytologic presentation. Acta Cytol. 1994;38(2): 218–22.
52. Pisharodi LR, Jovanoska S. Spectrum of cytologic changes in pregnancy. A review of 100 abnormal cervicovaginal smears, with emphasis on diagnostic pitfalls. Acta Cytol. 1995;39(5):905–8.
53. Frierson Jr HF, Covell JL, Andersen WA. Radiation changes in endocervical cells in brush specimens. Diagn Cytopathol. 1990;6(4):243–7.
54. Park JJ, Sun D, Quade BJ, et al. Stratified mucin-producing intraepithelial lesions of the cervix: adenosquamous or columnar cell neoplasia? Am J Surg Pathol. 2000;24(10):1414–9.
55. Hare AA, Duncan AR, Sharp AJ. Cytology suggestive of glandular neoplasia: outcomes and suggested management. Cytopathology. 2003;14(1):12–8.
56. Hirschowitz L, Sen C, Murdoch J. Primary endometrioid adenocarcinoma of the cervix with widespread squamous metaplasia–a potential diagnostic pitfall. Diagn Pathol. 2007;2:40.
57. Granter SR, Lee KR. Cytologic findings in minimal deviation adenocarcinoma (adenoma malignum) of the cervix. A report of seven cases. Am J Clin Pathol. 1996;105(3):327–33.
58. Hirai Y, Takeshima N, Haga A, et al. A clinicocytopathologic study of adenoma malignum of the uterine cervix. Gynecol Oncol. 1998;70(2):219–23.
59. Ishii K, Katsuyama T, Ota H, et al. Cytologic and cytochemical features of adenoma malignum of the uterine cervix. Cancer. 1999;87(5):245–53.
60. Hata S, Mikami Y, Manabe T. Diagnostic significance of endocervical glandular cells with "golden-yellow" mucin on pap smear. Diagn Cytopathol. 2002;27(2):80–4.
61. Hashi A, Yuminamochi T, Xu JY, et al. Intranuclear cytoplasmic inclusion is a significant diagnostic feature

for the differentiation of lobular endocervical glandular hyperplasia from minimal deviation adenocarcinoma of the cervix. Diagn Cytopathol. 2008;36(8):535–44.
62. Ballo MS, Silverberg SG, Sidawy MK. Cytologic features of well-differentiated villoglandular adenocarcinoma of the cervix. Acta Cytol. 1996;40(3):536–40.
63. Novotny DB, Ferlisi P. Villoglandular adenocarcinoma of the cervix: cytologic presentation. Diagn Cytopathol. 1997;17(5):383–7.
64. Chang WC, Matisic JP, Zhou C, et al. Cytologic features of villoglandular adenocarcinoma of the uterine cervix: comparison with typical endocervical adenocarcinoma with a villoglandular component and papillary serous carcinoma. Cancer. 1999;87(1):5–11.
65. Khunamornpong S, Siriaunkgul S, Suprasert P. Well-differentiated villoglandular adenocarcinoma of the uterine cervix: cytomorphologic observation of five cases. Diagn Cytopathol. 2002;26(1):10–4.
66. Choi Y, Kim H, Choi H, et al. Liquid-based cytology of villoglandular adenocarcinoma of the cervix: a report of 3 cases. Korean J Pathol. 2012;46(2):215–20.
67. Young QA, Pacey NF. The cytologic diagnosis of clear cell adenocarcinoma of the cervix uteri. Acta Cytol. 1978;22(1):3–6.
68. Hanselaar AG, Boss EA, Massuger LF, Bernheim JL. Cytologic examination to detect clear cell adenocarcinoma of the vagina or cervix. Gynecol Oncol. 1999;75(3):338–44.
69. Guidos BJ, Selvaggi SM. Detection of endometrial adenocarcinoma with the ThinPrep Pap test. Diagn Cytopathol. 2000;23(4):260–5.
70. Khalbuss WE, Pantanowitz L, Monaco SE. Cytomorphology of unusual primary tumors in the Pap test. Cytojournal. 2013;10:17.
71. McCluggage WG, Hurrell DP, Kennedy K. Metastatic carcinomas in the cervix mimicking primary cervical adenocarcinoma and adenocarcinoma in situ: report of a series of cases. Am J Surg Pathol. 2010;34(5):735–41.
72. Zhou C, Matisic JP, Clement PB, Hayes MM. Cytologic features of papillary serous adenocarcinoma of the uterine cervix. Cancer. 1997;81(2):98–104.
73. Zhou C, Gilks CB, Hayes M, Clement PB. Papillary serous carcinoma of the uterine cervix: a clinicopathologic study of 17 cases. Am J Surg Pathol. 1998;22(1):113–20.
74. Costa MJ, Kenny MB, Naib ZM. Cervicovaginal cytology in uterine adenocarcinoma and adenosquamous carcinoma. Comparison of cytologic and histologic findings. Acta Cytol. 1991;35(1):127–34.
75. Hayes MM, Matisic JP, Chen CJ, et al. Cytological aspects of uterine cervical adenocarcinoma, adenosquamous carcinoma and combined adenocarcinoma-squamous carcinoma: appraisal of diagnostic criteria for in situ versus invasive lesions. Cytopathology. 1997;8(6):397–408.
76. Ng WK. Thin-layer cytology findings of papillary adenosquamous carcinoma of the cervix. Report of a case with histologic correlation and molecular analysis. Acta Cytol. 2003;47(4):649–56.
77. Ulbright TM, Gersell DJ. Glassy cell carcinoma of the uterine cervix. A light and electron microscopic study of five cases. Cancer. 1983;51(12):2255–63.
78. Chung JH, Koh JS, Lee SS, Cho KJ. Glassy cell carcinoma of the uterine cervix. Cytologic features and expression of estrogen and progesterone receptors. Acta Cytol. 2000;44(4):551–6.
79. Ng WK, Cheung LK, Li AS. Liquid-based cytology findings of glassy cell carcinoma of the cervix. Report of a case with histologic correlation and molecular analysis. Acta Cytol. 2004;48(1):99–106.
80. Smith JH. Cervical cytology through the looking glass. Cytopathology. 2000;11(1):53–6.
81. Powers CN, Stastny JF, Frable WJ. Adenoid basal carcinoma of the cervix: a potential pitfall in cervicovaginal cytology. Diagn Cytopathol. 1996;14(2):172–7.
82. Vuong PN, Neveux Y, Schoonaert MF, Guettier C, Houissa-Vuong S. Adenoid cystic (cylindromatous) carcinoma associated with squamous cell carcinoma of the cervix uteri: cytologic presentation of a case with histologic and ultrastructural correlations. Acta Cytol. 1996;40(2):289–94.
83. Khoury T, Lele S, Tan D. Pathologic quiz case: an asymptomatic 79-year-old woman with an abnormal Papanicolaou test. Adenoid basal carcinoma of the cervix. Arch Pathol Lab Med. 2004;128(4):485–6.
84. Smith JHF. Other tumours and lesions of cervix, vulva and vagina. In: Gray W, Kocjan G, editors. Diagnostic cytopathology. 3rd ed. Oxford, UK: Churchill Livingstone Elsevier; 2010.
85. Waddell C, Chandra A. Glandular neoplasms of the cervix. In: Gray W, Kocjan G, editors. Diagnostic cytopathology. 3rd ed. Oxford, UK: Churchill Livingstone Elsevier; 2010.

Cytology of Other Neoplasms of the Cervix

7

John H.F. Smith

Abstract

In this chapter the appearance of neoplasms of the cervix other than glandular neoplasms as seen in cervical cytology preparations will be described.

Keywords

Neuroendocrine tumours • Transitional cell tumours • Soft tissue tumours • Carcinosarcoma • Lymphoma • Malignant melanoma • Metastatic tumours

Introduction

All the neoplasms of the cervix described in this tumour are uncommon and consequently description of their appearances in cervical cytology preparations is limited in the vast majority to individual case reports or small series. In addition in view of the relatively recent introduction of liquid-based cytology in cervical screening programmes the experience of the cytological appearances of these neoplasms is greater with conventional Papanicolaou cervical smears.

Neuroendocrine Neoplasms

As described in Chap. 6, the WHO classification of neuroendocrine neoplasms of the cervix is identical to the classification employed for pulmonary neuroendocrine neoplasms and varies from a well-differentiated tumour composed of small regular cells with a trabecular or solid streaming pattern typical of a carcinoid tumour, to a small cell carcinoma characterised by the presence of a monotonous population of small cells with scanty cytoplasm, ovoid or slightly spindled hyperchromatic nuclei, often exhibiting moulding, abundant mitotic and apoptotic activity, and in some cases, extensive crush artefact, nuclear fragmentation and necrosis [1].

The appearances in cervical cytology samples reflect the range of histological appearances.

In well-differentiated neuroendocrine neoplasms of the cervix (carcinoid tumour), the cells are usually in nests with round to oval mildly pleomorphic nuclei containing small punctate reddish nucleoli and finely granular chromatin. Cytoplasm is scanty and eosinophilic or basophilic and the cytoplasmic borders ill-defined (Fig. 7.1) [2].

Small cell neuroendocrine carcinoma (poorly differentiated neuroendocrine tumour) is characterised by sheet like clusters or dispersed small cells with finely granular chromatin, scant cytoplasm and absent nucleoli [3–5]. Nuclear moulding is typically present in conventional cervical

W.G. McCluggage et al., *Cellular Pathology of Glandular Lesions and Uncommon Neoplasms of the Cervix*, DOI 10.1007/978-1-4471-2210-4_7, © Springer-Verlag London 2014

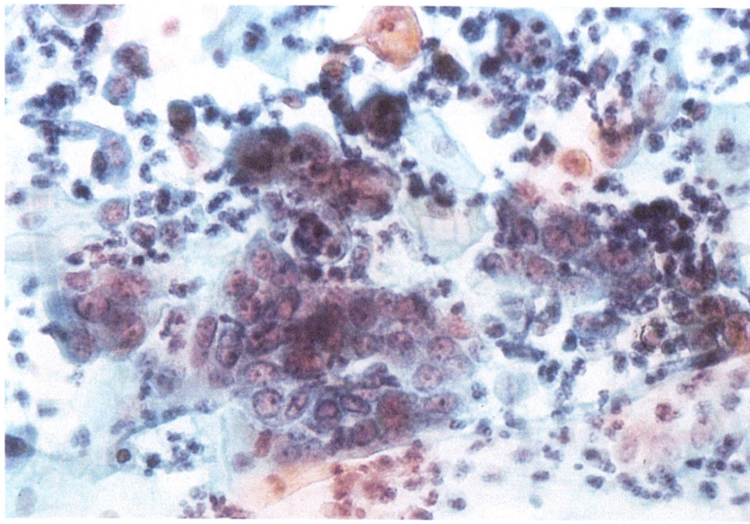

Fig. 7.1 Well differentiated neuroendocrine tumour in a conventional cervical smear showing a cohesive group of crowded cells with hyperchromatic nuclei and well-defined nucleoli (From Smith [55] with permission)

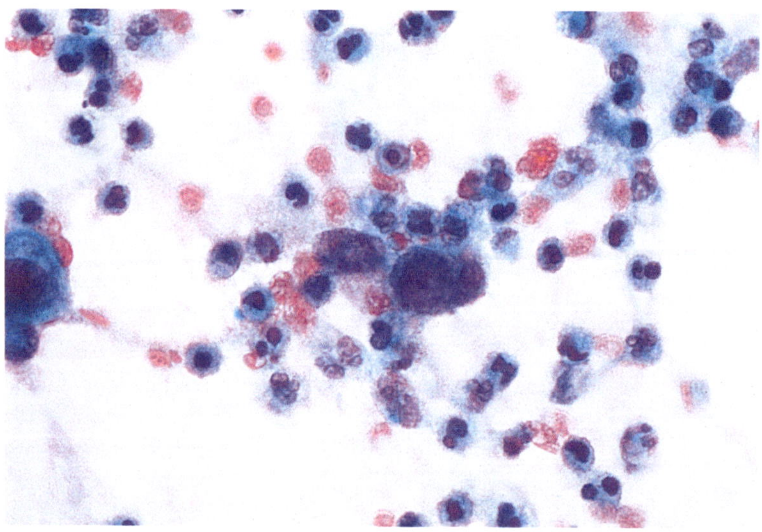

Fig. 7.2 Poorly differentiated neuroendocrine tumour in a conventional cervical smear showing marked tumour diathesis and a few small clusters of malignant cells with scanty cytoplasm and coarse granular hyperchromatic nuclei (From Smith [55] with permission)

smears of small cell neuroendocrine carcinoma but may not be conspicuous in liquid based cytology preparations (Fig. 7.2) [5, 6]. Cytological preparations from large cell neuroendocrine carcinoma are composed of large cells with relatively abundant or absent cytoplasm, coarse chromatin and prominent nucleoli. Mitoses may be frequent and smears may show palisading, moulding and abortive rosette formation [4, 7, 8]. A solitary case of neuroendocrine carcinoma of the cervix with psammoma body formation has also been reported [9].

The differential diagnosis of neuroendocrine neoplasms in cervical cytology preparations includes poorly-differentiated squamous carcinoma, adenocarcinoma or lymphoma and neuroendocrine neoplasms may coexist with the former epithelial neoplasms. If the sample contains two cell populations, because a squamous or glandular component is present, confusion with an adenosquamous carcinoma can arise or the neuroendocrine component may be completely overlooked. If small carcinoma cells are identified in a cervical cytology preparation, the possibility of metastasis from a pulmonary small cell carcinoma should be considered although metastases to the cervix are usually within the stroma and covered by intact mucosa, at least in the early stages; an appropriate history of lung tumour should be sought. It should also be noted that sparse cells from a small cell neoplasm of the cervix, whether of squamous or neuroendocrine type, are a well recognised cause of false negative cervical cytology reports [10, 11].

Transitional Neoplasms

The cytological features of six cases of papillary transitional cell carcinoma (squamotransitional cell carcinoma) of the cervix in conventional cervical smears, and nine cases in liquid-based cytology preparations have been described [12, 13].

In conventional cervical smears tumour cells with transitional features form cohesive groups in a multilayered fashion and have an oval or spindle shape with tapered ends. The nuclei are hyperchromatic, frequently display a wrinkled membrane, and have coarse and medium-sized granules, small or absent nucleoli, nuclear grooves and rarely pseudoinclusions. In all cases other cells with cytological appearances characteristic of squamous cell carcinoma were present and the background was necrotic or hemorrhagic [12].

Liquid-based cytology preparations of cervical transitional cell carcinoma often display moderate to high cellularity and contain three-dimensional, arborising, papillary clusters of basal or parabasal-like cells in which fibrovascular cores may sometimes be identified and basaloid cells are aligned horizontally at the epithelial surface. At high-power the appearance of the tumour cells ranges from bland-looking to high grade squamous intraepithelial lesions (high-grade dyskaryosis) and occasionally squamous cell carcinoma. Mitotic figures are commonly identified and tumour diathesis and dyskeratotic cells may be observed [13].

Mesenchymal Tumours

Smooth Muscle Neoplasms

Approximately 8 % of uterine leiomyomas (fibroids) occur in the cervix, making these the commonest benign mesenchymal neoplasms at this site. They are usually solitary. Although, if the overlying mucosa is ulcerated benign smooth muscle cells from the lesion may be present in cervical cytology samples, it has not been reported.

Embryonal Rhabdomyosarcoma

The cervix is very rarely the primary site of this aggressive tumour which typically presents in the reproductive years as a polypoid mass developing beneath the cervical surface epithelium associated with vaginal discharge.

The cytological features in a touch smear preparation of a case have been described by Matsuura et al. and consist of loose clusters of short spindle-shaped cells with elongated, scanty cytoplasm, and indistinct cell borders associated with tumour diathesis. The tumour cell nuclei are elongated or oval with a thin nuclear membrane, variable but usually fine chromatin and tend to have macronucleoli which are partly clear. The degree of cellular atypia ranges from mild to severe. Cross striations are rarely identified and without immunocytochemistry to confirm rhabdomyoblastic differentiation, distinction from other malignant mesenchymal neoplasms is difficult [14].

Myofibroblastoma

The appearance of this recently described tumour in cervical cytology preparations has not been documented to date, presumably because it arises from subepithelial mesenchyme and rarely causes ulceration of the overlying epithelium [15–17].

Other Mesenchymal Neoplasms

Other benign mesenchymal tumours of the cervix, namely haemangioma, schwannoma, neurofibroma, and lipoma are rare and the cytological findings have not to date been documented in conventional or liquid-based cervical cytology preparations.

Primary malignant mesenchymal neoplasms of the cervix are very rare; the most frequently encountered being leiomyosarcoma. Positive cervical cytology is rarely found in association with these tumours and even when abnormal cells are present it may not be possible to give a specific diagnosis. Cytological features suggestive of leiomyosarcoma are the finding of cell clusters or isolated neoplastic cells with oval to elongated, blunt ended nuclei showing fine granular chromatin with small nucleoli and delicate wispy cytoplasm. Stromal sarcoma of the cervix is usually a manifestation of direct spread from an endometrial stromal sarcoma. Features suggestive of endometrial stromal sarcoma are moderate or markedly cellular preparations composed of a mixture of single cells or stromal fragments in which small blood vessels may be identified. The individual tumour cells are spindle-shaped or epithelioid with minimal anisonucleosis and anisocytosis, fine granular chromatin with indistinct nucleoli, and scant to moderate delicate, amphophilic cytoplasm. The background usually includes blood and necrotic debris [18–20].

Mixed Epithelial and Mesenchymal Neoplasms

Carcinosarcoma (Malignant Mixed Mullerian Tumour)

This tumour is now generally accepted to be a metaplastic carcinoma [21]. In the majority of cases, carcinosarcoma of the cervix represents spread of tumour from the endometrium: in a series of 202 patients with cervical involvement by this tumour only one case was shown to be a primary cervical neoplasm [22].

The detection rate of malignant cells in cervical cytology preparations from histologically proven carcinosarcoma varies between 56 and 70 %. Most reports and series relate to tumours arising in the body of the uterus rather than the cervix. The histological blend of variable proportions of malignant neoplastic epithelial and stromal tissue, including in some cases heterologous elements showing rhabdomyoblastic or chondrosarcomatous differentiation, with undifferentiated small cells and spindle cells may be reflected in the cytological appearance in cervical cytology preparations, although the mesenchymal component is less commonly represented even in tumours with a predominant sarcomatous component, possibly because the latter does not readily exfoliate [23–25]. In a recent series of histologically proven uterine carcinosarcoma, 75 % of SurePath liquid-based cervical samples were originally reported as adenocarcinoma of possible endometrial origin. The cellular arrangement of the neoplastic epithelial cells is similar in conventional smears and liquid-based cytology samples and consists of neoplastic glandular cells in three-dimensional ball-like clusters, irregular clusters, and cohesive clusters or as dispersed individual cells. Tiny clusters of atypical glandular cells are easily overlooked in atrophic samples. Spindle-shaped malignant cells represent the sarcomatous component and these may show pleomorphism and multinucleation but more often resemble fibroblasts or fibroconnective tissue. The differential diagnosis of the sarcomatous component includes a spindle cell component of cervical squamous cell carcinoma. Heterologous elements are rare and are difficult to recognize with certainty in cervical cytology preparations (Fig. 7.3) [26].

Adenofibroma and Adenosarcoma

To date there have been no specific reports of the cytological appearance of adenofibroma or adenosarcoma in cervical cytology preparations.

Adenomyoma and Atypical Adenomyoma

Adenomyomas and polypoid adenomyomas of the cervix are rare. They comprise a mixture of benign endocervical glands and stroma composed predominantly of smooth muscle.

Atypical polypoid adenomyoma also rarely arises in the cervix. The glandular component in this entity is indistinguishable from endometrial intraepithelial neoplasia and there are usually conspicuous squamous morules.

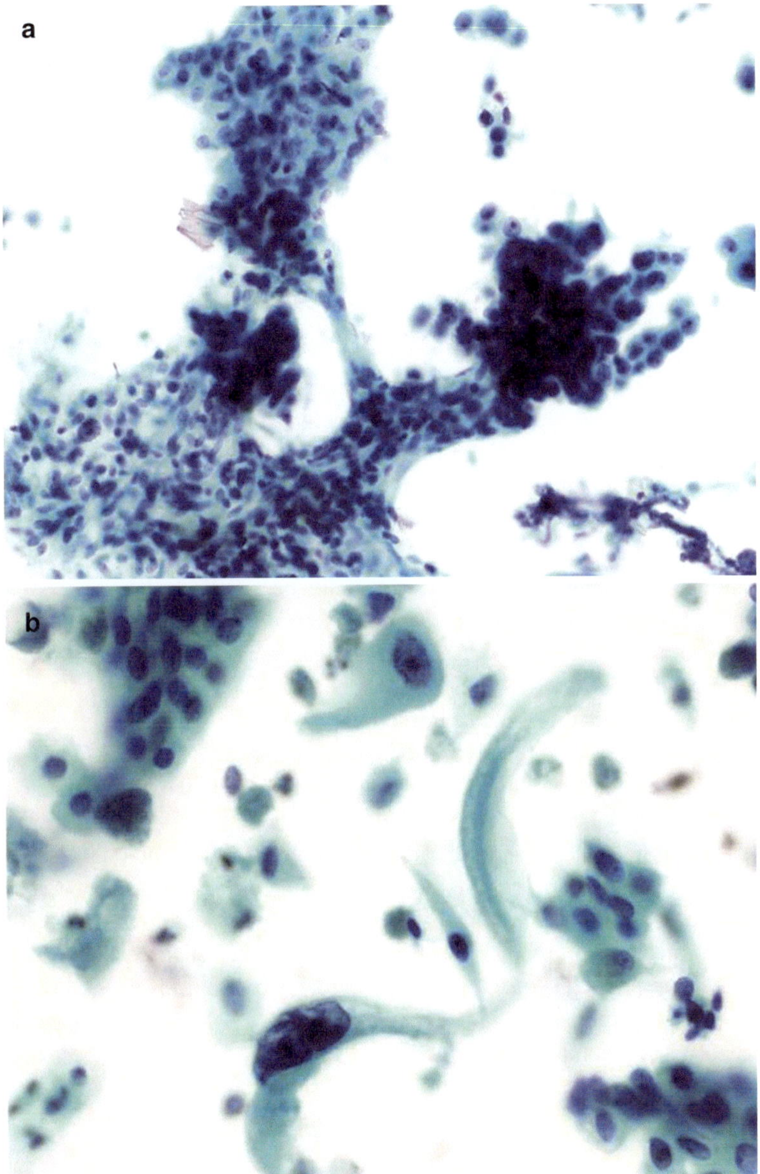

Fig. 7.3 Carcinosarcoma in a SurePath liquid-based cervical cytology sample. Three dimensional clusters of malignant epithelial cells associated with atypical spindle-shaped stromal cells (**a**) and an elongated malignant stromal cell with a malignant epithelial cell on an atrophic background (**b**) (From Gupta et al. [26]. With permission of Wiley Periodicals Inc)

The cytological features of both typical and atypical polypoid adenomyoma have been described in conventional and liquid-based cervical cytology preparations. In both cases cervical smears contained spindle-shaped smooth muscle cells, which in conventional smears may present as cohesive fragments with frayed edges revealing spindle cells with bipolar cytoplasmic processes, but whilst in the case of polypoid adenomyoma there were sheets and strips of reactive endocervical cells in an inflammatory background, in the case of atypical polypoid adenomyoma there were tightly packed, crowded clusters of atypical glandular cells [27–29].

Lymphoma, Leukaemia and Myeloma

Primary non-Hodgkin's lymphoma of the cervix is a rare but well-documented event with over 60 cases described in the world literature; it is usually of diffuse large B cell type and presents in middle-aged or elderly women with vaginal bleeding and a cervical tumour mass, which is then biopsied [30]. The finding of lymphoma or leukaemia in the cervix is more commonly a manifestation of secondary involvement of the female genital tract and has been observed in up to 40 % of cases with widely disseminated disease [31, 32]. Advanced Hodgkin's disease also may involve the cervix.

The cytological features of lymphoma of the cervix have largely been limited to single case reports, although a few small series have been reported. It is very rare for a cervical cytology sample to reveal abnormal lymphoid cells and such samples are typically normal or only show non-specific inflammation if the neoplastic cells are covered by intact mucosa; in the few reported cases with abnormal preceding cervical cytology samples, the abnormal cells have usually been interpreted as epithelial [30, 33–35]. There are also solitary case reports of cervical lymphoma in association with CIN 3 [36]. Lymphomatous cells on a cervical cytology sample must be distinguished from chronic inflammatory cells, small cell carcinoma, small cell severe dyskaryosis, endometrial carcinoma, poorly-differentiated adenocarcinoma, and sarcoma. Features favouring the diagnosis of lymphoma include single dissociated cells with prominent nucleoli, nipple-like projections on the nuclei, chromatin clumping at the nuclear borders and scant cytoplasm. Small cell carcinoma cells tend to be irregularly shaped and pleomorphic with indistinct nucleoli. Characteristic nuclear moulding and clustering may be present. Cells of small cell severe dyskaryosis may present in sheets as well as singly and individual cells may show evidence of keratinisation.

Subtyping of lymphomas in conventional cervical smears is not reliable but liquid-based preparations offer the possibility of immunocytochemical evaluation of the abnormal cells for phenotyping and accurate classification.

Reactive inflammatory cells will have a polymorphic appearance, being composed of a mixture of normal mature and immature lymphocytes, sometimes including plasma cells.

Myeloma rarely affects the female genital tract [37]. Atypical plasma cells have been described in the smear from a woman with postmenopausal bleeding in whom the diagnosis of myeloma had yet to be made. Myeloma cells appeared as large single cells with scant or deeply basophilic cytoplasm, hyperchromatic eccentric nuclei, some of which were multinucleate and had prominent large irregular nucleoli [38].

Leukaemic deposits in cervical stroma may occasionally be sampled by cervical cytology. The appearance of the cells varies according to the type of leukaemia. A leukaemic infiltrate may be mistaken for follicular cervicitis if the appropriate history is not available [39–41].

Melanocytic Neoplasms

Both benign and malignant melanocytic neoplasms occur in the cervix, of which blue naevus and malignant melanoma are the most common respectively.

Blue Naevus

In common with their cutaneous counterparts blue naevi of the cervix consist of spindle shaped or dendritic pigmented naevus cells situated in the ecto- or endocervical stroma. The overlying epithelium is intact, lesional cells are not exfoliated and therefore the appearance in cervical cytology samples has not been documented to date [42–44].

Malignant Melanoma

Primary malignant melanoma of the cervix is very rare. Most malignant melanomas of the cervix are the result of local spread from a primary vaginal tumour or metastasis from a distant site. The histological features are typical of melanoma at other sites, showing infiltration of tissues by epithelioid or spindle-shaped tumour cells with large pleomorphic nuclei and prominent nucleoli. Multinucleate forms are common and intracytoplasmic melanin is often present [45, 46].

The diagnosis of melanoma of the cervix may be suggested by exfoliative or fine needle

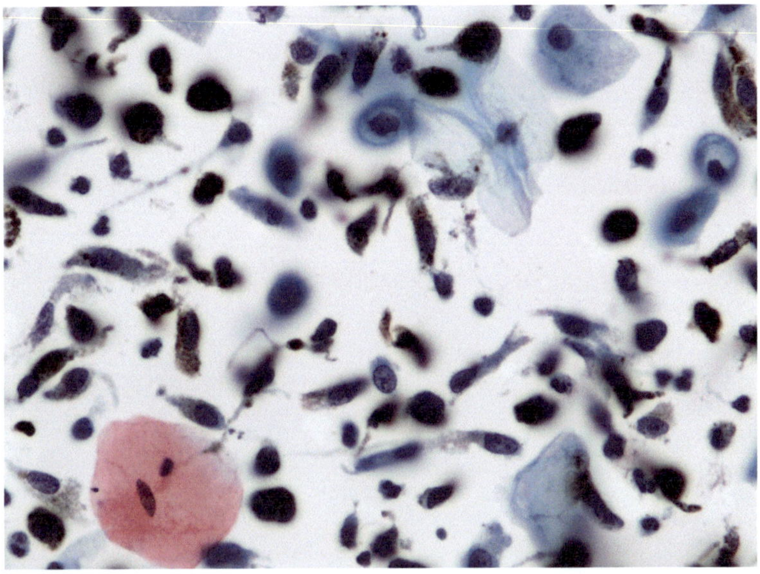

Fig. 7.4 SurePath liquid-based cervical cytology sample from a woman with primary malignant melanoma of the cervix. Dissociated pleomorphic malignant cells with abundant intracytoplasmic melanin pigment admixed with squamous epithelial cells

aspiration cytology and the cytological appearances reflect the histological appearances.

Although the cells may be arranged in loose groups and sheets, they typically occur singly and are epithelioid or spindle shaped with considerable cellular pleomorphism. The nuclei are pleomorphic and often eccentric, hypo- or hyperchromatic, bi- or multinucleate, and usually contain prominent nucleoli. The nuclear-cytoplasmic ratio is variable and nuclear moulding may be prominent. Intranuclear cytoplasmic inclusions, appearing as rounded intranuclear vacuoles, are a feature of some melanomas. The cytoplasm may be abundant and contain melanin pigment and the cell borders tend to be ill-defined with a lacy appearance [47–49] (Fig. 7.4).

Cellular pleomorphism is usually marked but melanoma cells can be small and uniform, blending with normal cervical cells on a smear, in which case they may be overlooked. The differential diagnosis also includes squamous carcinoma, adenocarcinoma and sarcoma. Spindle shaped melanoma cells may be misinterpreted as sarcomatous if the cells are exclusively of this type and no melanin is seen. A Masson-Fontana silver stain to detect melanin pigment may be helpful if pigment is not apparent on a Papanicolaou-stained smear. Immunocytochemistry, using antibodies to S100 protein or a more specific melanoma marker such as HMB 45, NKI C3 or Melan A, may be helpful if sufficient material is available.

Metastatic Tumours

Metastasis of carcinoma to the cervix is not uncommon and usually occurs in the presence of advanced disease. The cervical mucosa tends to remain intact so that tumour cells are not often seen in cytology preparations. The most common primary sites are elsewhere in the genital tract, the gastrointestinal tract, breast, kidney and rarely the lung. Tumour may also involve the cervix by direct invasion from the endometrium, bladder or rectum [50–54].

The cytological findings are variable, depending on the nature of the original tumour, the presence or absence of ulceration and the extent of cervical involvement by the metastasis. In general there are fewer abnormal cells than in smears from primary tumours of cervix. The cells are readily recognized as malignant, but tumour typing may be difficult unless distinctive features are present (Fig. 7.5a, b). Signet ring or goblet cell formation or large sheets of tall columnar vacuolated malignant cells palisaded along one edge may suggest an origin from the gastrointestinal tract (Fig. 7.5c) whilst neoplastic cells in a single file configuration with intracytoplasmic vacuoles is typical of metastatic lobular carcinoma of the breast (Fig. 7.5d) [54].

In conclusion, awareness of the patient's history should alert one to the possibility of metastasis but it is important to remember that patients with one tumour are also more likely to develop further neoplasms. If abnormal cells are seen in a cervical cytology sample from a patient with a known carcinoma, the original tumour histology should be reviewed and compared with the cytological findings.

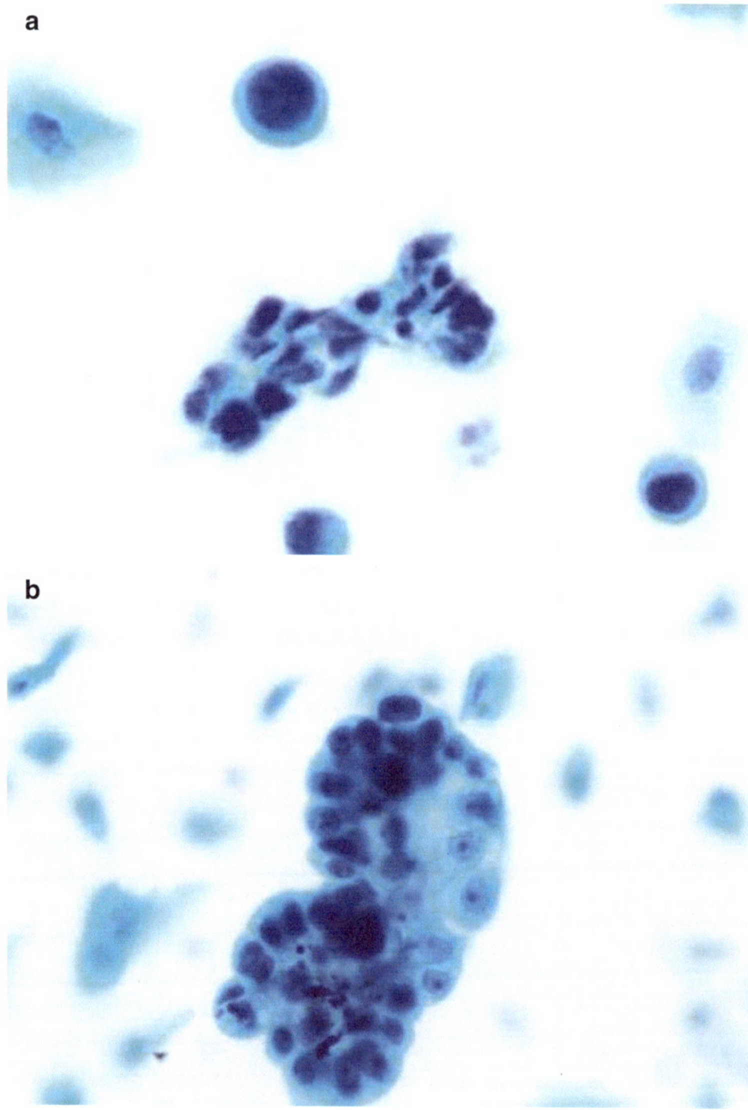

Fig. 7.5 Metastatic carcinoma in SurePath liquid based cervical cytology samples. (**a**) Scattered malignant cells with a high nuclear-cytoplasmic ratio in an atrophic background. This woman was known to have had a previous invasive ductal carcinoma of the breast. (**b**) A vaguely papillary group of malignant cells with a high nuclear-cytoplasmic ratio in a clean atrophic background. The patient was known to have had a previous invasive ductal carcinoma of the breast. (**c**) Large complex folded sheets of malignant glandular cells are present. The palisaded border of tall columnar cells with intracytoplasmic mucin vacuoles is unlike the usual appearance of primary cervical adenocarcinoma. This woman had had a prior resection of a rectal carcinoma. (**d**) Tumour cells in a conspicuous Indian-file arrangement with intracytoplasmic bodies from a patient with a known lobular carcinoma of the breast (From Gupta et al. [54]. With permission of Blackwell Publishing Ltd)

Fig. 7.5 (continued)

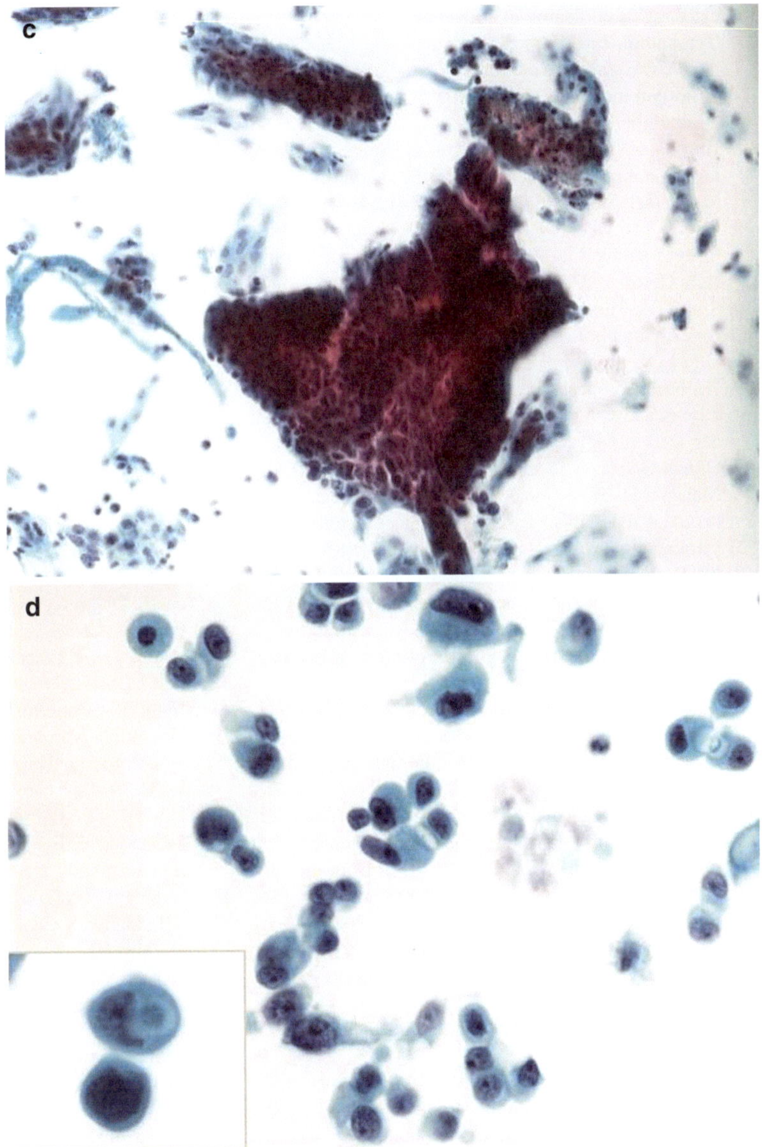

References

1. Albores-Saavedra J, Gersell D, Gilks CB, et al. Terminology of endocrine tumors of the uterine cervix: results of a workshop sponsored by the College of American Pathologists and the National Cancer Institute. Arch Pathol Lab Med. 1997;121(1):34–9.
2. Hirahatake K, Hareyama H, Kure R, et al. Cytologic and hormonal findings in a carcinoid tumor of the uterine cervix. Acta Cytol. 1990;34(2):119–24.
3. Reich O, Pickel H, Purstner P. Exfoliative cytology of invasive neuroendocrine small cell carcinoma in a cervical cytologic smear. A case report. Acta Cytol. 1996;40(5):980–4.
4. Li S, Zhu H. Twelve cases of neuroendocrine carcinomas of the uterine cervix: cytology, histopathology and discussion of their histogenesis. Acta Cytol. 2013;57(1):54–60.
5. Hoerl HD, Schink J, Hartenbach E, Wagner JL, Kurtycz DF. Exfoliative cytology of primary poorly differentiated (small-cell) neuroendocrine carcinoma of the uterine cervix in ThinPrep material: a case report. Diagn Cytopathol. 2000;23(1):14–8.
6. Ciesla MC, Guidos BJ, Selvaggi SM. Cytomorphology of small-cell (neuroendocrine) carcinoma on ThinPrep

cytology as compared to conventional smears. Diagn Cytopathol. 2001;24(1):46–52.
7. Lee WY. Exfoliative cytology of large cell neuroendocrine carcinoma of the uterine cervix. Acta Cytol. 2002;46(6):1176–9.
8. Kuroda N, Wada Y, Inoue K, et al. Smear cytology findings of large cell neuroendocrine carcinoma of the uterine cervix. Diagn Cytopathol. 2013;41(7):636–9.
9. Russin VL, Valente PT, Hanjani P. Psammoma bodies in neuroendocrine carcinoma of the uterine cervix. Acta Cytol. 1987;31(6):791–5.
10. Smith PA, Turnbull LS. Small cell and 'pale' dyskaryosis. Cytopathology. 1997;8(1):3–8.
11. Gupta N, John D, Dudding N, Crossley J, Smith JH. Factors contributing to false-negative and potential false-negative cytology reports in SurePath liquid-based cervical cytology. Cytopathology. 2013;24(1):39–43.
12. Ortega-Gonzalez P, Chanona-Vilchis J, Dominguez-Malagon H. Transitional cell carcinoma of the uterine cervix. A report of six cases with clinical, histologic and cytologic findings. Acta Cytol. 2002;46(3):585–90.
13. Ng WK. Thin-layer (liquid-based) cytologic findings of papillary squamotransitional cell carcinoma of the cervix. Review of cases over a 4-year period with emphasis on potential diagnostic pitfalls. Acta Cytol. 2003;47(2):141–8.
14. Matsuura Y, Kashimura M, Hatanaka K, Toki N, Sugihara K. Sarcoma botryoides of the cervix. Report of a case with cytopathologic findings. Acta Cytol. 1999;43(3):475–80.
15. Laskin WB, Fetsch JF, Tavassoli FA. Superficial cervicovaginal myofibroblastoma: fourteen cases of a distinctive mesenchymal tumor arising from the specialized subepithelial stroma of the lower female genital tract. Hum Pathol. 2001;32(7):715–25.
16. Ganesan R, McCluggage WG, Hirschowitz L, Rollason TP. Superficial myofibroblastoma of the lower female genital tract: report of a series including tumours with a vulval location. Histopathology. 2005; 46(2):137–43.
17. Stewart CJ, Amanuel B, Brennan BA, et al. Superficial cervico-vaginal myofibroblastoma: a report of five cases. Pathology. 2005;37(2):144–8.
18. Massoni EA, Hajdu SI. Cytology of primary and metastatic uterine sarcomas. Acta Cytol. 1984;28(2):93–100.
19. Wang X, Khoo US, Xue WC, Cheung AN. Cervical and peritoneal fluid cytology of uterine sarcomas. Acta Cytol. 2002;46(3):465–9.
20. Policarpio-Nicolas ML, Cathro HP, Kerr SE, Stelow EB. Cytomorphologic features of low-grade endometrial stromal sarcoma. Am J Clin Pathol. 2007;128(2): 265–71.
21. McCluggage WG. Uterine carcinosarcomas (malignant mixed Mullerian tumors) are metaplastic carcinomas. Int J Gynecol Cancer. 2002;12(6):687–90.
22. Silverberg SG, Major FJ, Blessing JA, et al. Carcinosarcoma (malignant mixed mesodermal tumor) of the uterus. A Gynecologic Oncology Group pathologic study of 203 cases. Int J Gynecol Pathol. 1990;9(1):1–19.
23. Barwick KW, LiVolsi VA. Malignant mixed mullerian tumors of the uterus. A clinicopathologic assessment of 34 cases. Am J Surg Pathol. 1979;3(2):125–35.
24. An-Foraker SH, Kawada CY. Cytodiagnosis of endometrial malignant mixed mesodermal tumor. Acta Cytol. 1985;29(2):137–41.
25. Snyder MJ, Robboy SJ, Vollmer RT, Dodd LG. An abnormal cervicovaginal cytology smear in uterine carcinosarcoma is an adverse prognostic sign: analysis of 25 cases. Am J Clin Pathol. 2004;122(3):434–9.
26. Gupta N, Dudding N, Smith JH. Eight cases of malignant mixed mullerian tumor (carcinosarcoma) of the uterus: findings in surepath cervical cytology. Diagn Cytopathol. 2014;42:165–9.
27. Ngadiman S, Yang GC. Adenomyomatous, lower uterine segment and endocervical polyps in cervicovaginal smears. Acta Cytol. 1995;39(4):643–7.
28. Baschinsky D, Keyhani-Rofagha S, Hameed A. Exfoliative cytology of atypical polypoid adenomyoma. A case report. Acta Cytol. 1999;43(4):637–40.
29. Chhieng DC, Elgert PA, Cangiarella JF, Cohen JM. Cytology of polypoid adenomyomas: a report of two cases. Diagn Cytopathol. 2000;22(3):176–80.
30. Chan JK, Loizzi V, Magistris A, et al. Clinicopathologic features of six cases of primary cervical lymphoma. Am J Obstet Gynecol. 2005;193(3 Pt 1):866–72.
31. Vang R, Medeiros LJ, Ha CS, Deavers M. Non-Hodgkin's lymphomas involving the uterus: a clinicopathologic analysis of 26 cases. Mod Pathol. 2000; 13(1):19–28.
32. Hanley KZ, Tadros TS, Briones AJ, Birdsong GG, Mosunjac MB. Hematologic malignancies of the female genital tract diagnosed on liquid-based Pap test: cytomorphologic features and review of differential diagnoses. Diagn Cytopathol. 2009;37(1):61–7.
33. al-Talib RK, Sworn MJ, Ramsay AD, Hitchcock A, Herbert A. Primary cervical lymphoma: the role of cervical cytology. Cytopathology. 1996;7(3):173–7.
34. King JA, Elkhalifa MY, Michael C. Malignant lymphoma identified on a cervical cytologic smear, with immunophenotypic analysis. Acta Cytol. 1997;41(4): 1228–30.
35. Matsuyama T, Tsukamoto N, Kaku T, Matsukuma K, Hirakawa T. Primary malignant lymphoma of the uterine corpus and cervix. Report of a case with immunocytochemical analysis. Acta Cytol. 1989;33(2):228–32.
36. Huang WT, Chuang SS, Eng HL, Huanga CC. Synchronous CIN 3 and cervical lymphoma: a case report and review of the literature. Pathol Res Pract. 2005;201(7):521–6.
37. Kang LC, Thomas DB, Wang J, Dunphy CH. Plasma cell myeloma presenting as abnormal uterine bleeding. Int J Gynecol Pathol. 2007;26(2):130–2.
38. Figueroa JM, Huffaker AK, Diehl EJ. Malignant plasma cells in cervical smear. Acta Cytol. 1978;22(1): 43–5.
39. Oliva E, Ferry JA, Young RH, et al. Granulocytic sarcoma of the female genital tract: a clinicopathologic study of 11 cases. Am J Surg Pathol. 1997;21(10): 1156–65.

40. Kazi S, Szporn AH, Strauchen JA, Chen H, Kalir T. Recurrent precursor-B acute lymphoblastic leukemia presenting as a cervical malignancy. Int J Gynecol Pathol. 2013;32(2):234–7.
41. Ikuta A, Saito J, Mizokami T, et al. Primary relapse of acute lymphoblastic leukemia in a cervical smear: a case report. Diagn Cytopathol. 2006;34(7):499–502.
42. Szumilo J, Patel A, Patel S, Burdan F. Blue nevus of the endocervix. Folia Morphol (Warsz). 2010;69(1):62–4.
43. Donofrio V, Terracciano LM, Boscaino A, De RG, Buffa D. Blue nevus of the uterine cervix. Pathologica. 1992;84(1092):539–45.
44. Patel DS, Bhagavan BS. Blue nevus of the uterine cervix. Hum Pathol. 1985;16(1):79–86.
45. Clark KC, Butz WR, Hapke MR. Primary malignant melanoma of the uterine cervix: case report with world literature review. Int J Gynecol Pathol. 1999;18(3):265–73.
46. Jin B, Goldsmith A, Budev H, Al-Abbadi M. Primary melanoma of the uterine cervix after supracervical hysterectomy. A case report. Acta Cytol. 2007;51(1):86–8.
47. Deshpande AH, Munshi MM. Primary malignant melanoma of the uterine cervix: report of a case diagnosed by cervical scrape cytology and review of the literature. Diagn Cytopathol. 2001;25(2):108–11.
48. Gupta S, Sodhani P, Jain S. Primary malignant melanoma of uterine cervix: a rare entity diagnosed on fine needle aspiration cytology–report of a case. Cytopathology. 2003;14(3):153–6.
49. Uzum N, Kose F, Ataoglu O. Metastatic malignant melanoma of the uterine cervix: first diagnosed on liquid-based cytology. Diagn Cytopathol. 2008;36(11):769–72.
50. Gupta D, Balsara G. Extrauterine malignancies. Role of Pap smears in diagnosis and management. Acta Cytol. 1999;43(5):806–13.
51. Haji BE, Kapila K, Francis IM, Temmim L, Ahmed MS. Cytomorphological features of metastatic mammary lobular carcinoma in cervicovaginal smears: report of a case and review of literature. Cytopathology. 2005;16(1):42–8.
52. Giordano G, Gnetti L, Pilato FP, Viviano L, Silini EM. The role of cervical smear in the diagnosis and management of extrauterine malignancies metastatic to the cervix: three case reports. Diagn Cytopathol. 2010;38(1):41–6.
53. Watkin E, Mejean-Lebreton F, Donne C, Devouassoux-Shisheboran M. Abnormal cervical cytology revealing a pulmonary adenocarcinoma. Cytopathology. 2010;21(6):403–6.
54. Gupta N, Dudding N, Smith JH. Cytomorphological features of extra-genital metastases in SurePath cervical liquid-based cytology: a series of eight cases. Cytopathology. 2013;24(2):123–8.
55. Smith JHF. Other tumours and lesions of the cervix, vulva and vagina. In: Gray W, Kocjan G, edtiors. Diagnostic cytopathology. 3rd ed. Churchill Livingstone Elsevier; 2010.

8 Colposcopy and Management of Glandular Neoplasia

John Tidy

Abstract

Glandular neoplasia of the cervix is a rare entity. Development of glandular neoplasia is associated with high risk human papillomavirus infection, most commonly type 18. The impact of cervical screening programmes in the detection and treatment of cervical glandular intra-epithelial neoplasia (CGIN) is unclear. Treatment of CGIN has become more conservative but concerns about skip lesions remain. High cure rates for CGIN by local excision are reported. Treatment of choice for early stage adenocarcinoma is surgery as radiotherapy may not be as effective compared with squamous cancers. Women with advanced adenocarcinoma of the cervix also have a worse outcome. Trials of new chemo-radiotherapy regimen are required.

Keywords

Glandular neoplasia • Cervix • Adenocarcinoma • Treatment • Surgery • Radiotherapy

Introduction

The greatest challenge when managing women with cervical glandular neoplasia is the rarity of the condition thus preventing a clinician from gaining extensive experience in the subject. Most publications report small number of cases and so extrapolating findings must always be done with some degree of caution. Colposcopy is important in the diagnosis of cervical neoplasia but unlike squamous lesions glandular neoplasia are almost never recognized on colposcopic examination hence management is very dependent on referral cytology.

Cervical Glandular Intra-epithelial Neoplasia

Incidence

In the year 2011/12 the English cervical screening programme reported 1,354 samples as showing ?glandular neoplasia out of a total of 3,457,752 cytology samples taken that year. Thus only 0.6 % of all the reported abnormal cytology samples fall within this category. During the same year only 0.8 % of the women referred to colposcopy were referred because of ?glandular neoplasia and of those who subsequently

W.G. McCluggage et al., *Cellular Pathology of Glandular Lesions and Uncommon Neoplasms of the Cervix*, DOI 10.1007/978-1-4471-2210-4_8, © Springer-Verlag London 2014

underwent excisional treatment for cervical neoplasia only 2.1 % of excised specimens contained high grade- cervical glandular intra-epithelial neoplasia (HG-CGIN) [1].

We know little about the incidence of borderline changes in endo-cervical cells within the English screening programme. Although well recognized by cytologists and colposcopists, this category was not recorded as an entity separate from squamous borderline changes. This situation has been rectified with publication of NHSCSP No1 3rd ed. ABC document in April 2013 and in future years we will be able to gain more accurate data on the incidence of this cytological diagnosis [2].

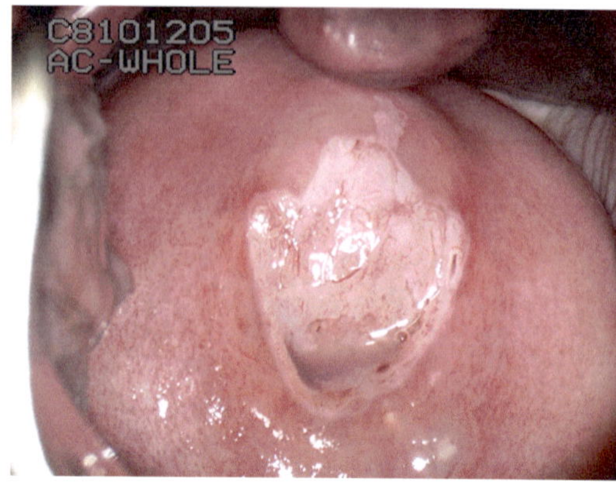

Fig. 8.1 Dense aceto-white changes affecting the columnar epithelium with fusion of the villi and abnormal blood vessel pattern

Aetiology

It is generally accepted that glandular neoplasia develops at the squamo-columnar junction rather than developing in endo-cervical cells high in the endo-cervical canal. Ibrahim et al. looked at cellular markers expressed at the squamo-columnar junction and found that the same population of reserve cells gives rise to both glandular and squamous neoplasia [3]. Cervical glandular neoplasia is associated with high risk HPV infection. HPV 18 is more commonly associated with this lesion as described in Chap. 3. It is unclear why HPV 18 may preferentially favour infection of endo-cervical reserve cells leading to glandular neoplasia. The fact that high risk HPV infection of the reserve cell population is common to the development to both squamous and glandular explains why many women with glandular neoplasia have co-existent cervical intra-epithelial neoplasia (CIN). In addition some women who are eventually found to have glandular neoplasia may have been referred to colposcopy with a screening cytology reporting only changes in squamous cells.

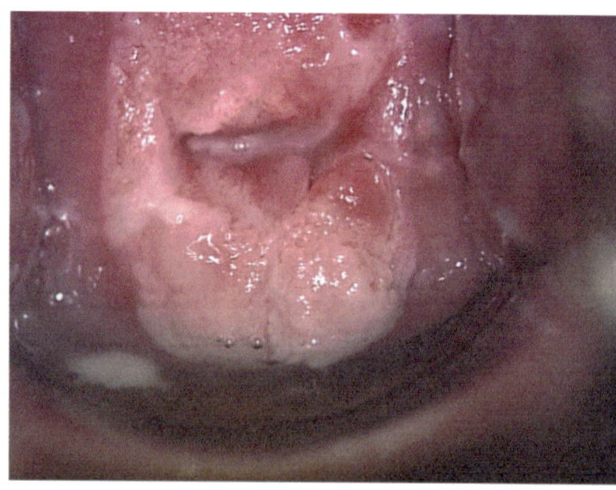

Fig. 8.2 Irregular lesion with the columnar epithelium with dense aceto-white changes

The Role of Colposcopy in the Diagnosis of Cervical Glandular Intra-epithelial Neoplasia

Glandular neoplastic lesions are located within the columnar epithelium of the endo-cervix so hampering full visualization of the entire at risk area by colposcopy even with the use of endo-cervical speculae. Features of cervical glandular intra-epithelial neoplasia (CGIN) are only present after the application of acetic acid. The two most commonly described changes are the presence of dense aceto-white columnar villi, especially if these changes are not adjacent to the squamo-columnar junction, and the finding of villi fused together (Figs. 8.1 and 8.2). Mosacisim or punctation are not usually found but atypical blood vessels can be seen and may raise the possibility of a micro-invasive cancer. Unfortunately these features are not always present and hence considered unreliable implying that colposcopists should not rely on the few features that have been described to either confirm or exclude the presence of CGIN [4, 5]. Between 47 and 87 % of women with pure HG-CGIN may have a normal colposcopic examination [6, 7]. These finding are similar to those reported by Pisal et al. who also reported with only 1 out 13 cases of HG-CGIN was diagnosed colpscopically [8]. National U.K. colposcopy guidance states that directed biopsies should not be used in the management of these cases [9]. Unlike squamous intra-epithelial neoplasia it is also not possible to assess if a lesion is low or high grade based on colposcopic features described above.

Although colposcopy cannot confirm or refute the presence of CGIN useful information can still be obtained as a result of the examination. The presence of any invasive cancer, as long as it is low in the endo-cervical canal, can be detected. Adenocarcinoma of the cervix shares the same features as squamous cancer; irregular surface either raised or ulcerated the presence of atypical blood vessels. The presence of any co-existing squamous lesions can be assessed and this may impact on how the abnormality is treated.

Management of Women with? Endo-cervical Glandular Neoplasia

Diagnosis

All women with an abnormal cytology sample showing ?glandular neoplasia should be referred to colposcopy. All reported series show high rates of significant disease including invasive cancer. Older studies also found cases of cancer of the endometrium, upper genital tract and other abdominal organs [5]. Modern classification system introduced over recent years has encouraged cyto-pathologists to try and differentiate endo-cervical glandular neoplasia from other glandular neoplasia.

Ullal et al. examined the performance of cytology and colposcopy in women with endo-cervical neoplasia [6]. While cytology had both a reasonable sensitivity (66 %) and positive predictive value (81 %) (PPV) colposcopy had only 10 % sensitivity but a high PPV (94 %). Even when colposcopy was reported as normal over 87 % had a significant lesion on the subsequent excised specimen. Talaat et al. reviewed 200 cases referred with ?glandular neoplasia over a 10 year period [7]. Pure HG-CGIN was a relatively rare finding with only 14 cases found out of 115 cases on intra-epithelial neoplasia, the most common finding was combined HG-CIN and HG-CGIN, 70 cases, and 30 cases of HG-CIN. 48 women were found to have invasive cancer, 28 cervical adenocarcinomas, 8 squamous carcinomas, 10 endometrial cancers and two ovarian cancers. The high incidence of significant disease within this category has led to the English cervical screening programme recommendation that women with this cytology abnormality should be seen in colposcopy within 2 weeks.

Endo-cervical Curettage

There are significant differences of opinion as to the role of endo-cervical curettage in the management of women with CGIN, while it is common practice in the U.S.A.; it is rarely performed in the U.K. The poor sensitivity associated with this technique linked to a variable but high rate of false negatives (59–78 %) has influenced the decisions of U.K. colposcopists not use this form of sampling [10–12]. In addition endo-cervical curettage is uncomfortable.

Treatment

The treatment of HG-CGIN must be by an excisional technique, which may be large loop excision of the transformation zone (LLETZ, LEEP), laser conisation or cold knife conisation. There is a wide range of opinion as to which method is best. It is best to try and remove a cylinder of tissue rather than a cone to minimize the risk of cross cutting the endo-cervical glands leading to an increased rate of incomplete excision. Some colposcopists favour using cold knife conisation as it does not damage the delicate endo-cervical tissue at the excision margin so providing better quality tissue for pathological assessment.

However, it can be difficult to minimize the size of the tissue excised using this technique leading to concern about removing too much tissue from the cervix. In addition this technique requires general or regional anaesthesia unlike laser conisation or LLETZ, which can be performed under local anaesthesia in a clinic setting. The depth of the excised tissue should be at least 1 cm above the squamo-columnar junction (SCJ) if it is visible, if the SCJ is not visible the depth of the excised tissue should be 2–2.5 cm. The depth of the excised tissue is significantly greater than for CIN, 0.8 cm if the SCJ is visible, or 1.5 cm is the SCJ is not visible. Van Hanegem et al. 2012 reviewed the management of 112 women treated for adenocarcinoma in-situ (HG-CGIN) with either cold knife cone biopsy or LLETZ [13]. The rate of negative margins was the same in both groups (79 % vs. 73 %). All women with positive margins underwent a further excision and the rate of residual disease was the similar in both groups (33 %). Some women with negative margins underwent re-excision but with no evidence residual disease. The depth of the excised specimen was much greater in the knife cone biopsy group but this did not reduce the incidence of positive margins. The use of LLETZ may be of greater benefit for young women, although some will need a second procedure the majority will be cured by the first excision.

Some experts remain concerned about the possibility of skip lesions; hence consider that negative margins within the excised specimen cannot completely exclude residual disease within the endo-cervical canal. Therefore there is still a role for hysterectomy as the primary management of women who present with glandular neoplasia and have completed their family. Some however recommend considering hysterectomy as completion of treatment once they have completed their family if they had earlier undergone conservative local excision. If follow-up cytology was normal during the interval between local excision and completion of their family the benefits of hysterectomy would only be to reduce the development of new disease rather than excision of any residual occult HG-CGIN.

Management of Women with Borderline Changes in Endo-cervical Cells

All women with an abnormal cytology sample showing borderline changes in endo-cervical cells should be referred to colposcopy. Unlike borderline nuclear changes in squamous cells there is a high incidence of abnormality, both squamous and glandular, associated with borderline changes in endo-cervical cells. In 2011 the English cervical screening programme introduced high risk HPV triage for all cytology samples reported as borderline, either squamous or glandular, and mild dyskaryosis. It is as yet unclear what effect this will have on the referral pattern as the English programme only started to record borderline changes in endo-cervical cells as a separate category from squamous borderline changes in April 2013 following publication of guidance from NHSCSP publication No1 (ABC) [2]. Studies have reported the presence of significant disease with in the category but rarely HG-CGIN. Patel et al. reported that 32 % of women had at least squamous high-grade intraepithelial neoplasia (HG-CIN) and 7 % had invasive cancer but only 4 % had HG-CGIN [8]. Other studies have reported the presence of high grade squamous lesions (10–33 %), invasive disease (1.8–22 %) and CGIN (10 %) [5, 14–17]. These studies are often small case series from individual colposcopy clinics or cytology laboratories using a variety of different cytological classification systems and hence must be viewed within this context.

Colposcopic examination will aid the diagnosis of invasive disease and CIN however it cannot confirm or exclude CGIN. Given the very low incidence of CGIN in this group a conservative approach to management is a reasonable option. Repeat colposcopic examination with cytology sampling should be undertaken 6 months later. If the repeat cytology is reported as showing borderline changes in endo-cervical cells excision of the transformation zone should be considered to confirm or exclude the presence of HG-CGIN.

The Role of Repeat Excision

Unlike squamous CIN where there is a lot of information about factors that influence repeat excision the data for CGIN is less abundant. Older data suggested that there was a high incidence of residual disease because of skip lesions but more recent studies suggest that the risk is much lower. Young et al. reported that the risk of residual disease was 55 % if initial excision margins were positive but only 13 % if they were negative [18]. In a large meta-analysis of 1,278 women treated for CGIN the incidence of residual disease was only 2.6 % in women with negative margins [19]. Kurina and al-Nafussi examined 121 cases of CGIN and found that if there was at least 3 mm of normal endo-cervical epithelium between the CGIN and the excision margin then there was no evidence of residual disease [20]. Li and Zhao in a recent review of 136 cases of AIS (HG-CGIN) found that at the time of hysterectomy the incidence of residual disease was 0 % if the prior conisation specimen had negative margins. There was only one case of recurrent disease in this group. In the group of women with positive cone margins 48.6 % had residual disease at hysterectomy [21]. The above data has confirmed that conservative management of completely excised CGIN is acceptable and now become the standard of care.

Management of Squamous Mucin Intra-epithelial Lesion (SMILE)

Although this is a variant of squamous intra-epithelial neoplasia it can be found co-existing with CGIN. There are no colposcopic features described for SMILE and it is best managed according the co-existing CIN or CGIN.

Follow Up of Women Treated for CGIN

All British cervical screening programmes recommend cervical cytology follow-up after treatment for CGIN. Concerns over the sampling and shedding of the endo-cervical canal has resulted in this group of women being excluded from using high risk HPV testing within the test of cure setting. Kitchener et al. reported a case of adeno-carcinoma that developed in a woman despite having negative cytology and negative for HR-HPV [22]. Intensive cytology follow-up, 6 and 12 months and a further 9 annual cytology samples is recommend. The presence of endo-cervical cells is a mandatory of the sample if it is to be reported as negative. In situations where the endo-cervical canal is stenosed due to conisation an additional endo-cervical brush sample may be required if the ecto-cervical brush cannot access the higher portion of the canal. A recent development in the English Cervical Screening programme has seen this recommendation change. Women will now have two samples taken, six and then 18 months after treatment. If the cytology is negative reflex HR-HPV testing will take place. If both samples are negative for both cytology and HR-HPV then the woman will be returned to normal re-call.

Invasive Adenocarcinoma of the Cervix

The number of cases of adenocarcinoma in England has remained relatively stable between 1989 and 2008, approximately 430–480 case per year, in the last year where data in available 2009 there was a reported 20 % increase incidence to 580 cases however it is unclear as whether this represents an trend or an isolated event [23]. The organised cervical screening programme in England, which was introduced in 1988, has reduced the incidence of squamous carcinoma of the cervix the programme appears to have had little impact in reducing the incidence of adenocarcinoma of the cervix. As a consequence the percentage of women with adenocarcinoma of the cervix has risen from 10 to 20 % of the total number of cervical cancers between 1989 and 2009. Adenocarcinoma appears to be slightly more common in women aged 35–50 years. Similar data has been reported

Table 8.1 Five year survival by stage for squamous carcinoma and adenocarcinoma [20]

Stage	Overall 5 year survival	
	Squamous carcinoma (%)	Adenocarcinoma (%)
1A1	97.9	92.8
1A2	94.6	96.8
1B1	90.5	86.8
1B2	79.5	65.3
2A	74.8	66.4
2B	67.4	55.9
3A	46.0	40.2
3B	44	23.7
4A	22.3	16.7
4B	9.3	13.0

from the SEER database of US cancer registries. Between 1988 and 2005 the incidence of adenocarcinoma and adeno-squamous carcinomas has increased from 21.3 to 24.1 % [24]. Overall survival is stage dependent. The last FIGO report found similar survival rates for early stage adenocarcinoma to those of squamous cancer but worse outcomes for more advanced adenocarcinomas (Table 8.1) [25]. Similar adverse outcomes for advanced adenocarcinoma and adeno-squamous carcinomas was also reported by Galic et al. whereas Katanyoo et al. found no difference in survival rates between locally advanced squamous and adenocarcinoma of the cervix [24, 26].

Early Stage Adenocarcinoma of the Cervix

Unlike micro-invasive squamous cancer of the cervix there are no reliable colposcopic features that allow the colposcopist to suspect the presence of the micro-invasive adenocarcinoma of the cervix. Larger cancers may be associated with an irregular surface within the endo-cervical canal, an ulcer within the endo-cervical canal or the presence of atypical blood vessels. The diagnosis of early stage adenocarcinoma is based on the pathological assessment of the excised tissue.

Local Excision

Conservative management by local excision is now regarded as the standard of care for women with early stage cervical squamous cancer (Stages 1A1, 1A2) however; clinicians have been more reluctant to offer this treatment for women with early stage adeno-carcinoma in part because of the difficulty for pathologists in agreeing how to measure early adenocarcinoma lesions. Factors influencing recurrence of early stage cervical cancer include completeness of excision, the presence of lympho-vascular space involvement (LSVI), spread to the cervical parametrial tissue and pelvic lymph node metastases. Blessing et al. reviewed both their own data but also the literature in the management of early stage adenocarcinoma [27]. There were no recurrences in the group treated conservatively by conisation. In the published literature the incidence of nodal involvement was 1.4, 3.0 % had LSVI but none of these cases were associated with nodal involvement and there were no cases of parametrial spread. These findings were confirmed by Reynolds et al. and Baalbergen et al. [28, 29]. Extensive surgery which included radical trachelectomy, hysterectomy and radical hysterectomy did no improve outcome. All the series with conservative management by conisation reported successful pregnancy outcomes. More recent data has also suggested that conservative management for small stage 1b1 cancers measuring less than 2 cm may also be feasible as these tumours are also associated with low rates of recurrence, parametrial spread and nodal involvement [30].

Stage 1B Adenocarcinoma

The standard of care for women with this tumour has been radical hysterectomy with pelvic lymph node dissection. However due to a combination of factors more women are being considered for radical trachelectomy and pelvic lymph node dissection, The trachelectomy may be performed either vaginally or abdominally and to date there is no data to demonstrate which is best. In the reported series the percentage of women treated by radical trachelectomy ranges between 27 and 53 % but some series also include women with stage 1A1 and 1A2 disease [31–33]. There is a trend for the need of adjuvant radiotherapy or completion hysterectomy in larger stage 1B1 tumours [32]. In a review of 412 cases reported in the literature the rates of recurrence and death (4.4 and 2.9 %) were similar those for more radical surgery [31]. The aim with radical trachelectomy is preserve fertility leading to a pregnancy with a viable outcome however it remains unclear how successful this is as the viable outcome rates published approach 50–66 % with a relatively high rate of premature labour and neonatal complications [31, 34]. In conclusion radical trachelectomy for small (<2 cm) stage 1B1 adenocarcinomas is gaining in acceptance with low rates of recurrence and death. The overall viable pregnancy rate may only be around 50–66 % therefore careful counseling is required.

Radiotherapy has been reported to be less effective when compared with radical surgery in the management of stage 1B adenocarcinoma. A Cochrane review found limitation with the studies in the literature. Many older studies compared surgery with radical radiotherapy and not chemoradiotherapy and others predate the use of MRI and more latterly positive emission tomography – computed tomography (PET-CT) scanning. The review concludes that for stage 1b adenocarcinoma of the cervix with no evidence of lymph-node involvement then radical surgery is the treatment of choice if patient co-morbidity permits [35].

Advanced Adenocarcinoma of the Cervix

The current standard of care for advanced cervical cancer is chemoradiotherapy usually incorporating weekly cisplatin. Most large trials have not been able to establish, due to the lower incidence of the disease, if the outcome for women with advanced adenocarcinoma of the cervix have the same outcome as women with squamous cancer. Tang et al. recently reported a large randomized trial comparing concurrent chemoradiotherapy with cisplatin with concurrent chemoradiotherapy with cisplatin and additional cisplatin and paclitaxel chemotherapy. The women randomized to receive the additional chemotherapy had longer progression free and overall survival [36]. Paclitaxel may be more active in the treatment of adenocarcinomas of the cervix. Rose points out in an editorial that more trials are needed to answer the question as to what is the based treatment of women with advanced adenocarcinoma of the cervix [37].

Rare Variants of Adenocarcinoma of the Cervix

The rare variants of this cancer type are described in Chap. 4. Most occur too infrequently for the acquisition of accurate outcome data and the clinical management is no different from that previously described. The only exception to this is villioglandular adenocarcinoma. Because this tumour rarely invades the underlying cervical stroma to any significant degree the reported rate of metastasis to the pelvic lymph nodes is much less than with other adenocarcinomas. In early stage cases (stage 1B) it has been suggested that pelvic lymph node dissection can be safely omitted hence reducing the morbidity of treatment but a recent large retrospective study suggested that although overall prognosis is good lymph node metastasis does occur [38].

Conclusions

Women with glandular neoplasia represent a small proportion of the women referred to colposcopy. Colposcopy cannot confirm or refute the presence of intra-epithelial glandular neoplasia. Treatment of HG-CGIN is by excision and follow-up up is increasingly conservative with re-excision only being offered to women with positive margins. Conservative management of women with HG-CGIN and early stage cervical adenocarcinoma is increasingly relevant and acceptable provided the disease is completely excised. More trials evaluating the role of chemoradiotherapy in the management of advanced cervical adenocarcinoma are required to ascertain the optimal therapeutic strategy

Acknowledgments I am grateful to Narindra Pisal, Consultant Gynaecologist, Whittington Hospital, London for the colpo-photgraphs of CGIN.

References

1. Cervical screening programme – England 2011–12. Health and Social Care Information Centre, Screening and Immunisations team; 2012.
2. NHSCSP No1 3rd ed. Achievable standards, Benchmarks for reporting, and Criteria for evaluating cervical cytopathology; 2013.
3. Ibrahim EM, Stewart RL, Corke K, Blackett AD, Tidy JA, Wells M. Upregulation of CD44 expression by interleukins 1,4 and 13, transforming growth factor -β1, estrogen, and progestogen in human cervical adenocarcinoma cell lines. Int J Gynecol Cancer. 2006;16:1631–42.
4. Lickrish GM, Colgan TJ, Wright VC. Colposcopy of adenocarcinoma in situ and invasive adenocarcinoma of the cervix. Obstet Gynecol Clin North Am. 1993; 20:111–1224.
5. Cullimore J, Scurr J. The abnormal glandular smear: cytologic prediction, colposcopic correlation and clinical management. J Obstet Gynaecol. 2000;20:403–7.
6. Ullal A, Roberts M, Bulmer JN, Mathers ME, Wadehra V. The role of cervical cytology and colposcopy in detecting cervical glandular neoplasia. Cytopathology. 2009;20:359–66.
7. Talaat A, Brinkmann D, Dhundee J, Hana Y, Bevan J, Irvine R, Bailey S, Woolas R. Risk of significant gynaecological pathology in women with glandular neoplasia on cervical cytology. Cytopathology. 2012;23:371–7.
8. Pisal NV, Sindos M, Desai S, Mansell E, Singer A. How significant is a cervical smear showing glandular dykaryosis? Eur J Obstet Gynecol Reprod Biol. 2003; 108:209–12.
9. NHSCSP No 20 2ed. Colposcopy and Programme Management; 2010.
10. Denehy TR, Gregori CA, Breen JL. Endocervical curettage, cone margins, and residual adenocarcinoma in situ of the cervix. Obstet Gynecol. 1997;90:1–6.
11. Azodi M, Chambers SK, Rutherford TJ, Kohorn EI, Schwartz PE, Chambers JT. Adenocarcinoma in situ of the cervix: management and outcome. Gynecol Oncol. 1999;73:348–53.
12. DeSimone CP, Day ME, Dietrich CS, Tovar MM, Modesitt SC. Risk for residual adenocarcinoma in situ or cervical adenocarcinoma in women undergoing loop electrosurgical excision procedure/conization for adenocarcinoma in situ. J Reprod Med. 2011;56: 376–80.
13. van Hanegem N, Barroilhet LM, Nucci MR, Bernstein M, Feldman S. Fertility-sparing treatment in younger women with adenocarcinoma in situ of the cervix. Gynecol Oncol. 2012;124:72–7.
14. Mohammed DK, Lavie O, de B Lopes A, Cross P, Monaghan J. A clinical review of borderline glandular cells on cervical cytology. BJOG. 2000;107(5): 605–9.
15. Finall R, Olafsdottir R. Outcomes of cervical liquid-based cytology suggesting a glandular abnormality. Cytopathology. 2009;20:367–74.
16. Jadoon BA, Kehoe S, Romain K, Celland C, Sundar SS. Analysis of outcome in women with borderline glandular change on cervical cytology. Eur J Obstet Gynecol Reprod Biol. 2009;147:83–5.
17. Patel A, Thampy N, Hemming D, Naik R. A clinical review of borderline glandular cells reported on liquid-based cervical cytology. BJOG. 2010;117:1051–9.
18. Young JL, Jazaeri AA, Lachance JA, Stoler MH, Irvin WP, Rice LW, Andersen WA, Modesitt SC. Cervical adenocarcinoma in situ: the predictive value of conisation margin status. Am J Obstet Gynecol. 2007;197:195.
19. Salani R, Puri I, Bristow RE. Adenocarcinoma in situ of the uterine cervix: a metaanalysis of 1278 patients evaluating the predictive value of conisation margin status. Am J Obstet Gynecol. 2009;200:182e1–5.
20. Kurian K, al-Nafussi A. Relation of cervical glandular intraepithelial neoplasia to microinvasive and invasive adenocarcinoma of the uterine cervix: a study of 121 cases. J Clin Pathol. 1999;52(2):112–7.
21. Li Z, Zhao C. Long term follow-up results from women with cervical adenocarcinoma in situ treated by conization: an experience from a large academic women's hospital. J Low Genit Tract Dis. 2013;17:452–8.
22. Kitchener HC, Walker PG, Nelson L, Hadwin R, Patnick J, Anthony GB, Sargent A, Wood J, Moore C, Cruickshank ME. HPV testing as an adjunct to cytology in the follow up of women treated for cervical intraepithelial neoplasia. BJOG. 2008;115: 1001–7.
23. Cancer statistics registrations. Series MB1, No. 41. London: ONS; 2010.
24. Galic V, Herzog TJ, Lewin SN, Neugut AI, Burke WM, Lu Y-S, Hershman DL, Wright JD. Prognostic significance of adenocarcinoma histology in women with cervical cancer. Gynecol Oncol. 2012;125:287–91.
25. Quinn MA, Benedet JL, Odicino F, Maisonneuve P, Beller U, Creasman WT, Heintz AP, Ngan HY, Pecorelli S. Carcinoma of the cervix uteri. FIGO 26th Annual Report on the Results of Treatment in Gynecological Cancer. Int J Gynaecol Obstet. 2006;95 Suppl 1:S43–103.
26. Katanyoo K, Sanguanrungsirikul S, Manusirivithaya S. Comparison of treatment outcomes between squamous cell carcinoma and adenocarcinoma in locally advanced cervical cancer. Gynecol Oncol. 2012;125: 292–6.

27. Bisseling KC, Bekkers RL, Rome RM, Quinn MA. Treatment of microinvasive adenocarcinoma of the uterine cervix: a retrospective case study and review of the literature. Gynecol Oncol. 2007;107: 424–30.
28. Reynolds EA, Tierney K, Keeney GL, Felix JC, Weaver AL, Roman LD, Cliby WA. Analysis of outcomes of microinvasive adenocarcinoma of the uterine cervix by treatment type. Obstet Gynecol. 2010;116: 1150–7.
29. Baalbergen A, Smedts F, Helmerhorst TJ. Conservative therapy in microinvasive adenocarcinoma of the uterine cervix is justified: an analysis of 59 cases and a review of the literature. Int J Gynecol Cancer. 2011; 21:1640–5.
30. Al-Kalbani M, McVeigh G, Nagar H, McCluggage WG. Do FIGO stage 1A and small (≤2 cm) 1B1 adenocarcinomas have a good prognosis and warrant less radical surgery? Int J Gynecol Cancer. 2012;26: 291–8.
31. Shepherd JH, Spencer C, Herod J, Ind TE. Radical vaginal trachelectomy as a fertility sparing procedure in women with early-stage cervical cancer-cumulative pregnancy rate in a series of 123 women. BJOG. 2006;113(6):719–24.
32. Abu-Rustum NR, Neubauer N, Sonoda Y, Park KJ, Gemignani M, Alektiar KM, Tew W, Leitao MM, Chi DS, Barakat RR. Surgical and pathologic outcomes of fertility sparing radical abdominal trachelectomy for FIGP stage 1B1 cervical cancer. Gynecol Oncol. 2008;111(2):261–4.
33. Helpman L, Grisaru D, Covens A. Early adenocarcinoma of the cervix: is radical trachelectomy safe. Gynecol Oncol. 2011;123:95–8.
34. Kim CH, Abu-Rustum NR, Chi DS, Gardner GJ, Leitao MM, Carter J, Baraket RR, Sonoda Y. Reproductive outcome of patients undergoing radical trachelectomy for early-stage cervical cancer. Gynecol Oncol. 2012;125:585–8.
35. Baalbergen A, Veenstra Y, Stalpers L. Primary surgery versus primary radiotherapy with or without chemotherapy for early adenocarcinoma of the uterine cervix. Cochrane Database Syst Rev. 2013;(1):CD006248. doi:10.1002/14651858.CD006248.pub3.
36. Tang J, Tang Y, Yang J, Huang S. Chemoradiation and adjuvant chemotherapy in advanced cervical adenocarcinoma. Gynecol Oncol. 2012;125:297–302.
37. Rose PG. Are the differences in treatment outcome for adenocarcinoma of the cervix different enough to change the treatment paradigm? Gynecol Oncol. 2012;125:285–6.
38. Lataifeh IM, Al-Hussaini M, Uzan C, Jaradat I, Duvillard P, Morice P. Villoglandular papillary adenocarcinoma of the cervix: a series of 28 cases including two with lymph node metastisis. Int J Gynecol Cancer. 2013;23:900–5.

Index

W.G. McCluggage et al., *Cellular Pathology of Glandular Lesions and Uncommon Neoplasms of the Cervix*,
DOI 10.1007/978-1-4471-2210-4,

MIX
Papier aus verantwortungsvollen Quellen
Paper from responsible sources
FSC® C105338

If you have any concerns about our products,
you can contact us on
ProductSafety@springernature.com

In case Publisher is established outside the EU,
the EU authorized representative is:
Springer Nature Customer Service Center GmbH
Europaplatz 3, 69115 Heidelberg, Germany

Printed by Libri Plureos GmbH
in Hamburg, Germany